To Peter
Szego — you know
better than I how good it was —

WHO KILLED THE QUEEN?

MCGILL-QUEEN'S/ASSOCIATED MEDICAL SERVICES STUDIES IN THE HISTORY OF MEDICINE, HEALTH, AND SOCIETY

SERIES EDITORS: S.O. FREEDMAN AND J.T.H. CONNOR

Volumes in this series have financial support from Associated Medical Services, Inc. (AMS). Associated Medical Services Inc. was established in 1936 by Dr Jason Hannah as a pioneer prepaid not-for-profit health-care organization in Ontario. With the advent of medicare, AMS became a charitable organization supporting innovations in academic medicine and health services, specifically the history of medicine and health care, as well as innovations in health professional education and bioethics.

Who Killed the Queen?

The Story of a Community Hospital and How to Fix Public Health Care

HOLLY DRESSEL

McGill-Queen's University Press
Montreal & Kingston • London • Ithaca

© Holly Dressel 2008
ISBN 978-0-7735-3340-0

Legal deposit second quarter 2008
Bibliothèque nationale du Québec

Printed in Canada on acid-free paper that is 100% ancient forest free
(100% post-consumer recycled), processed chlorine free

This book has been published with the help of a grant from the Queen
Elizabeth Foundation

McGill-Queen's University Press acknowledges the support of the Canada
Council for the Arts for our publishing program. We also acknowledge
the financial support of the Government of Canada through the Book
Publishing Industry Development Program (BPIDP) for our publishing
activities.

Library and Archives Canada Cataloguing in Publication

Dressel, Holly Jewell
Who killed the Queen? : The Story of Community Hospital and How to
Fix Public Health Care / Holly Dressel.

Includes bibliographical refererences and index.
ISBN 978-0-7735-3340-0

1. Hospital closures – Canada. 2. Medical care – Canada. 3. Queen
Elizabeth Hospital (Montréal, Québec) 4. Hospital closures – Canada –
Case studies. I. Title.

RA395.C3D74 2008 362.10971 C2007-906411-6

Typeset by Jay Tee Graphics Ltd. in 10.5/13 New Baskerville

Contents

Introduction

This book was originally conceived to commemorate the life and death of a small but famous Montreal hospital, the Queen Elizabeth. Much of the history of this community hospital, established in the late 19th century, is typical of hundreds of other hospitals across Canada, but the Queen Elizabeth was also the site of a worldwide transformation in the practice of anesthesiology and the birthplace of many innovations, such as Canada's first Intensive Care Unit and first use of pre-operative antibiotics. Its sudden closing in 1995, as part of the widespread hospital closures and health care cutbacks of that period, caused enormous bitterness and distress – emotions specific in some ways to its local community but also typical of feelings across the country. Given this interplay between the general and particular, it became clear that it would be necessary to discuss the Queen E, as it was affectionately known, in the context of the history of Canadian hospitals and the health care system as a whole.

In North America, the most common academic approach to the study of such large subjects is to attack the general theme – for example, the history of public health care – and then illustrate points with particular examples, such as the experience of this or that hospital, influential personality, or legislative event. In Europe, and especially in France, the opposite approach is more common. That is, students take one very particular case, study it in detail, and then relate it to its complete context, going from the particular to the general rather than the other way around. Having experienced this method of teaching while in university in France, I learned to appreciate its efficacy and it seemed to be a useful way to look at the history of one hospital while

also investigating the much broader context that was ultimately responsible for both its birth and its early death.

This is therefore a somewhat unusual book. It includes both entertaining and amusing descriptions of particular historical events and
unique personalities as well as rigorous, well-documented analyses of
the broad economic, philosophical, and political contexts that nur-
tured or challenged the people and institutions described. It lays out
the history and the efficacy of our national systems of hospital and
health care – how they came about, and how they compare with other
such systems. Because my study of the Queen E and the broader context in which it operated suggests ways of evaluating the effectiveness of
hospitals and the health care system in general, I have provided primary and secondary references to enable readers to judge the arguments made here.

Given the political and social importance of health care, this book,
although well supported by the data, will undoubtedly be controversial.
This was not my intention when I took on the project, but, as my
research proceeded, it became clear that information about such vola-
tile and politically charged subjects as surgical wait times, the cost and
effectiveness of private versus public hospital systems, the actual results
of mixed private and public-system care, and the current· state of
national health care as interpreted by international statistics, as well as
the influence of international banks and private corporations on Canadian hospital and health policies, is surprisingly abundant and consistent. Because I had the luxury of a long period of research and could
approach the subject without preconceptions or outside interference of
any kind, this book shatters myths and establishes some shocking historical connections. One of these connections goes very far to explain not
only why the Queen Elizabeth Hospital, after more than a hundred years
of exemplary service, was summarily closed in 1995 but why hundreds of
other hospitals and thousands of hospital beds were closed all across
Canada during the same period, with repercussions on our health care
system that have never been adequately analyzed or understood.

Who Killed the Queen? is intended to be a seminal source of knowledge
and research options, as well as a political and philosophical challenge
to the reader. It will also, I hope, provide a great deal of reading pleasure. The family most closely associated with the Queen Elizabeth Hospital, the Griffiths, contained two doctors who could just as well have
become journalists. The diaries, letters, papers, autobiographies, and
even annual reports written by A.R. Griffith, who helped found the

hospital in 1894, and his son Harold, a world-renowned anesthesiologist, are unmatched in the annals of medical literature. Most hospital histories have to make do with a few newspaper stories from the late 19th or early 20th century and a couple of interviews to supplement the dry, bare-bones fare of annual reports and medical board minutes. I had access to not only over a hundred years of the latter documents but also reams of chatty, highly descriptive, emotionally revealing, and extremely candid papers from two doctors who were also hospital administrators and whose careers covered the 1890s through to the 1970s.

A.R. Griffith's writings provide both personal anecdotes and details about the life of a hospital that began as a centre for homeopathy and eventually gave rise to incredible medical advances, including having been a major pioneer in laparoscopic surgery. Harold Giffith's writings start around 1918 and chart scientific research at the Queen E in a breezy, pictorial writing style that makes even his annual reports read like entertaining family letters. Seldom, if ever, have the vicissitudes, triumphs, and worries of Canadian medical practitioners and hospital administrators been so clearly expressed. Even if the only papers we had from Harold were those on the developments in the knowledge and practice of anesthesiology, they would still be invaluable. His family letters, World War I diaries, lay sermons, when joined with his father's similarly open, honest and often humourous descriptions of early medical conditions, paint an unequalled historical picture of medicine at the time. The bulk of the Griffith papers, amassed during research for this book, are being given to McGill University to become the Queen Elizabeth Hospital of Montreal Archive, where they will be available to future researchers.

Added to information from the Griffiths are the testimonies of a small sample of the many hundreds of people who worked devotedly in the Queen E from the 1940s until its closing, and who are now able to compare its practices with those they have encountered since. Their extreme openness about their work stems from loyalty and affection, but also from the freedom conferred by the hospital's closure. It was made clear at the outset of this project that if the research uncovered flaws in the way the hospital worked, even very serious ones, they would not be glossed over. No one, including the Board of Directors who initiated this project, expressed any problem with that, perhaps because they felt that, although any institution is going to have flaws, the Queen E was an institution of which they could be proud.

Although this book has been organized as a single narrative whose arguments support one another, its length and the varied topics it covers make it possible to read certain sections on their own. Chapter 1, "Serving the Queen," is largely made up of interviews with the people who worked in the Queen Elizabeth Hospital of Montreal until its closure and who are therefore best able to describe what it was like. Their stories of its high levels of professionalism, unusual egalitarianism, and great parties always became tangled up, however, with their emotional distress and bitterness over the loss of this hospital. Nearly all the informants interpreted the Queen Elizabeth's closure as a local tragedy engineered by provincial authorities, but, given the hospital's fiscal stability and international reputation at the time, they found the unreasonableness of such a closure the most painful part of their loss. Although they knew that hospitals in other parts of Canada had been closed around the same period, none of them saw hospital bed closures as a national problem, rather than a provincial or even a municipal one. Why the Queen E, and many other exemplary hospitals, were closed in the mid 1990s has remained a mystery even to the people most involved in their administration. "Serving the Queen" is therefore set up somewhat like a murder mystery: who was the victim and why is the death a tragedy worth investigation?

The second chapter, "Growing a Culture," follows from the first chapter's conclusion that the Queen E was a exemplary and comparatively successful medical institution. But such a judgment makes no sense without a picture of the way the hospital actually worked in the context of other such institutions over the past 100 years. Thanks to the rich material available concerning the Queen Elizabeth's first incarnation as the Homeopathic Hospital of Montreal and references to North American hospital history, both the particular features of the Homeopathic/Queen Elizabeth and the way it compares to other hospitals can be fully presented. Chapter 3, "Family Medicine," pursues the historical story begun in chapter 2 by looking at the childhood and career of the Homeopathic's most illustrious doctor, Harold Griffith, who carried on his father's administrative work while revolutionizing the practice of anesthesiology and helping found it as a new specialty, feats for which he is still honoured today. The story of anesthesiology itself is one filled with errors, deaths, eccentricities, and dark comedy.

The fourth chapter, "Medical Bills," gets to the basics of what makes hospitals work – funding. Unlike the U.S., in Canada charitable hospitals were not separate from private ones, so the public-private partnerships being discussed today were the norm in the country until the 1960s and 70s. Chapter 4 discusses the challenges of paying for modern medical care and explores how hospitals throughout the world, including the Queen Elizabeth, have coped with ever-growing public demands and professional expenses. Neither the author nor the hospital board funding this book had any particular bias towards public or private funding methods at the outset of the work – this chapter was intended to provide the most reliable data available so that a general reader could get a clear overview of different funding options around the world. The statistics, mostly provided by the UN as well as by national statistical organizations, very clearly illustrate which funding methods are by far the most efficient, both in terms of guaranteeing general health throughout a country's population and in keeping costs as low as possible. It turns out that similar data has been available to researchers for decades: the same studies are carried out again and again, and the results are always the same. Particular interests – economic, political, and philosophical – have, however, argued against the evidence presented by this now enormous mass of scientific data – and continue to do so.

Chapter 5, "The Queen Must Die," returns to the murder mystery. Now that we know what a hospital is, both in general and in the particular history of the Queen E, and have some understanding of the professional and economic challenges the Queen E and other hospitals face, who or what was responsible for its demise? Specific pressures were brought to bear on this and all hospital systems in the late 1980s and early 1990s, pressures based on professional theories that favoured less institutional and more community care, coupled with economic and political interest in increasing private participation. It was also a period of mass government borrowing, which resulted in record national deficits. Chapter 5 reveals that the number of hospitals and hospital beds closed in Canada over about a four-year period was so large that government charts and statistics themselves show that the entire health system was in serious danger of breaking down. In fact, although this period is generally unrecognized or discussed within the country itself, Canada is frequently used in international studies to study the effects of extremely sudden and wide-spread hospital closures on the health system of an industrialized country.

"Social Pathologies," the sixth chapter, deals with the extremely difficult issues that hospitals and health systems, regardless of methods of payment, now face. Philosophical questions about the right of wealthy individuals to obtain better treatment than their fellow citizens are only one small part of current challenges. Particularly important is how to deal with the unprecedented power and influence of the pharmaceutical industry, which today has larger profits than any other industry, including oil and weapons. Other private, vested interests, such as the HMOs and health corporations of the U.S., also exert alarming influence on those in the health professions or doing research in these areas, as well as on governments, making it even more difficult for hospital professionals to deliver services, not to mention deciding what services are appropriate to give. These influences are not new – all of them played a part in the mass closures of the 1990s and continue to affect everything from drug efficacy trials to pre-med education and journalistic integrity. They are, however, coming under increasing scrutiny, with louder calls for better control.

The last chapter of the book, "Long Live the Queen," shows how the best parts of a successful institution, even if, like the Queen Elizabeth, it no longer exists, can be applied to help determine present and future hospital care priorities. The book ends on a positive note, with inspiring success stories from around the world, buttressed by appropriate studies. These examples show that hospital care and the overall health of the general public can be maintained without the huge investments demanded to provide modern drugs and technologies – investments that would bankrupt the public systems that make hospital care available to most Canadians in the first place. The short afterword is intended to enable readers to identify methods of health and hospital care management that can be reliably used over the long term to provide them and their children with the health care they need.

Acknowledgments

This book is dedicated to Dierdre M. Gillies, Dr Harold Griffith's protégé in anesthesiology and a great teacher and specialist in her own right. She conceived the idea of having a book written to commemorate the story of the Queen Elizabeth Hospital of Montreal ten years ago and devoted a good part of her energy in the last months and weeks of her life to make sure it would become a reality.

This book is also dedicated to the late Robert Bourne, who spent his career at the Queen Elizabeth Hospital as a gastroenterologist. Bob was a son of Wesley Bourne, McGill's famous professor of anesthesiology who established the university's first department of that specialty and was also a friend and lifelong colleague of Dr Harold Griffith. Bob presided over the early research and helped with many of the interview arrangements for this book. His enthusiasm for the project, terrific encouragement to the researchers, and help in dealing with all the little problems as they arose was wonderful and greatly missed after his death in 2006.

This book would not exist without the unsurpassed energy, support and many professional contacts – to say nothing of the sweeping philosophical, academic, and medical expertise – of Dr John Hughes, a well-known Montreal family medicine practitioner formerly at the Queen Elizabeth. Dr Hughes organized everything from funding sources to publication, as well facilitating access to all the people, archives, and institutions required. We only hope he approves of the result. Miranda Smith did substantive editing of a manuscript that was grievously long and in places meandering, with the greatest good humour and an enormous, growing interest in the subject. For her patience with my rusty footnote form and overuse of adjectives, I am eternally grateful.

Montreal researcher Ken Hechtman took on the unenviable job of reading and summarizing one hundred years of medical board minutes. This took physical as well as mental strength, since they were all piled up in sealed boxes in a cramped, airless closet. Despite his strong habit of journalistic cynicism, even Ken fell under the charm exerted by the ingenuous writing of the Griffiths. I am indebted to him for his sardonic turn of phrase in his many, many notes on the material, which I have not been able to resist quoting. I also thank my old friend Jim Latteier, who always takes the time to criticize my books at an early stage. In this case, his knowledge of medical history and terminology helped me avoid some serious errors; any errors or omissions that remain are, of course, entirely my own.

I am especially grateful to everyone at McGill-Queen's for their unfailing kindness, patience, and remarkable flexibility regarding a book quite unusual to their usual editing and publishing methods, particularly Philip Cercone and Joan McGilvray. Without Ligy Alakkattussery, I never could have amassed the illustrations or kept my spirits up during the inevitable delays! I profoundly thank all the Queen Elizabeth and Calgary General doctors, nurses, employees, and activists who so generously gave me time, expertise, and loans of material. I apologize to the many, many Queen Elizabeth people whose stories would have been just as good as the ones I collected had I not run out of time, space, and energy. I particularly wish to apologize to people like Queen E alumnus Francesca Lanza and Jewish General ER nurse Pascale Audy, who in the latter case loaned me books and in both instances gave wonderful interviews that I loved but which we ended up having to cut from the book entirely for space reasons. I particularly apologize for how long it all took, due to my own health and other problems over which I had little control.

Dr Franco Carli and his successors in the Harold Griffith Chair of Anesthesiology at the Royal Victoria Hospital provided easy and unlimited access to all their material, and Dr Carli provided me with an essential insight into Harold Griffith's great discovery about curare, which made all the difference to a layperson's understanding of that feat. Marianna Bilotta, Cynda Heward, and Carolyn Dooge at the St Mary's Hospital Foundation, which administered the needed funds, could not have been more friendly, sympathetic, and responsive in time of need. Thank you all! I also wish to express my great appreciation for the now-disbanded Board of the Queen Elizabeth Hospital, which met one last time to launch this project and which waited for this book for five years with understandable impatience coupled with very charitable kindness. As a serious journalist, I also thank them for making it clear from the outset that I was at liberty to do as I saw fit with the research material.

And of course, I particularly thank the Griffith family, from Jim Griffith's son-in-law Albert Nixon to his surviving daughter, Betty Griffith Jennings; Harold's two daughters, Barbara Clark and Linda Mary Jacobson, and his many grandchildren, most notably John Alexander Clark, and Tom and the late Ken Jacobson. This extended family not only loaned me (as it turned out, for several years) some of the family's most prized possessions, they more than once opened their country home to our research. I also wish to thank Gordon Burr, chief curator of the McGill University archive, for finding the time to visit and access the scattered collections pertaining to the Queen Elizabeth Hospital, and for having the taste and perspicuity to recognize the importance of granting this material its own archive.

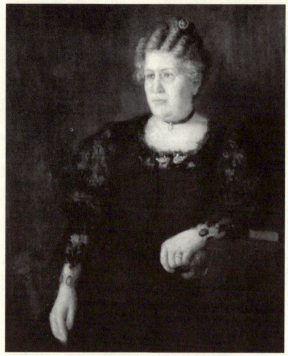

Georgiana Duff Phillips, known as the "Foundress of the Hospital" and "Our Patroness," ca. 1894

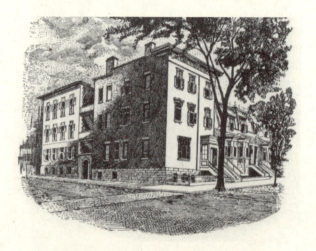

Artist's rendering of the first house on McGill College, bought for the Homeopathic in 1894.

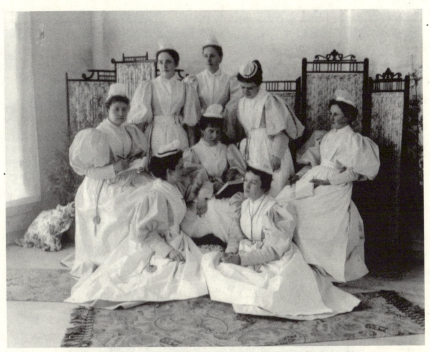

Phillips School of Nursing, graduating class, 1896

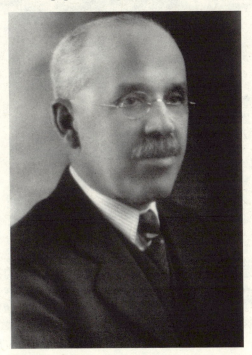

Dr A.R. Griffith, circa 1925

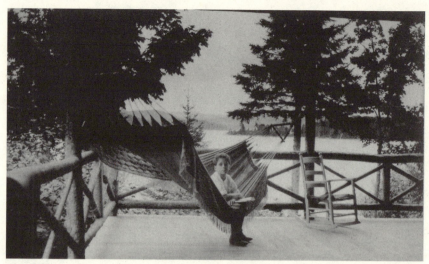

Arthur, the youngest of the four Griffith brothers, on the porch of their
Laurentian cottage at Lac des Iles, around 1910

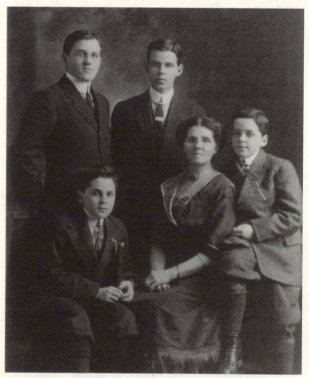

Mary Milne, and her four sons, Harold and Hugh, the
two eldest, and young Jim and Arthur, around 1912

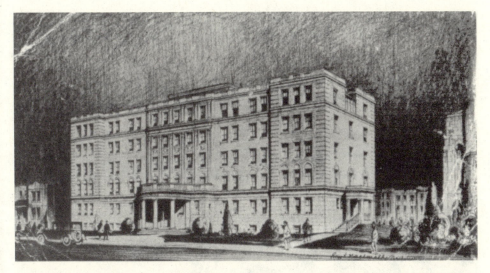

The new building housing the Montreal Homeopathic Hospital, on Marlowe Street in the Montreal suburb of Notre Dame de Grace, opened in 1926

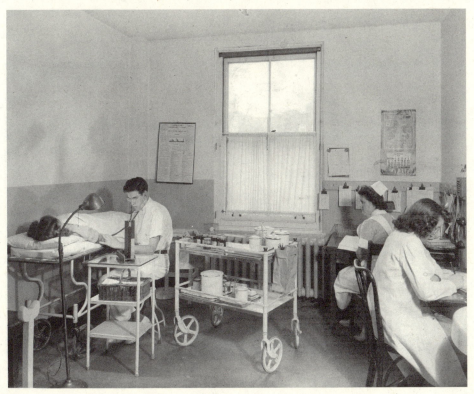

Homeopathic Treatment Room in 1940

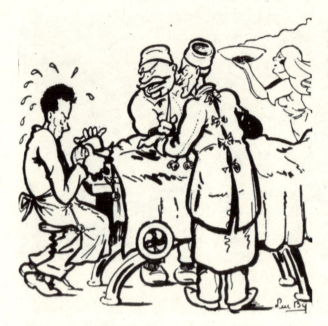

Harold Griffith's favourite cartoon depicting his job in its earliest years

LES JOIES DE L'ANESTHESISTE

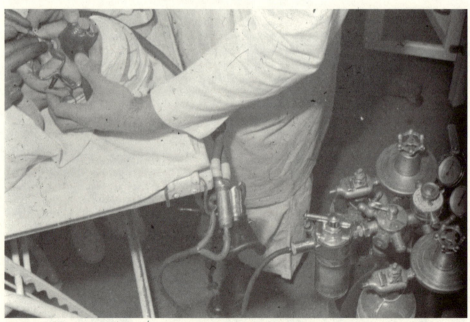

The complicated apparatus of anesthesiology, 1950s

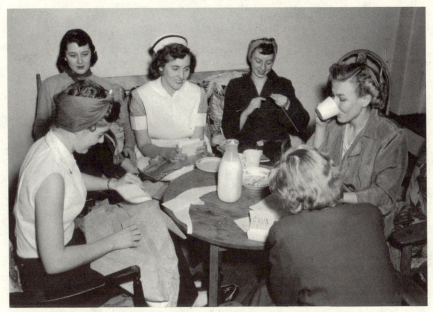

Nurses relaxing together at home in the Queen E's Phillips School, late 1940s

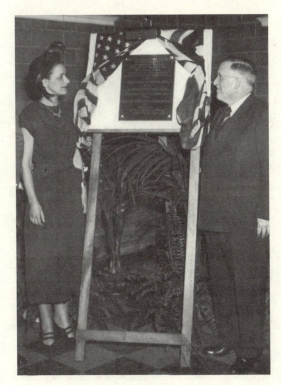

Dr Harold and Enid Johnson at the unveiling of a placque honouring their work on curare, early 1950s

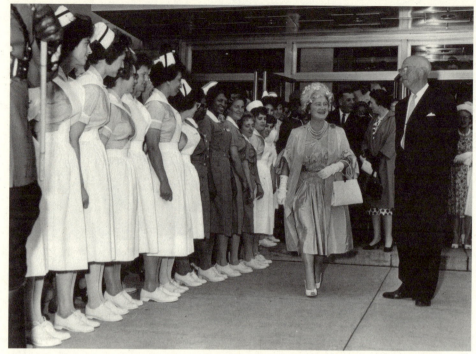

The Queen Mum christening the hospital re-named for her in 1955 – the Queen Elizabeth Hospital of Montreal

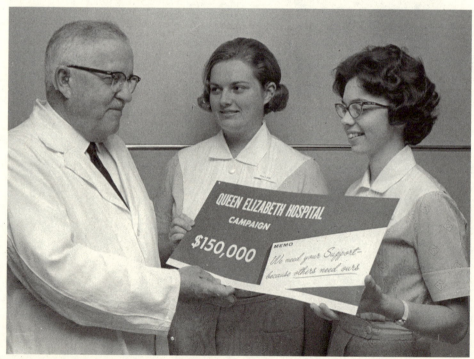

Dr Harold kicking off an early 1960s fundraising campaign, with nurses Sandra Hunt and Roberta Reynolds

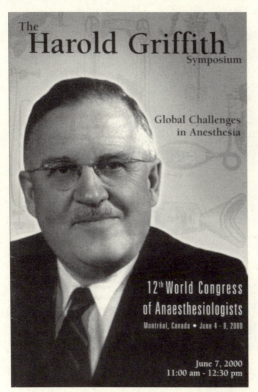

Harold Griffith advertising "the Harold Griffith Symposium" for the 12th World Congress of Anaesthesiologists held in June of 2000

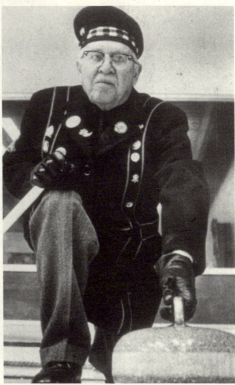

Dr Harold still curling late in life

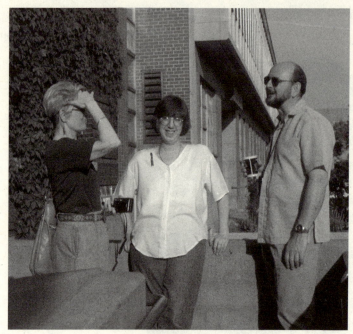

From left to right, Leona King, nurse, Lorna Titterton (ER head nurse Pat Titterton's sister), and Dr John Hughes, a party in the late 1980s

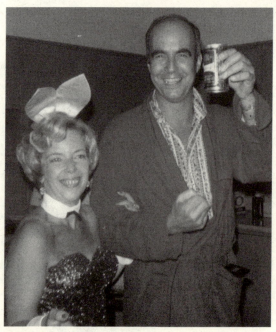

Nurse Judy Trainor and Dr Fred Weigan at a Queen E costume party, mid-1980s

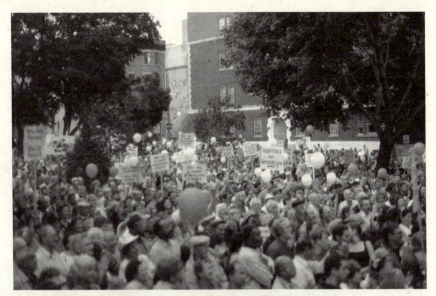

One of many marches to try to save the Queen, June, 1994

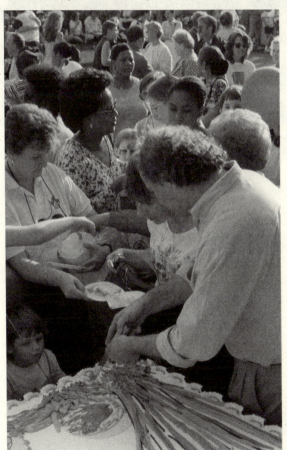

Left to right, Maria Bybel, head of Social Services, Dr Judy Levitan and Dr Don Smith dividing up the cake at the very last party, 1995

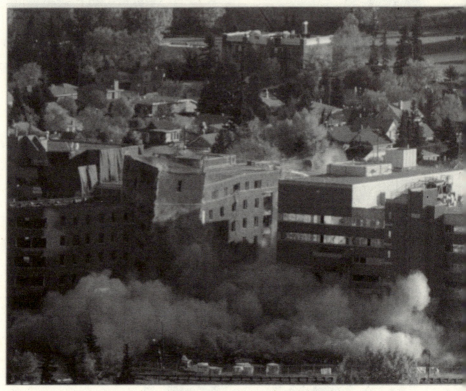

The Calgary General Hospital being blown up by the Alberta government, 4 October 1998. Photograph by David Moll. Reprinted with permission of the *Calgary Herald*.

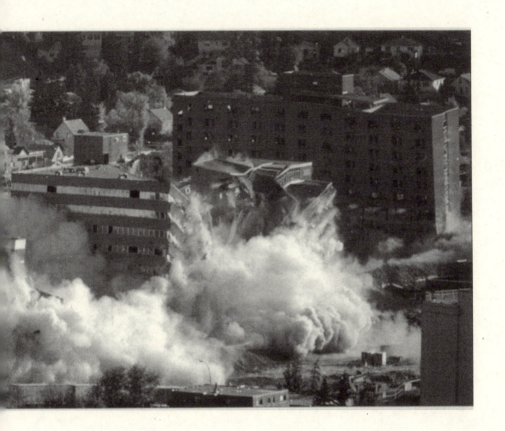

WHO KILLED THE QUEEN?

Serving the Queen

The approaching disaster of closing our precious hospitals should be recognized for what it is – a long-term plan to dismantle our superb system of health care.

Samuel Levy, chief of biochemistry, QEH[1]

Who gave you the mandate to ransack Montreal's hospital network?
opposition Liberal leader to Quebec Premier Jacques Parizeau[2]

When the Quebec government announced that nine, and then eight, hospitals in the Montreal area were going to be summarily closed for budgetary reasons in 1995, health care in Montreal was forever changed. In fact, although few Canadians have realized this even today, hospital care all across the country was being violently downsized during this period. A largely unanalyzed and widespread initiative to cut hospitals and hospital care in almost every province continues to haunt Canadian efforts to maintain an effective and humane universal health care system. But in 1995, when Montreal experienced the first closures, the news set off what seemed to be primarily a local wave of shock and disbelief in all the hospitals and communities affected. The most violent reaction came from the Montreal borough of Notre Dame de Grace, west of downtown. This was the location of one of Montreal's oldest and proudest community medical institutions, the Homeopathic Hospital of Montreal, as it was first named. It became the Queen Elizabeth Hospital in 1955, its re-christening complete with a visit from its namesake, the Queen Mum.

The loss of the Queen Elizabeth Hospital was significant not only for Montrealers but also for anyone interested in Canadian hospital care and in analyzing the scope and severity of the closures that hit the health system in the mid-1990s. Although only one of the hundreds of such institutions and thousands of beds affected across the country, the

Queen Elizabeth is typical of the institutions that were lost: most were small hospitals well integrated into their communities. For that reason, studying how it worked and what happened when it closed is instructive about the whole country. Of course, like any such institution, Montreal's Queen Elizabeth Hospital was unique. This was particularly true because it had been an extremely successful medical facility so that its closure illustrates both the severity and the desperation of the sudden and sweeping bed closures. It is thus a very good microcosm for looking at the macrocosm of hospital care in Canada.

The Queen Elizabeth or "Queen E," as it was affectionately known, although small and primarily serving a single borough in Montreal, Notre-Dame-de-Grace, had been the birthplace of revolutionary innovations in medical procedures. It was widely appreciated for its tradition of holistic care and was considered by many professionals to be a model institution that was unusually egalitarian and accessible to both staff and patients. It was also unusually accessible to its constituency. As one of its doctors, surgeon Fred Weigan, said, "Location, location, location was why the Queen E was so successful! It was spectacular – so suited to its catchment area: Victoria Street on the east, to Ville St. Pierre on the west, down to Verdun, and up to southern Ville St. Laurent. Three hundred thousand people, 12 percent of Montreal's population at the time. The Reddy [Memorial Hospital] or the [Montreal] General served those east of Victoria Street. We were one block from the north-south and east-west arteries of Decarie and Sherbrooke – so accessible! There's studies now of people-flow, and there's no significant flow between north of Montreal's Metropolitan freeway and south of it. That ease of access always took my breath away – and there was a huge parking lot."

This well-situated old hospital was the birthplace of a globally significant revolution in anesthesiology just after World War II. One of its founding doctors, Harold Griffith, developed the new materials and techniques that made possible the life-saving surgical techniques we take for granted today. This same community hospital pioneered new techniques in upper-respiratory surgery and laparoscopy, today's widespread method of using minimally invasive surgery that employs fibre-optic cameras and imaging. It was also the originator of Canada's first surgical recovery room and its very first Intensive Care Unit, and it pioneered the use of pre- (as opposed to post-) operative antibiotics in this country in the 1980s. To understand the significance of the closure of such a hospital, along with many others much like it, it's useful to investigate its particular characteristics and successes.

In the case of pre-operative antibiotics, Ron Lewis, the surgeon responsible, had come to Montreal from a tiny town on the Caribbean island of St. Lucia, via New York City. He did part of his McGill residency training at the Queen E and rapidly embraced the little hospital, where the feeling was mutual; his gifts were received by the Chief Surgeon at the time, Cam Darby, with delight, and Lewis was given every opportunity to flourish. Lewis says, "[Our studies] turned out to be so conclusive, so quickly, that one surgeon, who at first didn't want us to experiment on his patients by giving them possibly unneeded antibiotics before surgery, almost immediately tried to get out of having his patients be any part of a non-antibiotic-taking control group! Of course, other places were doing this kind of thing, but we were the first Canadians to conduct proper studies on antibiotic prophylaxis and publish them."

Laparoscopy was developed by a number of surgeons in the 1970s at the same small Montreal hospital. One of the lead investigators, Joe Mamazza, today runs the MIS or Minimally Invasive Surgery department at St. Michael's in Toronto. Mamazza claims that he could never have developed this revolutionary surgery technique at one of the larger teaching hospitals. "To be open to exploration, I would say you need the kind of team-approach camaraderie that prevailed at the Queen E, which frankly worked better than most health institutions in this country. The future bodes ill for the kind of breakthroughs we were able to make in the fifties, sixties, seventies, and eighties at these small hospitals. At the Queen E, I had almost unlimited access to the operating room, which you don't see in big hospitals that deal in, say, trauma or obstetrics."

Dodie Gibbons, an ER nurse who spent most of her long career at the Queen E, was present at the first laparoscopic surgery. "It was so amazing! I could hardly believe it was possible." She credits Ron Lewis with the fact that, "Our hospital was the first for prepping bowel operations with antibiotics in order to decrease post-op infections. We also had the first female resident surgeon. Other hospitals in town where I worked not only didn't have firsts; they weren't even up to date." Worst of all, in Gibbons' view, was the fact that, "the nurses [at other hospitals] weren't interested in learning more about health care; they just went through the motions."

Besides encouraging continual education of both doctors and nurses, the Queen Elizabeth was famous for, of all things, the quality of its cafeteria food, its after-hours sports teams, and its great parties. These apparent details were part of a long tradition of making the hospital as delightful a place to work as possible. Dodie adds, "At the Queen E., not only were you stimulated by the atmosphere of professionalism, the doctors knew how to make learning attractive, even fun. For example, John Zidilka would have lunch meetings with the nursing students. He'd say, 'Today we're going to discuss red blood cells, so we'll have red wine.' White wine was for white blood cells, and if he was talking about plasma, they'd have brandy!"

Mary Owen, a Queen E-trained nurse now working at St. Mary's in Montreal, explains why the hospital was so popular with its staff. "Rather than the usual hierarchical levels of management, the Queen E was a visionary place – more linear. Doctors and nurses worked as a *team*. I've yet to find that relationship in any other hospital. That's what caused me the greatest difficulty when I went elsewhere. Nurse turnover was very low at the Queen E. Respect was reciprocal. You were interested in learning; they were interested in teaching. I know doctors who spent hours teaching us things that supposedly we didn't *have* to know, like interpreting blood gases. Carl Svboka spent hours of his off-time teaching this stuff. It wasn't considered vital to our training, but, say you're monitoring a critical patient. If you know more about blood gases, you can read the apparatus and know better when to get a doctor."

Derek Marpole is a specialist in cardiology at the Royal Victoria Hospital in Montreal; he used to do rounds at the Queen E. He feels that medical teaching was very good there, "largely because everyone got along so well. The rotating trainees from other hospitals, like the General, just loved working at the Queen E. because they were given more responsibility. They were guided, of course, but they were given opportunities that the big bureaucracies didn't afford them, which was both gratifying and helped them learn fast." Marpole thinks the systems that can be available in smaller hospitals, with "good supervision but no interposed layers of residents between the attending and the patient," is by far the best way to train young doctors.

Orthopedic surgeon Larry Lincoln, who spent only four years at the Queen before it closed, used those years to pioneer cheaper, less invasive techniques such as laparoscopic knee surgery using only a local anesthetic. He echoes Marpole. "I trained at McGill and came to the

Queen E on rotation to the medical floor. I did an elective in hematology before I specialized. It was a lot of fun to train at the Queen as a student because it was personable and small, only 200 beds ... The staff mixed with you and treated you as an equal. They made learning and practicing fun. The atmosphere was so different from the teaching hospitals! They're just like being in the military where a student is a private on the bottom rung. And it wasn't just the students who were treated more humanely; the patients were too."

He agrees with Dodie Gibbons about the Queen E's high level of professional teamwork. "The nurses at the Queen E were pretty close to being equals with the doctors in terms of influence, respect, day-to-day ordering of priorities – everything! The surgery nursing staff I worked with was tremendous. We meshed so well as a group. Sometimes nurses in other hospitals I've worked in aren't so interested, aren't as competent. And nothing is more frustrating than trying to work with a nurse who doesn't care about what's going on, who wants to be somewhere else! Of course," Lincoln adds, "that's understandable. It's not an easy job; they're not well paid ... it's a tough life ... But at the Queen E the nurses followed what you were doing with great attention, even got ahead of you, they were so interested! They got the same pay and worked the same shifts. But somehow they fed off each other to get this attitude. They were of very high quality and we all worked as a team. That's one of the other things that attracted me to work there. It felt like a different world."

BUILDING A TEAM

Teamwork improves patient care. When we make big plans for our society's health care, these kinds of considerations are being completely left out of the equation.

Pat Titterton, ER Nurse

Pat Titterton, whose time at the Queen Elizabeth spanned more than 30 years and who was the head nurse of the ER for many of them, tells a story about how medical personnel learn to tell whether they're part of a team or not, and what that does to morale. After the Queen Elizabeth closed, one of her most experienced and dedicated colleagues moved to a similar small hospital. Early into her new position, this nurse, with decades of experience, asked to see a patient's x-ray that she had just brought to several doctors. The doctors asked why she wanted to see it.

She answered, tactfully (because she'd been reading x-rays for years), 'I thought I could learn something.' And they responded, 'Oh, it's not necessary for *you* to know any of this.'" Not only is such a response diminishing and demoralizing, "It's ridiculous," says Pat. The requirements for being a good nurse are always in flux, and there's always more to learn, as anyone even slightly aware of the history of the profession knows. "It was a doctor who taught me how to take blood," Pat says. "In the 1960s and 70s, only doctors started IV and took blood samples. But at the Queen E, they taught us to do both because it was so time-consuming to have to wait for them to do it. Technically, we weren't supposed to be doing it until it legally became a 'delegated act.' Now, of course, it's a normal part of a nurse's repertoire, and nurses are much faster at it. Being able to read x-rays in the ER, believe me, is knowledge a nurse could use."

Dodie Gibbons, an Intensive Care nurse for 30 years as well, says, "You aren't allowed to look at X-rays in other hospitals. At the Queen E, we'd be looking right over the doctors' shoulders. We'd of course carry them around and because we were interested in our patients' conditions, we'd look. We were never prevented from growing professionally. I taught things to the interns and residents, and that was normal! We all sort of grew together. It was a very forward-looking hospital. When it closed, it was very hard for its nurses to go to different hospitals and go back to not being treated with respect. At the Queen E, I could say to any doctor, 'You know, I don't like Mrs. Smith's looks today. Something's wrong.' And, that doctor would order more tests. At [larger hospitals like] St. Mary's or the [Royal] Victoria, they'd either ignore a comment like that or they'd act like you were overstepping your professional boundaries."

The Queen E was unusual in that its doctors did more than encourage their nurses to be part of the team; they disciplined newcomers who didn't grasp the concept. Mary Owen says, "I was working with this young intern, and I was trying to get him to take a patient's chest pains seriously and call a resident. He simply refused, so finally I called the senior resident, Marcel Fournier. I went over the intern's head, which in most hospitals would have gotten me into trouble. Fournier came, saw the patient, and then said to the intern, in front of me, 'I've got some advice for you. You can learn a lot from nurses. If an Intensive Care or ER nurse tells you to do something, I suggest you do what she says.'"

Although many doctors will tell stories about how common it is everywhere to be dressed down by nurses for such things, the nurses say there are fewer and fewer people coming up in the profession who have been made to feel confident enough to do so. The point that Larry Lincoln made earlier is important. It takes more work and energy to be a really good nurse than to just show up physically. Why were the nurses at this particular small hospital so eager to shoulder responsibilities that weren't supposed to be theirs? In part, as Mary Owen says, "I think we did all that because we did get so much respect from the doctors that we wanted to learn more, not make any mistakes, and really contribute to the whole process."

Pat Titterton says that the shared concern for the patient is in fact the foundation of achieving professional teamwork in any hospital setting. "We had a few doctors who were snobs but for the most part, the doctors were very approachable. When you had a doctor who wasn't nice to the nurses, we wouldn't go out of our way either. But for a doctor who acts like you're all a team, working towards the same goal – half their work would be done by the nurses!" Ron Lewis, their chief of Surgery, concurs. "In the OR, I was a stickler for how things should be done, which naturally meant small altercations with nurses. But I never met an OR nurse at the Queen E who didn't shine above any nurse elsewhere by a country mile. The very best nurse at the [other hospitals where I've worked] would have been the worst at the Queen E. Where I am now, you take what you get. Why? It was partly a culture of multitasking, and only someone who knows what you're doing in the operation and is paying attention can do that." As Lewis puts it, "If you're about to cut a knot, it's obvious you're going to need scissors. You'd be surprised how few nurses follow along enough to notice that! At the Queen E, they were with you, even ahead of you, they were so good. It was nurses working with you rather than having some contest of egos. I told someone the other day, when you hold out your hands to have a nurse put on the gloves, you can tell whether this is going to be a collaborative effort or the meeting of two totally different universes who happen to be in the same room."

Mary Owen says, "I think that ultimately a culture of reciprocity has to come from the administration, from the top right down. The Queen E administration, for example, had a very visionary idea of what the goal of all our work should be. There was an old admonition that was a serious motto in that hospital: 'Nurse, you have the entire care of this patient.' We took that seriously and so did the hospital; nursing was as important as doctoring. I think it's what hospital nursing *should* be. At the other hospitals I've worked, it's a simple hierarchy. Administration, doctors, then the lowly nurses and the rest of the staff even further down. So you do what you're told, even if you think it might be wrong, and it's the doctors who have the responsibility for anything that happens. Of course, some nurses are able to stand up for themselves and their own vision of the job, but many are hesitant by nature, they're young, or they've become bitter."

It's not surprising that few people are able to assert their own ideas and take responsibility for suggestions that could affect a patient's survival if they're discouraged from doing so. Because the staff at the little Queen E was given respect, certain kinds of basic, common-sense actions never had to be justified. "For example," Pat Titterton says, "when I was a student in Emergency, in those days you would be all alone manning the ER. A train had run over a man's foot and it was really a mess; I'd never seen anything so terrible. You're supposed to call an intern, but you have to wait until they arrive. I looked around and saw the chief of surgery, Dr Goodall, by the front door with his coat on and about to leave for the evening. So I left the ER, me, a student nurse, and simply grabbed him and said, 'You have to help me! You can't leave me alone with this!' He came right in and helped; he never talked about protocol or made me feel for an instant like I shouldn't have done that."

Most workplace efficiency experts will affirm that in order to be well established, teamwork has to be extended beyond the work place. At this and other small hospitals like it, receptionists and nurses, nurses and doctors, even surgeons and cafeteria workers got together on their off hours and had fun, through sports teams and parties organized at the hospital. Nurse Mary Owen became such close friends with Judith Levitan, a General Practitioner, that they would trade clothes; Mary had bikinis and fancy beach outfits, and once a year Judith would take off for Club Med and borrow them, in the time-honoured way of girl-friends everywhere. When Mary had a heart attack two years ago, she described how several old Queen E doctors, specialists, and nurses showed up in her hospital room. "Mary Rona, who used to be at the Queen E, called and came to visit; she was fantastic. Not professionally, you understand, but as friends." Is this kind of thing common in other hospitals? Television shows like *ER* and *Scrubs* make you think it is. "No," Mary says, "it's rare. I don't think many doctors and nurses are comfortable enough with each other to be as close as we were. I think it was because the Queen E was so small that we knew each other." Yet, many of the hospitals people now complain about are not much bigger.

Mary says, "Yes ... and the scary thing is, even when they're bad in comparison, they still give better care than most of the big ones."

Mary says, "the doctor/nurse relationships from that era have lasted, even past closing. I've tried to figure out why we were so happy at our work. My family asks me too. 'What was so special there that you liked it so much, that you miss it so much?' I think it was respect – on all levels, from the highest to the grassroots. We had it from the beginning under Harold Griffith, of course, but Mario Larivière, our last general director, was still carrying that on. He wanted to hear from people; his office was open. He wanted nursing decisions to be in the hands of nurses, not government appointees, bureaucrats, or board members. It really was a vision of how to manage a place as well as how to provide care for the patients, so much so that we talk about it today in our nursing meetings. We had an advisory committee back in 1997 to look at the tremendous problem of shortages because girls aren't going into nursing any more. What attracts people is being of service, but in a professional and respected way, not in a constant crisis! Patient-focused care is what we envisioned, what we tried to give, what would serve the community, and [what] still attracts nurses today. It requires respect from all involved, and it requires the funding to do it right."

HAVING FUN

People would fix the taps in the scrub room so they'd spray all over you. The doctors sent a dead bee down to pathology on a gurney. Their note read that it had died from 'abnormal causes (a shoe), and needed a post-mortem.'

ER nurse Dodie Gibbons

How can institutional teamwork be achieved? Modern business gurus provide reams of advice, and brand-new theories are always being broken in and touted by some group or other. But few people look at existing institutions and deconstruct how successful ones got that way. At efficient and beloved hospitals such as the Queen Elizabeth, the key methods used by the staff and administration to maintain a productive work atmosphere were alarmingly simple – and seemingly off-subject. One major source of that institution's high morale was the cafeteria. Besides offering good food, it was not divided hierarchically. Everybody ate and drank together and mixed up tables, disciplines, and levels of employment every day. Moreover, from its inception, staff members at the old hospital were expected to take part in the institution's organized parties and sports teams, which means they got to know each other outside of the work context. In order to promote equality and empowerment, parties, dinners, and team sports as well as a friendly atmosphere that encouraged familiarity, horseplay, and practical jokes were an integral part of the hospital's routine. The administration also made sure that staff never missed educational opportunities and that participants received adequate funding, even in periods of serious belt-tightening. Although such policies sound more serious, they fit into the same category as good food and baseball. It's a seldom-admitted fact that for many people, the stimulation of continuing to learn is the main way to have fun at work.

Mario Larivière was the hospital's last director general. After it closed, he became the director general at the Hôpital St. Eustache, which is located in a large suburb west of Montreal. He retired early – not long after he was interviewed in 2004. Being a DG is very similar to being the CEO of a corporation. Larivière served as the DG for four major Quebec hospitals over his career. At the Queen E, as elsewhere, he was responsible for the budget, the hospital's relationship with the government, its day-to-day running efficiency, and the allocation of all resources. He had such a good managing record that no matter whether the Liberals or the Parti Quebecois were in charge, he was regularly flown in to take over a hospital that found itself in trusteeship. Larivière, a warm, handsome man in his early fifties, estimates he has worked in various advisory capacities for about 80 percent of Quebec's urban and rural hospitals, but that his all-time favourite medical institution was the Queen Elizabeth. He takes on a higher colour as he talks about his years there.

"I love talking about the Queen E," he says. "There were so many parties! People had a passion for the place, and they could celebrate! I would have stayed so much longer. Every month we had a physician's lunch together, a huge buffet at the Badminton club, with the staff meeting after. The Queen E made parties and dinners out of the hard and often boring work of deciding budgets and protocol, every single week. There were those kinds of events and also employee and retirement and holiday parties, auxiliaries' teas, and you went to them all. There was a really huge Christmas dinner and party for the entire hospital staff every year as well. The kitchen was great, the best in Montreal, and they specialized in really great food for parties."

These benefits were more than luxurious frills. They seem to have seriously improved patient care. Surgeon Fred Weigan learned about a large variety of medical styles by working in all kinds of hospitals all over the world. After the Queen E closed, he went to the OR of another Montreal hospital for two years and then worked in Third World hospitals for Médicins sans frontières (Doctors Without Borders). "A typical scenario at the Queen E," Weigan says, "We're all at the weekly lunch. I'm a GP. I'm smart and competent, but I'm not a cardiologist with a specialty in hypertension. So I ask a colleague, who is all that, about this new drug, Robaxycene, that I've heard about and am thinking of prescribing, and he says, 'Oh Jesus, Fred, don't touch it, there have been four deaths!' "Wow. Thanks, Bob. Have some dessert?' That kind of regular interplay saves lives! On top of that, every Wednesday we'd have special presentations, to make sure really important innovations or dangers didn't slip by us. It was one happy family, because we ate together and talked all the time."

Derek Marpole, a specialist like Wiegan, agrees. "The rapport between the specialties was very good at the Queen E. Anesthesia was very important, of course. They more or less ran the ICU [Intensive Care Unit] with the nursing staff. But most importantly, family medicine was not looked down on at all, the way it so often is in the big teaching hospitals. Lots of small hospital ERs are run by GPs, and at the Queen E they were particularly good – good doctors, nice people!" Of course, Montreal's big teaching hospitals have occasional dinners and parties that are attended by all the staff, but attendees describe them as being very different. Marpole says, "There used to be an annual dinner for attendings and house physicians at the big hospitals, but they got so malignant! Why? Well, it was that master-slave relationship. There were skits where the underlings, the house staff, interns whatever, would try to get revenge for the demeaning way they were treated every day, and the events got downright libelous. So the whole thing was shut down. They would have skits at the Queen E celebrations too, but they were fun. Sometimes the chiefs of staff and administrators would get up and lampoon themselves!"

George Subak, chief of the Queen E's large and respected Department of Psychiatry says, "There was a lot of camaraderie between all the doctors at the Queen E, even those of us in psych and the rest. The Queen E didn't have that famous gulf and animosity between psychiatry and the other specialties you so often find elsewhere. We got consults in the ICU, in gastroenterology – constantly. There was a good feeling that you had a valuable input into their specialties and vice-versa, not this, 'We don't care about psychiatry attitude.' We had some strong allies in administration that helped make that happen: John Hughes, Mario Larivière, Albert Nixon. I had great satisfaction working at the Queen E."

Dodie Gibbons remembers the mid-1980s hospital softball team. "They were wonderful games," she laughs, "Imagine: everyone was there, playing and laughing, falling down, getting muddy – kitchen and laundry workers, nurses, doctors, orderlies, even some administrators! Because of those silly games, the specialists and GPs were always available to each other and to us nurses. You could talk to an internist over wine or baseball without having to pay money for a consult or a referral. It's so hard at the other hospitals I've worked at to even *speak* to a specialist; there's simply no proper social situation or opportunity, on top of the general discouragement against nurses having ideas. At the Queen E, we all went by first names. I could go up to any cardiologist or chief of staff and voice my concerns or questions about my patients – feel free to ask their opinion about procedures."

Dorothy Mapes is from an earlier period. She finished her studies before World War II, when the hospital was still run as a largely private institution by the Griffith family. Even back then, the hospital's weekly staff lunch meetings were a tradition. "That was my time to learn things – you'd get one-on-one with doctors or speakers every Wednesday, plus once a year we'd have a world-renowned speaker." She also mentioned the morale-building great food. "It was very good – and free until the 1950s; after that, we nurses had to pay a very small charge." There were also meetings of all the head nurses. Discussion periods dealt with problems or exciting new procedures that might be showing promising results. "It was a means of communication and learning, held once a month – a way of getting input from everyone in nursing. And there were all the other meetings where you'd get to know the rest of the staff."

Pat Titterton has albums of party and sports photographs showing how well the Queen E knew how to keep on having fun, right up to closure. "I think this made a big difference professionally as well as socially. At conferences we were always up to date; sometimes we were ahead! We'd be surprised; we knew we were just a little community hospital, but we'd go down to a huge place like the Boston General, and we were right up there with the big, formal institutions in terms of innovations and knowledge." On one occasion, the Boston General was giving a conference for emergency staff. Pat says, "Very few ER nurses except ours were invited; no nurses from the big Montreal hospitals like General or the Vic were there. I think that's because we really worked side by side with the doctors in our ER and understood what was going on. Everyone, seven or eight of us emergency doctors and nurses, would keep each other informed. A doctor working on a patient would call out, 'Pat! Come over here, look at this! Do you see what I'm doing?' You'd learn a lot, and on a daily basis. I know they don't do that at other hospitals."

Dodie Gibbons concurs. During Pat's and her tenure, the game was softball. Joe Mammazza quotes Dr Gay Goodall from an earlier era laughingly: "He said, only partly joking, 'Unless you play squash, you can't do general surgery at the Queen E!'" In Larry Lincoln's day, it was hockey, and before he was born, the doctors and administrators were meeting each other for badminton and curling. Harold Griffith, one of the hospital's major progenitors, made sure that his first Jewish physician, Eli Katz, was admitted to the Westmount Curling Club so they all could play together. As we'll see ahead, he had been carefully trained by his doctor father, A.R. Griffith, the hospital's founder, not only how to practice medicine but also how to have fun.

NURSING SCHOOL

If I were very ill and I had a choice to make between a good doctor and a good nurse – I'd take the good nurse. Because she'd make sure I got good care from the doctors, as well as good nursing.

Mary Owen, RN

The older I get, the more I appreciate nurses – and the less I appreciate doctors!

Surgeon Fred Weigan

From its founding moment in 1895 until 1978 – that is, for ninety-five years – the Queen Elizabeth hospital, like almost every other early community hospital in Canada, was as much a training school for nurses as it was a facility to receive patients. Most of the nurses in the prime of their career when the hospital closed in 1996 – the head nurses of the ER, the ICU, and the medical floors – had been trained in its school, which had closed only 13 years before. Most city hospitals, not just in

Montreal but across the country, had their own nursing schools in the early days. Prior to the discovery of the importance of sanitation, and especially prior to the discovery of antibiotics and the new surgical techniques that only became possible after the risk of sepsis was removed, hospitals were places the sick went to be *nursed* far more than they went to be doctored. At that time, doctors performed tasks that are now firmly considered nursing: bathing foreheads, changing dressings, sitting by the bedside waiting for changes in breathing rates or fevers. Nurses did more of the scut work: winding bandages, drawing blood, doing the terrible and unending clean-ups. Still, their presence, to say nothing of their free labour, was so vital to the healing process that they absolutely had to live in the building, so as to be on 24-hour call.

The Queen E, or rather, the Homeopathic Hospital as it was then known, was quite literally built around its nurses' school and for those 95 years was home to thousands of young women who came in as girls of nineteen or twenty and left as trained professionals – in the very first profession widely open to women. Upon leaving, many of the nurses who didn't marry doctors went no further than the same building in which they had trained and remained there for their entire careers.

The Homeopathic was a markedly female institution for reasons that extended beyond this constant physical presence of the nurses living inside its walls. The first hospital building was the outright gift of a local woman devoted to the new science of homeopathy, Mrs. Georgiana Duff Phillips. Quickly following in her footsteps, a Women's Auxiliary of like-minded, well-off local women became the hospital's most dependable source of funding. The Auxiliary continued to provide a significant amount of the hospital's discretionary income well into the modern era, when Albert Nixon, director general between 1971 and 1989, was still turning to this women's group, as to a faucet, whenever he needed money for a new machine or even for a new wing. Physical presence and economic clout at least partly explain the unusually egalitarian position of its nursing staff *vis-a-vis* its physicians, right up to its closing day.

The earliest nurses are long since gone, of course. But some, who go back at least halfway to the founding day, are still going strong. Dorothy Mapes, for example, attended the Homeopathic Hospital's Nursing School between 1937 and 1940. Aside from being away at McGill briefly and doing private nursing up north in Temiskaming, her entire career was there. By 1940, she was well installed in her profession; the war was on in Europe, and the young women of her school's class took on the very serious duty of serving on the Home Front. She very quickly became head nurse. "Under normal circumstances," she says, "that would have taken a lot longer; you would have had to wait for someone to die off!" Later on, she became supervisor, then assistant director of nursing, and finally associate director of nursing. That was a job that required her to plan budgets and allocate personnel. "With the increasing constraints of government management, that got worse and worse. We started with public donations, but when the government came in, in the 1960s, we lost control over salaries and much of the budget."

Dorothy says, "In those early days, "it wasn't the government but the chief surgeon who was God, and the head nurse really was the Virgin Mary. We also had a 'lady superintendent' whose job was difficult to describe. She was a kind of prestigious hospital housekeeper who checked for dust as people entered, saw to wine glasses for the important patients, gave a sort of tone to the place." Despite her always-escalating responsibilities, Dorothy's salary was $50 a month, which even in those days wasn't enough for her to have her own place. "It was enough," she says, "to pay my share of rent, hydro, and so forth in an apartment with four roommates. We still had that great canteen and ate for free at work. We were aged 17 to 21. Gradually things changed; two got married. The remaining two of us old maids kept the apartment and stayed there for ten more years. In those days, we lived and worked together and were very good at getting along, and I still hear from them all."

Dorothy's career spanned both the 50th anniversary of the founding of the nursing school and its sad demise, so she had to deal with the first waves of student nurses trained in CEGEPs, Quebec's two-year post-secondary colleges, away from hospital practice. Although the way this has played out has differed slightly from province to province and from country to country, in general, the hospital-tied nursing schools of the 19th century became attached to colleges or universities in the late 20th century, so changes in training became more standardized for all nurses in North America. Pat Titterton and others talk about how difficult it is, under the present regime, for young students to go from classroom theory to the stress and mess of sickroom realities. "It was very traumatic for people who came from CEGEP," Dorothy agrees. "And we wondered, when we first got them, what are they learning? It didn't seem to be at all what they needed. They would be taught some basic principles, but it wasn't like the kind of apprenticeship training we had. I would imagine there are far more drop-outs from the profession today because they get thrown into the real world of hospitals with no concrete preparation. The most important thing about our training was to work as a team, which is a lot easier to learn if you know each other so well."

Of course, the nursing shortage, not just in Quebec but in all of Canada, has become a regularly recurring social problem. None of the results of these pedagogical changes – removing schools from hospitals, instituting mostly theoretical courses in colleges, closing the hospital schools – have been properly tracked by government studies or discussed in the political arena. Mario Larivière says, "Remember in 1997, only seven or eight years ago, they were actually paying nurses, specialized nurses, to quit! ... We [administrators] said, 'Good heavens, please don't do this! We don't have enough nurses as it is!' The government didn't listen. We lost 7,000 nurses, some in the prime of experience – irreplaceable! Pat Titterton is a good example; she wasn't ready to retire. There were no jobs offered in her specialty – she was a magnificent ER nurse – and yet she was paid money to leave, instead of to stay!"

Because of shortages and the scheduling problems they entail, the way nurses manage a hospital ward has entirely changed. Family physician John Hughes says, "You used to have the head nurse – the spider in the web who knew everything, who went to bat with everyone necessary in order to look after the patients in her wards. Below her, you had the charge nurse, responsible for each individual patient. After that, you had the nurses' assistants, volunteers, and so forth. But today the same nurse doesn't see the same patient two days in a row because the nursing-patient ratio was pushed so far you can now only have a generalized pool of doctors and a pool of nurses. This is not designed for the patients' well-being but for the welfare of the financial bottom-line; obviously, you'd get better care with more people with clearer responsibilities and some personal identification with certain patients."

Pat Titterton says that today, nurses in training only do what are called in French "stages" – maybe eight days out of a month working on the floor in hospitals. "But in the nursing school days, we were down in the wards every day. When we got the CEGEP-trained nurses, we found they needed full supervision for at least a year, whereas the in-house ones were ready to be left on their own a year earlier. What does that cost the system?" She described the life of a beginning student at the

Queen E's school. "From the very first day of class they sent you up to change water jugs at 7 a.m. Gradually, you moved from water jugs to emptying bedpans and giving bed baths. One or two girls might have quit then. You're as vulnerable as anyone else to disgust and fear. Or you should be."

Titterton, who was the head of the Queen E's very active Emergency Room, reminisces on her own experience. "From the time I was very young, I always wanted to be a nurse," she says, "but I was sick at the sight of blood, so I thought I couldn't be one after all. [Eventually,] I applied at all three hospitals, the Queen E, the Royal Victoria, and the Montreal General. The latter were cold, unfriendly; they seemed uninterested in me. But at the Queen E, I made a connection, and because of that I felt I could confide in them; I admitted that I was really nervous because I was squeamish about blood and suffering. You know their response? They said, 'Oh, you'll make an excellent nurse!' They told me having that kind of reaction meant I was empathetic with sick and wounded people. They said, 'We want people like that.' I was so encouraged! And there was another consideration that doesn't seem like much but meant a lot in those days. The Queen E paid their senior nurses $50 a month. All hospitals took advantage of the labour of their in-house student nurses, but only the Queen E paid them even a token amount for it."

Pat agrees that it's a shock for young girls when they begin dealing with wastes and sick bodies, but, as she points out, "If you had a bad day, you could talk about it before you went to sleep – not go home all alone and upset with no one to confide in who understood what was bothering you. In the school, we were assigned Big Sisters who were one year older, and they took their role seriously and helped us."

Dorothy Mapes agrees that the intangible benefits of working and living in the hospital, knowing your colleagues so very well, cannot be overestimated. "It was part of our work routine in my era, too. We'd get together as soon as our shift was over and of course we'd talk about our day. That way you could compare notes, see if things were really as bad (or good!) as you had been thinking. You'd learn from the more experienced ones, who'd say, 'Well, I would've done this or that,' and you'd try that next time. Today, student nurses are much more isolated because it's unlikely that, even if they do manage to bond with someone in the classroom, they will end up in the same hospital." Dorothy says the various nursing schools in town in her era also had methods of enabling individuals in different hospitals to get to know each other.

"The Royal Victoria and the General had their own schools as well. They were all proud of their schools, and tightly knit. But at the Homeopathic, we really did feel that we were the best. Inter-hospital sports teams used to bring us all together too. In the war years, of course, there was a higher percentage of females playing the games, and to a great degree, we were running the whole hospital."

Although the school was still thriving, Mapes says that, "By the 1960s, you could feel the heavy hand of government. There was a constant push to *cut* the number of nurses, not recruit them; there was no money to pay them and they became very hard to get. People were specializing, too, as ER or ICU nurses, say, so that was an added complexity. Some people only wanted to work in surgery, not medicine, because medicine had a lot of chronic care and in surgery, of course, people tend to get better, so the work is less demoralizing. We found it hard to fill our shifts, like the midnight to 8 a.m. Because there was a shortage, that rare available nurse could say, 'Look, I'll do days but not nights or afternoons.' So staffing got more difficult. And we had gotten new machines that people had to learn to use. We had courses for heart machines given by the company on the hospital's time, but there was always something missing in terms of staff."

During this period, Dorothy had moved up the ladder to become associate director of nursing, and had also ended up teaching. "In 1947, 48, and 49, I left to go to McGill. I took a degree in teaching and supervision. It was financed by one of our nursing school alumni, and I arrived back just as the Queen E got a new director of nursing, Miss Bryant. We two became the entire nursing school's Teaching Department. I did sciences, she did arts. I spent the first year being about a day ahead of my students – six to twelve girls! Today, all these years later, we still get together for lunch every year." Dorothy got no extra pay for her teaching responsibilities. She says, "The situation for nurses, if not the pay, actually kept getting worse every decade. The 1970s were the worst in my career for a shortage of nurses. There was more government control, which brought in even more difficulties with staffing. Women were also beginning to have their own ideas about what they wanted to do in their professions. And finally, unions came in. That made us all become employees, instead of colleagues."

Pat Titterton points out that since country-wide unionization of nursing, there are a lot of complex details to take into consideration when trying to rate whether working under each provincial government's aegis has improved or harmed the profession. "For example, Quebec's wages for nurses are lower, but the benefits are superior. You get two weeks' vacation the first couple years, then pretty soon, you're up to a month. You get thirteen paid holidays, sick days, and you can also get a Christmas bonus. But we had something that went well beyond all that at the Queen E: we had the chance to learn and expand. We had the Griffith Education Fund, set up to benefit nurses; you could apply to it in order to attend conferences or improve your skills in any way. Your immediate superiors would approve or disapprove of a trip or a course; naturally, we tried to keep expenses within the interest in the fund. There's nothing like that now."

One example Pat gives of how supportive the Queen E was to nurses' ongoing education and professional growth is when the Canadian Nurses' Association called her in the early 1990s and asked her to create a new national ER certification exam. She realized she would have to leave work for five days, so she went, with some trepidation, to the director of nursing to ask for the time off. "And my director said, 'This is so great! We'll pay your salary while you're gone! Phone them right back and say you're coming!' That's real support." She adds, "Sometimes the Queen E staff would take the initiative and tell us, 'your Association is having a conference; does anyone want to go? Tell them to apply and we'll sign for it.'" These were conferences where nurses could learn new procedures like ACLS [Advanced Cardiac Life Support], or how to read ECGs, what was new in the use of certain drugs, and so on. "Our head nurse of ICU knew that nurses as well as doctors need these courses. She said, 'We're having to do these things!' So we were sent off to take them. I got to take, for example, the ACLS course with two nurses, then we trained our own team, doctors and nursing educators, so we all had this advanced cardiac course. You go to any other hospital, you'll find nobody else did that. Dodie Gibbons said they told her at the new job she took, following closure, that she had to have CPR to work in their Emergency Room. She told them, 'Well, no problem. I even have my ACLS.' They didn't know what she was talking about and made her take CPR, anyway, a kindergarten course in comparison."

This continuous education for the nurses was paid for by a special fund, the Griffith Educational Fund, which was set up by the Griffith brothers, Harold and Jim, for this purpose in 1966. It funded continuing education trips for doctors and interns as well, but including nurses was one of its most unique attributes. It was so well-managed that nearly ten years after the demise of the hospital, the fund was able to

subsidize not only this book and a formal archive of the hospital's materials, it also founded two Chairs at McGill: the Queen Elizabeth Hospital of Montreal Foundation Chair in Pediatric Anesthesia in 2004,
almost ten years after the Hospital was closed, and the much older Harold Griffith Chair in Anesthesia Research that oversees anesthesiology
at all of the McGill teaching hospitals.

Queen Elizabeth nurses achieved national firsts in both medical and
surgical treatment because of their ongoing training opportunities as
well as the responsibilities they were routinely given. Pat Titterton
remembers when the Canadian Nurses' Association was devising certification processes for various specialties. "They already had them in
things like psychiatry, but they decided to create a certification for ER
nurses. They sent me a pamphlet with all the requirements, and I
decided to go for it. I told the staff and left the information around.
Eight out of our staff of twelve signed up to take it. At that point, the
Association said only nine nurses in the entire province were taking the
exam! 'So, since you've packed the test, can we have it at your ER?' It
was very rigorous, an eight-hour exam, three hours in morning and five
more in the afternoon. Even the pass mark was very hard. You had to
get 75, not 60. All my nurses passed, but it didn't get them better work
because no one demanded such a high level of expertise! After closure,
one of the nurses who was certified in this demanding specialty went to
St. Mary's; they put her on the geriatric ward."

PATIENT-CENTRED CARE

The patient is the focus of care and nursing plans are built around the
patient. Other places are disease-centered, with guidelines for stroke,
cardiac, and so on. We were taught to adapt to the patient – not
everyone reacts the same just because they have the same disease or
injury.

                                        ER Head Nurse Pat Titterton

Of course, every hospital likes to emphasize their capacity to care more
about people than about money, and most emphasize their desire to
put the patient at the centre of their activities. However, there can be a
big difference between the touchy-feely public relations television
spots trying to attract customers to a private hospital in the U.S. and
the way that individual patients actually experience their treatment.
Measuring the feeling of the overall patient experience is particularly

difficult in the all-public setting of countries like Canada, France, or Great Britain because there are no distracting bells and whistles of "special arrangements." These hospitals lack softly-lit, wallpapered, private rooms with a view, for example. Generally, they have no private rooms at all. Public hospitals all sport the same bare-bones atmosphere of undecorated pale-green walls and spongy institutional blankets; they use the same gurneys and beds and the same tired or distracted figures, swathed in blue or green, are moving around their grotesquely bright, neon-lit halls. So when you're down to the real basics, how are people made to feel, day-to-day, and what exactly does the former staff of the Queen E *mean* when they say they centred their activities around the patient? There are no reliable statistics that enable anyone to measure an institution's performance in such areas.

The Queen Elizabeth was still called the Homeopathic Hospital when Dorothy Mapes, associate nursing director, trained there. Its atmosphere retained much of the Edwardian era flavour of the institution's first days, preserving a world where the nurses reigned supreme over the wards. It was the nurses who had the power to create the entire tone of patient care, and they all knew it. In that respect at least, hospitals haven't changed much. As Mary Owens put it in 2004, "I believe nurses are the center of any hospital. I speak mostly for the ER, but nurses are out there every day. They're the ones with the patients. They're the ones who know what is going on." The early days of hospitals attracted people to medicine as a calling and a duty as spiritual as it was social. Health professionals still took the ideal of having charity and compassion for the sick very seriously.

As for the Homeopathic, "It was a good place," Mapes says. "People were nice to other people. In our case, that was part of what we learned as students – part of the way nurses were supposed to look after people, look after their patients. They aren't objects. I had the great good fortune to have a post-World War I teacher, a woman who was very gifted at teaching us how to treat a person with dignity." In the days before antibiotics, machines, and skilled surgery, patient care meant comforting someone who was likely to be suffering for quite awhile. Hospital stays extended for weeks and months, even for obstetrics. Mapes explains, "We were trained to do the things that make a stay in a hospital more bearable. The head nurse would always ask one question about a bed-bath: 'Did you put the patients' feet in water?' That was her way of saying, 'Did you do a good job? Did you make it as pleasant an experience as possible?' We all carried around these little bags with powder, sponges, and so on. We gave a good bed-bath, complete, sensitive – you know, making sure to pull the screens around and give privacy, even if the person wasn't aware. She also made it clear that we should take the opportunity to teach people hygiene. This was the 1930s and 40s; a lot of people still never cleaned their teeth, for example, or took care of their feet properly. So we, as health professionals, were supposed to use their stay in hospital as an opportunity to help them learn these things."

Mario Larivière likes to describe how caring about the little things made the Queen Elizabeth so unusual in his experience, almost 50 years later. "I remember a typical example. Here's an elderly patient, not poor, but alone and mildly ill after his wife's death. The doctor he had before his discharge went in person to his house to see how he was – which was the kind of thing the Queen Elizabeth doctors did. The doctor realized he was malnourished and not in a position to do much about it, so he arranged for him to take his meals at the hospital cafeteria, which was as good as a hotel, I must say, the best in the city. So here was this old man, at a cost to the province of about $5 a day, socializing, getting out, getting fed – imagine what all those services would cost the taxpayer in a foster home! The staff at that hospital was like that – dedicated to the mission of the hospital, to help the patients. And they knew what their population needed."

Pat says that no one at the Queen E was surprised at the size and vehemence of the community reaction during the fight to save the hospital. "We fully expected that kind of turn-out; I think there should've been even more. We were like parts of a family. When someone came into the ER, they were treated like a human being. People wrote us letters, called, and came in person to thank us for treating them that way."

Mario Larivière, the outside convert, says, "Everybody was proud to work there; many even lived in the community, in fact hardly ever left it. The most important thing was that these professionals – specialists, nurses, staff, general physicians – all worked together very well and all recognized that one goal: the patient comes first. Most hospitals say that; but do they do it? Here's a story of a typical reaction I witnessed. A patient showed up at five p.m. He said he thought he had an appointment for blood work, but that department was closed; everyone had gone home. He was talking to me. I'd been there a couple years, so I didn't know what to tell him. He'd come a long way on the bus; I was saying 'It's too bad, we're sorry,' when a technician who was off duty happened to walk by and heard me. She told him, 'Come with me, I'll

take your blood and do it for you.'" Many other former Queen E people have similar stories. GP Judith Levitan talks about Francesca Lanza,
who worked the admissions desk at the Queen E. "Someone came by
with a specimen for the lab. Francesca started explaining where to take
it. He looked confused. After three minutes, she just said, 'I'll take it
for you.' That was no big thing for her. Where could you go to get that
kind of attitude today?"

Judith Levitan is a former Queen E doctor. She's pretty, intense, and
currently a member of the board of the Royal Victoria teaching hospital. She says that there are such clear benefits to people having caring
and humane experiences that she doesn't understand how that central
goal could have been lost. "Being treated badly makes people fearful,
anxious, defensive, even angry and uncooperative – how does that save
time and money? Trying to get people out rather than in, even if they
need care, that's what hospitals do now." She worked for another hospital following the closure of the Queen E, but she couldn't stand the
lack of that central directive, patient care. "In the hospitals where I
worked after closure ... I've had patients come up and grab my arm and
say, 'Get me out of here!' It's not so much that they will die or get
sicker, although with *C. difficile*, that's changing too. But really, it's the
peripheral things. It smells bad, it's noisy, frightening, unnecessarily
uncomfortable, or even painful. For example, one night I was doing
admissions and there was a little old lady there where I was working. I
spent some time with her. Eventually she told me, 'My intravenous is
really hurting.' It was stuck in the fold of her wrist. So I went to look for
her nurse, who was listening to a ghetto blaster and eating popcorn. I
told her the old lady's IV was hurting her. She replied, 'Is it working?' I
said, 'Yes, but it hurts her.' I'll never forget her answer. She said: 'We
don't do that here. If you want to change it, do it yourself.' Imagine.
'We don't do that here – we don't care about unnecessary suffering.' I
helped the old woman, but I quit. I haven't worked on a ward since."

We are at a huge disadvantage in judging how health care is managed because there's no mathematical model – the only model modern
managers recognize – for assessing how a patient is actually treated
beyond simply assessing whether they live or die. The hollowness at the
core of our current system, which is a lack of an inspiring and edifying
central goal like the Queen E's "patient-centred care" in the context of
the exceedingly difficult, demoralizing, and messy work of trying to
keep sick people alive, may be doing far more harm than we can imagine to our health professionals as well as to their patients. Judith

Levitan goes on, "If I haven't been able to settle since the Queen E closed, it's because I'm not used to working where you're not allowed to make decisions when serious problems come up." She adds, "[Today, I am] surprised to hear good stories about hospital stays. People used to go into hospital to feel safe and cared for. Now they're terrified, and they really shouldn't even be in there without an advocate, an aggressive relative or someone to make sure they really *are* cared for."

GP John Hughes says one way to assess at least the most basic level of the quality of care and comfort in a hospital would be to simply keep track of "bedpan time," that is, how long people have to wait for help to get to the washroom or for bedpans, and rate the hospital accordingly. Judith says, "I've heard of cases where people *beg* for bed pans – they're only asking to be handed a bed pan, not even for an orderly to help them to the bathroom – and they're told to mess their bed and it will be changed eventually! Imagine what that does to their comfort, their self-esteem, their ability to believe they can get well!" Hughes agrees that if you can't get help with such daily needs, you're not getting the quality of care you deserve, regardless of whether or not you survive the experience.

THE FIGHT

What was awful was that after two years of work, we'd turned the place around, solved the beds issue, gotten out of deficit, and been rewarded with that CT Scan, the brand-new ER. We had hope; we had all the proper constituents to grow, we had proven success, backing of the community, everything. They closed the wrong hospital.

Director General Mario Larivière

The announcement of the closure of this object of extravagant loyalty and praise came at one of the many high points of its existence. There had been terrific struggles when it was first founded in the 1890s as an upstart hospital staffed by homeopathic doctors who had been denied access to the established Montreal General and the new Royal Victoria. And all along, it had faced periods of hardship and near-bankruptcy. But by 1995, after four years in the hands of their popular new director general, Mario Larivière, the Queen Elizabeth Hospital of Montreal was fully on course. The Quebec government had just funded a brand-new ER that the doctors and nurses had been able to design themselves. Moreover, in apparent recognition of two years of perfectly balanced budgets, Quebec was preparing to award them a long-coveted CT scan. So it was a staggering shock to hear, with no warning, that the newly expanded hospital was slated for closure. Beginning in September of 1995, a continual outpouring of denial and disbelief, rage, sorrow, and desperate attempts at compromise – all the classic stages of human grief – erupted from both the community and the hospital's large staff. There were even death threats, which in some cases actually came true; four psychiatric patients committed suicide in despair at losing the hospital's walk-in clinic.

The Queen E was not alone. Seven other hospitals across the city and, although few people actually absorbed the implications of the fact, many, many more across the country were in the same situation. In the nearby Montreal suburb of Lachine, chief admitting officer Geri Armstrong and paymaster Micheline Racicot organized to try to save their hospital, the Lachine General, by amassing 20,000 signatures out of a town population of only 35,000 people! Patricia Bush and Linda Sherrington, in wheelchairs, who took part in their mile-long march in June, were from the nearby Kahnawake Mohawk reserve and said the Lachine hospital was the most convenient one for natives. "At the Lachine General, they treat you like family; you're not just another number!" And back at the Queen Elizabeth, switchboard operator Nicole Aquin was overwhelmed with more calls than the hospital had ever received. "Some people, elderly people," she reported to the newspapers, "are crying on the phone, wondering what's going to happen to them."[3]

Because of the legal morass involved in figuring out who owned what at partially private institutions where equipment, supplies, and even additions and wings had often been donated by individuals, the governments involved had to pass various laws establishing its rights to the spoils. In Quebec, Bill 83 gave Health Minister Jean Rochon new powers. He was allowed to withdraw the permits of public or private hospitals. "In essence," as the *Montreal Gazette* explained, "[Bill 83 gave] the government the power to shut down hospitals and liquidate their assets." Even with these unprecedented and arguably highly undemocratic powers, all hospital property could not be alienated; protagonists were promised a legal nightmare of months in court figuring out who owned what and/or whether to "liquidate" holdings at auction. The result was often the kind of waste that Eli Katz later described where state-of-the-art equipment was mothballed during the court battles and was never again integrated into the system.

Of course, little if any of the economic costs and wasted resources this fight entailed was figured into the projected savings that closing hospital beds was supposed to bring to the government, and it seems puzzling that the revenue-hungry government bodies seem to have paid so little attention to this elementary addition and subtraction. It helps to remember that the middle 1990s was also the era in which the economic theories of a decade before, championed by Prime Ministers Brian Mulroney and Margaret Thatcher as well as by President Ronald Reagan, were being consolidated with what can only be called religious zeal. The message of this revolution, actually termed by its protagonists "a New World Order," seems in retrospect to have demanded a good deal of pure faith. It included the implementation of legislation and regulations supporting the basic policy that governments – whether in Canada, France, the U.S., or Britain or even the developing world – would no longer willingly sponsor any form of social welfare. In nearly all cases, governments would begin to take the side of the liquidation of public assets and their management for corporate profit.

Owen Ness, then on the Queen Elizabeth Board of Directors, says that one of the Quebec government's decisions – to close two rehabilitation (long-term care) facilities, the Catherine Booth and Villa Medica – was a pure mistake. "The Regional Board had intended to only close acute-care beds but knew so little about the English hospitals that they closed the wrong one!" Whatever the reasons, when the decision was announced, the media reported that the government's plan to close 291 beds at these two institutions – a savings of $22 million – would be offset by increased in-home services for people in need of rehabilitation and convalescent care, at a cost of only $4 million. Dr Catherine Lounsberry, director of professional services at the Catherine Booth, pointed out at the time that, "those in-home services simply don't exist yet! In any case, even the best home-care programs can't replace a team of doctors, nurses, and therapists monitoring a patient's progress around the clock."[4]

Peggy Curran, of the *Montreal Gazette*, was one of the rare local journalists to call the government's often-cited economic savings argument into question. She wrote that "the decision to shut the rehab centre doesn't make sense on any level, particularly the health board's stated goal: preparing patients to go home sooner and healthier." Curran quoted nurse Katherine Fitz-O'Neill, who said that the patients, who were recovering from amputations, joint replacements, fractures, heart

attacks, and neurological difficulties, were on average 72 years old.
"Most ... live alone, or have an elderly spouse. They need help toileting
or transferring from bed to chair. You can't tell them to cross their legs
and hold it for eight hours!" Fitz O'Neil wondered how the government was going to save money sending nurses and doctors out to people's homes several times a day.

The occupancy rate in such hospitals is always very high – the
Catherine Booth's was at 97 percent and they were turning away 600
patients a year. A few months later, very quietly, the Catherine Booth
was taken off the chopping-block; it was the only Montreal city hospital
to be saved. It continues to operate today, although its budget and size
were slashed at the time by 20 percent. Since then, cuts have been even
greater. By 2003, this once-popular English maternity and rehab hospital, like most of the other remaining hospitals in Montreal, had
endured so many budget cuts that basic operations, including housekeeping, were seriously understaffed. Lack of proper sanitation led to
rampant hospital-borne infections, especially *C. difficile*, which infected
the weakened, elderly patients at the Catherine Booth at one of the
highest rates in the province. Ninety people died unnecessarily there
in one year and 1000 deaths in a single year were caused by other *C.*
difficile outbreaks in similar hospital situations across Quebec.[5]

KILLING OFF SWEET OLD LADIES

The fiscal conservatism of the 1990s has turned hospitals from political
sacred cows into fatted calves on the altar of balanced budgets.
                                        Dale Eisler, Macleans, 1997[6]

At the same time Montreal hospitals were fighting for their lives, so
were other Canadian landmark health care institutions. The Calgary
General Hospital, located downtown, was nicknamed "the grand old
lady." It had opened in 1890 and eventually grew to be three times
larger than the Queen E. It was also the city's major teaching hospital.
However, the old lady's age, teaching status, size, and even the fact
that Calgary had no other ER in the inner city, were not enough to
save her from closure in the mid-1990s. Shocked doctors, nurses, staff
and patients began a monumental fight for their hospital when the
government doomed the institution in July of 1994, about a year
before the Queen Elizabeth received its death sentence. Calgarians
supported an even larger and longer citizens' protest than the fight

for the Queen E but managed to save the big hospital from closure for only an extra year.

As in Quebec, the Alberta government insisted much of the money saved from closing three of its capital city's hospitals would go back into the system, in this case to reconfigure the old structure and support other hospitals. But after the General was empty and its staff and equipment scattered, there was still so much public pressure to re-open that the government actually *blew up the hospital*, in the faces of massed protesters, blanketing the city with dust that was deemed dangerous to the public health. The pit in the middle of downtown that had been the Calgary General was, as a *Maclean's* article describing its last days noted, "the biggest North American hospital ever to shut down and have its functions, equipment, staff and patients integrated into existing hospitals."[7] Its closure left Calgary "the only large city in Canada without a downtown emergency department," something this greatly expanding oil boom-town still lacks. Today, all three functioning emergency departments are, at best, 15 to 25 minutes from downtown. Many preventable deaths have been blamed on these distances and the resulting lack of 24-hour surgical staff, and lawsuits have been filed. Within less than a year of blowing up the building, the government itself admitted that there were no longer enough hospital beds available in the city and began to enthusiastically talk about building an expansion to the remaining hospitals – as if they hadn't destroyed viable institutions only months before.

By 1996, hundreds of hospitals and thousands of beds across the entire country were gone. In Montreal alone, seven hospitals with hundreds of beds each had been closed: the Queen Elizabeth, the Lachine General, the Reddy Memorial, St. Laurent, Ste. Jeanne d'Arc, Bellechasse, Guy Laporte, and Gouin-Rosemont. St. Michel Hospital was converted from acute to long-term care. Moreover, all hospitals across the province received substantial cuts. Few provinces escaped similar fates.

In Toronto, between initial death threats in 1995 and final closures in 1999–2000, seven hospitals were lost to the city, including the popular Wellesley, the Salvation Army Grace, Riverdale, and Runnymede. Wellesley was one of the most vitally required institutions because it was a specialized orthopedic and arthritic hospital. "Just about every other hospital in the Toronto area" was also subject to financial restructuring that involved loss of beds and personnel.[8] Fifteen of the city corporation's 39 operating hospitals, or *nearly 40 percent of the care available to*

Torontonians, disappeared with restructuring. Beginning in 1995 and under Conservative Premier Mike Harris, Ontario also cut a staggering $2 billion from its health care budget province-wide. The public was told that these Ontario closures and cutbacks were based on the need "to get spending under control." Eight hundred million dollars of this money was taken from hospitals, resulting in thirty-five hospitals closed across the province, 7,000 fewer beds available, and a new waiting list of 18,000 people, "mostly seniors and disabled" waiting for chronic-care beds.[9]

Elsewhere in Canada, four hospitals in Halifax were merged into that city's Queen Elizabeth II, and a similar integration of health services bloated the Regina Hospital in Saskatchewan's capital. Again, it was claimed this radical restructuring would lower health care costs. By 1999, *no fewer than 52 hospitals had been closed across the province of Saskatchewan.* Most were small, rural hospitals with very few beds, but their loss forced seriously ill people and seniors in rural areas to take on the rigours of travel on top of worsened conditions when they needed help.

Although most of the employees affected – including the nearly 10,000 people employed at the Queen Elizabeth – were promised immediate jobs, the government admitted that only three-quarters of them had any real job security. As the interviews above show, many trained workers never found jobs that were anything like the ones they left. This means that the governments' actions resulted not just in fewer beds for the sick but also in the loss of irreplaceable professional experience within its health care system. Across Canada, from the Maritimes to British Columbia, *between the years 1994 and 1997, Canada lost 20 percent of its hospital beds.* This was such an unprecedented retraction of health care services in an industrialized country that Canada has become a focus for World Health and UN studies on what hospital closure does to a health care system.[10]

Within Canada itself, however, the extent of these hospital bed closures has never become an item for national discussion. To this day, most Canadians are unaware of their dubious status in international studies – that is, as the industrialized world's leader in sudden mass hospital closures. Our only competitors are Kyrgyzstan and Kazakhstan. Part of the reason for this ignorance lies in the fact that, in spite of their scope and ubiquity, all these closures were and continue to be treated as local issues – largely because health care is seen in Canada as a strictly provincial jurisdiction. In Alberta, opponents at the time of the closures, such as former Alberta Health Department researcher Kevin Taft, believed that one reason why public health and economic data were not properly analyzed was media complaisance with the official versions of why the closures were necessary in the first place.[11] An analysis of the articles reporting on the issue throughout the early 1990s does show that the majority of newspapers and television reporters across the country almost always simply repeated the government's message that Canadian health care costs, particularly in Alberta and Ontario, were "out of control." Few journalists actually crunched any numbers. In Quebec, the reports added the concept that hospital beds were not only too expensive, they were old-fashioned and unnecessary. The public in most provinces was generally told by both governments and the media that these extremely rapid closures – none of which was preceded by impact studies, preparation of alternative facilities, or community involvement – simply reflected a natural progression towards fewer beds and that, in any case, savings from closings would enrich a new system of CLSCs, private clinics, and home care. Governments emphasized that health care systems of the future will focus on services rather than institutions. "The conventional wisdom is that admission rates are high and lengths of stay are too long, so that if you make greater use of outpatient clinics, home-care programs and various community resources, you could greatly reduce inpatient care and hospitals could be eliminated," was how one article quoted a health care economist's summary. The press largely repeated the same idea, over and over, across the country.[12]

Despite the similarity of each locality's situation and the epidemic of closures over this short period, virtually no mass media treated the issue as a national one. Generally, coverage rarely went beyond the municipal, so much so that it's now difficult to tell how many hospitals were affected, even within each province. The media in Montreal was typical in that, with only a few exceptions, reporters seldom postulated any other reason for closure beyond the one cited by government officials or mentioned any hospital closures besides those in their own city. Even the most careful and suspicious writers, such as Peggy Curran of the *Montreal Gazette*, tended to treat the problem as local, despite the simultaneous anguish about hospital closings in Toronto, Halifax, and Calgary.[13] In most stories, reporters cited studies about the "glut" of hospital beds and quoted prominent experts who were claiming that "financial constraints and changing medical practices ... justify a shift

in direction – better home-care services for the elderly, same-day surgery, and shorter hospital stays."[14]

The rare articles that did recognize that the tendency to move
towards closures and cutbacks was national as well as local generally
quoted health care experts such as Ottawa health economist Douglas
Angus, who was saying that the proposed closings, "fit a national trend
toward *more streamlined medical services and that people should get used to it.*"
It was Angus's report, in fact, that had concluded, fatally for many hospitals, that, "Canada's public health-care costs could be trimmed 15
percent without jeopardizing care."[15] The public was then reassured by
promises of investment in new kinds of health care, as in the following
Gazette quote: "Part of the saving would be used to meet a $190 million
budget cut imposed by Quebec over the next three years, and part
would fund improved home care and surgical techniques that shorten
hospital stays."

It's worth noting that, more than a decade later, the promises made at
the time of the original hospital cutbacks that the money "saved" would
"free up funding for community-based services" are still being used in
the debate about privatization and also in the continuing arguments in
favor of closing yet more hospitals. Michael Hurley, president of the
Ontario Council of Hospital Unions, reiterated in an interview in April
of 2006, "The cuts [keep being] made, but community-based services
have [still] not benefited."[16] In fact, since the beginning of the massive
cuts to hospitals over ten years ago, virtually no reliable studies have
been carried out in Canada by federal, provincial, or independent bodies to seriously assess whether any of these objectives have been attained.
There are also no clear accounts of where the millions of dollars citizens
were told were "saved" by these measures really went. This mystery lies at
the heart of the demise of community hospitals such as the Queen Elizabeth and has become an integral part of the story of their existence. But
at the time of the cutbacks and for quite a few years afterwards, people
were entirely caught up in crisis management, not cool analysis.

THE FIVE STAGES OF GRIEF

Denial, Anger, Fear, Bargaining, and Acceptance

Elizabeth Kubler-Ross

In Montreal, as elsewhere in the country, there was a great deal of popular and administrative resistance to the closing of each community

hospital. Marches and demonstrations in support of keeping the city's eight threatened hospitals open were at their height in September of 1995, but the Queen E's were by far the most passionate and vociferous. From the time of the first announcement until the very last gasp in September of 1996, literally tens of thousands of supporters and the staff participated in musical fund-raisers in the park, mass marches in the city streets, and rallies and protests in government offices. The hospital got 135,000 signatures on a petition, hired outside economists and experts, organized crowded and passionate community meetings, wrote outraged letters to the media, and filed four lawsuits.

Even when ignored by the government and beaten, they found the spirit to throw a massive good-by party for the public, featuring a cake the doctors and nurses made themselves. It incorporated 234 eggs and 63 pounds of butter, and, in typically off-beat style, was decorated with a four-colour swamp scene of reptiles and amphibians – to showcase the hospital's colours of green and yellow and, some suspect, as a reference to the government and their minions. They had also had an equally ebullient in-house farewell. "At one point, to get under budget, I had to cut the party and food budget, and I was so sorry!" Mario Larivière says. "But when we got that terrible news that we were closed for sure, I said, next September the doors will lock, but this Christmas let's make a party no one will ever forget. Everything was free – gifts like alcohol, suits, trips, restaurants, good-by presents from our suppliers. We got ready for fun. We had Nez Rouge [Quebec's designated driver service] and a security agent to make sure anyone who needed a ride got it. A buffet like you've never seen, a DJ, games ... it was something to remember!"

Like everyone else, Larivière, the hospital's director general, simply hadn't been able to believe the news that in June of 1995 the Queen Elizabeth, along with other large, important, and venerable city health institutions, was slated for almost immediate closure. Horrible as the prospect was for city hospital care in general, he was sure that with flexibility he and his staff would be able to convince the government to let the Queen E, out of all the threatened hospitals, stay open. Like a healthy person suddenly diagnosed with a lethal disease, everyone echoes his sentiment that it all seemed like a dream, a horrible mistake that just needed a little energy to put right. After all, their hospital's books had been balanced perfectly; they had just opened that new ER; and they had also just been given $3 million for the new CAT scan by the same government now seeking their end. The staff can be forgiven

for thinking they were merely pawns in a political game and that the
government intended to save them at the last minute to cloak the
demise of, say, four or five of the original eight by the reprieve of the
two or three really good ones.

By and large, hospital protagonists entirely bought into or found
themselves forced to address the government and media claims of cost
overruns and the "modern" movement towards homecare. Mario
Larivière was even ready to admit that, "Of course, [our hospital had]
some problems. We had too many long-term care patients in the acute-
care wards, for example. And no doubt there were a few hospitals too
many for the city's size – maybe two or three – certainly not seven!"
Larivière admits that when he had first arrived at the Queen E, three
years before, he had found that, like many other small hospitals, this
one had some problems. "They needed to reinforce their already
strong community service aspect, and to organize the building better –
it had grown up in a thoughtless way at times. They needed to end the
isolation of certain powerful sectors such as anesthesiology and orthopedics. But I have to say that the board, with John Hughes and Owen
Ness on the selection committee, knew they were in for this kind of
thing when they hired me. They knew they needed an outsider to help
them with the government, and they knew there would be a price to
pay when an outsider came in who had the power to make them
change some of their ways. They really loved the place, but they were
centered on themselves and they were beginning to realize they
needed an external view. They were good, but they needed an outsider
to remind them they still had room for improvement."

Larivière emphasizes that this is "always the danger in any community hospital: isolation and internal influences. There isn't a clear line
between your profession and your family, which can be both good and
bad. There were even lots of romances, that kind of thing, that had its
own effect on operations. That can be bad and create conflicting interests and intrigues; it can keep people apart as much as it may get them
together! But their real problem in the late 1980s was simply that their
decision-making structures were not sufficiently organized. They
needed to realize that the world changes and that an institution needs
regular external input, in financial and organizational as well as professional matters. It needs to send its people out to learn not just how to
do medicine. They were very good at that. But they needed to see how
other hospitals operate and bring others in to assess their management
methods; they needed to allocate funds to do that." What stunned him

about closure was that when the bad news came, all these problems had been dealt with and the budgets were balanced.

Orthopedic surgeon Larry Lincoln, who was among the fiercest fighters for the institution in its very last days, speaks for many when he says, "I was so incredulous when I heard they were going to close us that I simply wouldn't credit it. We should have been the last place the city could afford to lose. I only got involved in the fight to save it after John [Hughes], Owen [Ness], and Mario gave up. I think our goose was always cooked, but I had been so much in denial I didn't get involved at first." George Subak, chief of Psychiatry, says that Lincoln wasn't alone. For example, the head of the hospital's Radiology Department continued to travel to Europe and Japan to get the latest expensive versions of computerized tomography and have them installed in the new ER, secure in his belief of a last-minute reprieve, even as other chiefs, such as Dr Subak in Psychiatry, considered the voluntary suicide of their own departments as a possible way to save the life of the larger institution. According to Subak, even after much of the staff "realized that the hospital was doomed, that [kind of] radiology work being done in the ER continued to go on almost until the very end. The reason people carried on as normal, spending money and making future plans for their departments, is that out of all the hospitals up for closure, so many of us thought that *surely* they wouldn't sacrifice the Queen E."

Meanwhile, other departments, like his own, had already gone "into high gear, devising scenarios to save money, to save the hospital at large. The Regional Boards of Health, the Regie regionales, which were local bureaucracies between us and the government, were, of course, trying to divide and conquer. They implied that if we closed certain departments, like psychiatry, they'd keep the hospital. Of course, psychiatry is very vulnerable. You can live without it; people don't immediately die like they do of a heart-attack. And we in psychiatry even agreed! 'Close us, save the hospital!' But that was the kind of self-destructive idea that plays into their hands. How can we be a community-based hospital if we transfer these people from our community elsewhere? And the rest of the administration didn't like singling out a single department for closure either, so it wasn't finally done."

"It was shameful," Larivière says, not only of the sudden, drastic announcement, but of the government's methods in dealing with the shocked hospitals. "They closed too many, and they also closed the wrong ones. They were never straight with us. And their decisions made no sense. They kept St. Mary's, supposedly to serve NDG, but it's very hard to get to and not popular. So they created problems of accessibility, among many other things, partly because their decisions were so sudden and not based on actual studies. They liked the idea of diagnostic equipment, machines, to replace mixed care. In short, they didn't understand or believe in the mission of community hospitals."

When all these cuts began, the government had to have some kind of rationale for their choice of which institutions to destroy, but, as Larivière says, in terms of their stated purpose to improve and streamline medical care, they also went about this task in an oddly backwards manner. "They made up their minds to close these places so incredibly rapidly, without ever looking into their actual operating efficacy, and then designed criteria for closure based on whatever excuses they could find in some past detail of behaviour. For example, they seized on a single misunderstanding about occupation rates as an excuse to put us on their list. In order to be good and get under budget, the hospital had closed one unit because of reduced population in the area. But the director general at the time didn't modify the permit for number of beds. So although we explained the situation, the fact that on paper we appeared to have too many beds was used as an excuse to sign our death warrant."

The people most implicated in the death of the Queen E give a lot of reasons why it was selected for closure in the first place. This often-mentioned mistake in the hospital's accounting system, which took place in the late 1980s, may have provided Quebec bureaucrats with base criteria for deciding which might live and which might die but doesn't explain why seven hospitals in the Montreal area had to close so suddenly. Larivière says, "For me, the earlier problem of being in the red wasn't the real reason we got the axe. The region's deficit – Montreal in general – was why." He's talking about the fact that Quebec's sagging credit rating on the New York stock exchange was having a big influence on government behaviour at the time.

We now know that from the late 1980s and into the mid-1990s, the province was being pressured by the big American lending institutions to which it owed money to economize in order to preserve Quebec's high credit rating. Quebec bureaucrats were told that they had too many beds per capita, for example, too many students on scholarship, too many government employees in general – all money that could be used to service debts and make the province more attractive to investors. During a crippling nurses' strike as early as 1989, analysts noted that one reason the Quebec government was so anxious not to give in to nurses' demands was "the province's foreign debt."[17] The nurses were striking because they were over-worked and wanted help, but the province's preoccupation was to lower its numbers of health care workers, not raise them.

That year, Moody's, a powerful Wall Street bond-rating firm, had threatened that Quebec bonds would be downgraded from double- to single-A status if cuts were not immediately made in spending. The government, not unusually, had tried to gain popularity by borrowing from large banks to fund expansive programs. Now it sought to fix its financial overdrafts by cuts in social spending. When provincial governments go too far into debt, their ability to get buyers for the bonds that finance many of their activities becomes dicey. In fact, getting downgraded even from a Triple-A to a Double-A status is practically a diplomatic incident; it can shake a government to its foundations. This kind of behind-closed-doors budgetary crisis situation has vastly increased since the implementation of a globalized economy in the late 80s and early 90s. In June of 1999, for example, "the Japanese government took the unprecedented step of calling a Moody's representative before their parliament's Lower House committee to explain why the debt agency cut the credit rating of the world's second-largest economy."

Business reporter Dale Jackson explained in a *Globe Investor* article that the methods the financial giants like Moody's or Standard & Poors use to determine the economic risk and lending status granted to a country don't always make sense, but they have dampening to devastating effects on both economic growth and social programs. In the Japanese case cited above, "the new rating [had] placed Japan below Botswana – an African nation whose largest creditor is Japan." That certainly doesn't make sense, but technically, there was nothing Japan could do about the situation beyond asking for explanations. Moody's and Standard & Poor's are the most famous debt-rating agencies in the world. Business analyst Dale Jackson explains that, "Moody's ... 800 risk analysts stretch the corners of the globe looking for debt issues significant enough to rate. They also provide a vital service by linking borrowers with lenders."[18]

Throughout the 1980s, we know that several such linking services had rated many provincial governments so highly that Quebec, Alberta, and Ontario in particular had been able to issue bonds and spend money with abandon. However, by the early 1990s, the good times were coming to an end and the bond raters were switching tactics. Since even a slightly lower credit rating has terrific implications for a provincial government, the new demands were very powerful. "For the issuer [of the bond,] it means higher borrowing rates and a loss of credibility. For the investor, it's the difference between getting a return on your investment and getting diddly-squat."[19] In the late 1980s or mid-1990s, as today, any country, let alone a province like Quebec, would be very threatened by the possibility of lower ratings and would likely have reacted with panic, focusing on a rapid program of spending cuts in order to service the debts and retain its favoured lending status.

About the only explanation that makes sense in this whole situation is the strong possibility that provincial governments, both in Quebec and elsewhere, didn't take the money they saved by cutting back hospital services to spend on roads, schools or even their own pork-barrel schemes. They most likely spent it servicing their debts to the big New York banks or the International Monetary Fund to stabilize their credit ratings. The anti-globalization rallies so common in the late 1990s and early 21st century brought these shadowy government practices into the headlines, mostly in the context of Third World debtor nations. In the poor countries of the world, hospitals and social services have often been "rationalized," that is, radically down-sized, by order of financial entities like the World Bank and the IMF so that the original loaners, the big banks, could be repaid. But because the whole process is secret, North Americans tended to be unaware that similar liquidations were going on in countries like Canada. Unlike in the Third World, here they were more masked by local politics and greater general prosperity. At least, unlike countries in the former Soviet Union and Africa, Canada still had a few hospitals left after the downsizing.

So the central discussion occupying most of the protagonists' energies at the time – that their governments would be applying the savings they realized from closing the old hospitals towards creating new and more modern systems – was probably never genuine. The argument that their beloved hospital was unneeded or inefficient was also untrue. It seems most likely that the money everybody was arguing about was simply no longer the province's to spend in any case. Details ahead demonstrate that this money was very likely already spoken for, probably by an international lender like the International Monetary Fund (IMF) as well as national ones like the New York Stock Exchange. The Queen E, along with many other hospitals in the provincial and

Canadian health system, was being liquidated so the province would have the money – at least on its books – to pay off those debts. Such an explanation for an otherwise irrationally under-researched and unprecedented overhaul of an entire country's hospital system goes far to explain the extreme rapidity with which the hospitals met their doom: *The provinces had to get their finances in order before the next fiscal year.* If their stated reasons of system reform had been true, at least three to five years would have been a rational political timeframe for such radical measures to be undertaken and for new structures like ACCs, or even inadequate ones such as expanded CLSCs, to be put into place. As Mario Larivière explained, ACCs, or Ambulatory Care Centres, were "all supposed to go in – at Sacre Coeur, at Maisonneuve, and at the Montreal General. They would have been separate buildings close to the hospitals, with savings to patients and for the government, because they would have eliminated the need for full hospitalization for many procedures. *But we never got them,* and people are still fully hospitalized, at great cost, for the smaller, faster procedures that these ACCs were supposed to handle. I mean before, you'd be in hospital for two weeks for an appendectomy. Today, with laparoscopy, you can be out the same day and home in your own bed. But instead of reinvesting those savings in a cost-effective way, they kept them!" Even a minimal timeframe wasn't granted because those in the know realized the whole question was not about health care efficiency or reform – it actually concerned trade balance and financial ratings.

In order to understand the history of a community hospital like the Queen Elizabeth, it was once necessary to be very familiar with the history of its actual community and catchment area and then its municipality. Secondarily, one had to understand something about the province that eventually took over the institution's funding. Finally, it was important to include certain national policies, such as Canada's decision to have fully public health care. Today, however, in order to comprehend why a local hospital has gurneys in its corridors, we sometimes need to know about American and international lending and rating agencies and even international trade treaties that involve NAFTA, the IMF (International Monetary Fund), and the World Trade Organization. Chapter Five is dedicated to analyzing the power these bodies now wield over formerly local policies and formerly economically sovereign governments and their social programs. The current financial situation, as it affects Canadian social services, is not only unprecedented for the historian but has left even large federal institutions in powerful countries, such as France and the U.S., with few defenses. So, while it may seem strange to lump the death of a small hospital – or two, or 20 percent of the national total – in with how provincial or national governments borrow from international lenders, no one can deny that all these activities are closely entwined today.

THE DANGER OF HAVING AN ENLARGED HEART

The QE revolved around a great pride in its character as a servant of the community. It was a living organism, it conferred an identity. The people who were hired fit in with that.

Dr Joe Mammazza

What makes the mass closures of the mid-1990s so suspect in terms of international debt is the speed with which they were implemented. All the hospitals affected reported great shock concerning how little time they were given to respond to the sudden and unexpected charges that they were wasteful and inefficient. In fact, the whole sweep of closures across Canada – with thousands of beds and scores of institutions summarily destroyed – took less than two years. Most high-level government lending records, including dealings with global trade organizations like the International Monetary Fund, remain secret. However, a pressing need for speed does accord with the idea of debt foreclosure. In order to qualify for more loans or better status, a government's financial books would have to be rapidly balanced. The demands of creditors and rating agencies are urgent and non-negotiable. Resources would naturally have to be liquidated with great rapidity if the deadlines they set for payment are to be reached.

At the Queen Elizabeth, surgeon Fred Weigan recalled how the province's social safety net was greatly affected several times by similar financial crises in the past. Referring to mass bed closures, he says, "That's not without precedent. In 1988, the salaries of all public workers were cut by 20 percent. That was, in fact, mandated by the Chase Manhattan Bank, which had decided Quebec was a credit risk. There was no real proof that it was, but it gave rise to their having to borrow more and ending up with a huge provincial deficit." So, if faced with a rigid order to close a specific, non-negotiable number of beds from people in New York who were holding the province's purse-strings, the only choice the provincial government would have had to make was: which ones?

The ex-director general of the Queen Elizabeth Hospital, Mario
Larivière, thinks that the local, community hospitals, even highly innovative ones like the Queen E, would have been at the greatest disadvantage under economically mandated bed closure demands. "The
government would want to save the teaching hospitals in order to
attract specialties that, in theory, would bring more prestige and funding from industry and the private sector." Publicly, there was endless
talk of "fiscal responsibility" and "debt reduction" throughout this
whole period, but no province or politician actually cited their province's or the country's international debts as the actual reason why they
were closing hospital beds. They did imply that because such things as
the CBC, educational institutions, and hospitals had "spiraling," or "out
of control" costs, cutting them back would be the logical place to find
funds to service "the growing national debt" and take "hard fiscal medicine" to improve the economy. Politicians, whether Liberal or Conservative, also made the exercise sound as if it were a political party policy
aimed at balancing the budget, either provincially or federally, rather
than an urgent liquidation mandated by those holding that debt. Consequently, everyone, including outspoken critics like economist Linda
McQuaig or pollster Angus Reid, treated the matter as errant national
policy – that is, as if Canadian politicians still had a choice about
whether or not to pay back their creditors.[20]

As we will see in Chapter Five, the major international entity that
deals with the speed at which national debts must be repaid is the International Monetary Fund. They made their power to demand instant
repayment very clear in their 1994 and 1995 *IMF Reports to Canada,*
which, like all IMF dealings with national governments, were secret and
have become only partially available recently, many years later, under
access to information laws. Although the two reigning Canadian political parties at the time, the Liberals and Conservatives, found that
national health care services that are enshrined by law are a particularly difficult thing to cut, both managed to do so, much as they continue to do so today. These umpopular politicial actions are partially
explained by the *Reports* discussed ahead.

At the time, however, the excuse for cutbacks in all sectors, including
health, was not only to service the debt everyone was so concerned
about but to get rid of waste and make those services sleeker and more
modern. Mario Larivière says, "They claimed the reason for the closures was that we had more hospitals than we needed and by removing
them from the system, we would benefit the remaining ones. As health

care evolved, the CLSCs and Ambulatory Care Centers would do more, and we wouldn't even need those beds once the CLSCs were better managed. That was a laugh, wasn't it?"Although Quebec's CLSCs, the province's regional health clinics, are better organized today than they were ten years ago, they have not really become the mid-level health care institutions promised by the government in the early 1990s, save for a few exceptions in large cities. Most of them outside Montreal or Quebec City still do not have doctors dependably available at any time, let alone around the clock, and none of them has "airway management," the capability that actually defines a hospital. Airway management means having the equipment and specialists to anesthetize a patient and perform emergency procedures. Because these clinics lack this capability, those who are worried that they or the person they're responsible for might be having a heart attack, internal bleeding, or another serious problem cannot waste time going to a CLSC, even one of the rare urban ones that's open all the time and has doctors on call. These patients and worried relatives therefore flood Emergency Rooms across the province.

Because people often do have problems requiring real hospitalization, many end up on stretchers and gurneys in hallways. The hospital beds that Montreal and many other cities used to have to accommodate these people have not been replaced by more efficient back-up services simply because the back-up services envisioned by the provincial bureaucracy when money was so tight weren't hospital beds. So even though the rapidity of the closures mitigated against the quick solutions that were promised, CLSCs never had the capacity to become as useful as expected. Full-fledged hospitals have services that clinics can never hope to challenge.

The argument that so many hospitals and beds weren't going to be needed anymore was always fairly disingenuous, even if bureaucrats can be partially forgiven for not understanding how medical systems actually work. Back in the 1990s, many studies that demanded "increased efficiency and productivity" from government-funded social programs like hospitals had gained great popularity with government bureaucracies. In determining the primary objective of our hospital systems, the discussion had become less about giving the best clinical care to the patient and more about providing the best care for the least amount of money. Today, many embittered health workers will say that from the funding governments' point of view, our prime objective has become not public health but the balanced financial functioning of the hospital corporation within the balanced financial functioning of the provincial and national budgets. And in fact, over the years, the managing of hospitals has gradually gravitated from the first objective towards the last.

The most telling example of this tendency is termed "per forma." This is an accounting term that refers to the idea of utilizing all your resources at least to the level of 90 percent. It is almost universally used in Canada as a measurement of whether an enterprise is functioning acceptably or whether it needs to be punished or redesigned because it's being fiscally mismanaged. It's the mark that condemns a hospital with the economic sin of "inefficiency." If we're talking about a hospital, per forma requires that 90 percent of its beds should be full; its OR and ER should both be working at 90 percent capacity; 90 percent of its nurses, doctors, and surgeons should be as busy as they can be; its cafeteria and laundry, its pharmacy, labs, and technical facilities, should all be operating at 90 percent capacity, and so forth. Higher is even better, and one of the reasons the Queen E caught the auditors' eyes when they were looking for hospitals to close was that they appeared to have more than 10 percent of their beds empty, at least on paper. Two years before closure, they had committed the sin of not being "per forma."

But what does this figure, developed in the sphere of factory production and economic seminars, mean in a medical context? Dr John Hughes says, "Dealing with the output of machines or factory workers is fundamentally different from dealing with a natural system, which a hospital necessarily is." Hospitals have to reflect natural systems – the rhythms of the human body and the pulses of the ills that befall it. These do not respond to economic theory but, literally, to nature. Any number of studies have proven, and any number of doctors and nurses will tell you, that even in the 21st century, births continue to peak during full moons with a smaller jump at new moons. So do injuries and accidents. ERs are predictably crowded at certain times of the year, depending on geography. Human illness still corresponds to seasonal changes in temperature and precipitation, and old people die in droves in northern climes in the months of November and April.

Hughes says, "If you're dealing with a natural phenomenon and you're aiming for above 90 percent utilization, you will be in trouble 50 percent of the time, which is about how often our ERs are in crisis now. What is it about managerial training that makes it impossible for these corporate managers to understand that they're not dealing with economic systems here? It should be obvious that if you're operating at almost 100 percent capacity in a natural system, that is, a system that fluctuates widely, then around 50 percent of the time you're going to go over-capacity. That's just mathematics. Going over-capacity for even a nanosecond on a space shuttle will destroy it. It can do the same thing to a patient." The only reason, he says, that patient mortality due to this one managerial concept isn't much higher, "is the guts and spirits of the men and women trying to save people in spite of it. What we desperately need to do is to educate both managers and the public about the protean and cyclic nature of health events!"

We're far from that. Mario Larivière's St. Eustache community hospital had 170 beds when the Queen E was closed, with an occupancy rate of 85 percent. Now it has 220 beds crammed into the same building, *all* occupied, bringing it well beyond 120 percent normal capacity – which provides an idea of what a bad weekend must be like. Despite the crisis situation that returns to plague Canadian ERs every flu season and peaks alarmingly every two or three years, in Quebec as elsewhere, governments are always talking about closing thousands more short- and especially long-term-care hospital beds. This, combined with a rapidly aging population, would overload ERs even more spectacularly. And, whenever a government is faced with a budgetary shortfall, it still seems to think that hospital beds are expendable. In the winter of 2007, the ER chief at the Jewish General, mentioned in a *Montreal Gazette* article as having "perhaps the best-run ER in Montreal," referred back to John Hughes' analysis of natural systems, saying, "When people see an occupancy rate of 120 percent, they have a tendency to think it's not that bad. But it's extremely bad – it's awful! What we have here is a total disaster."[21]

Added to this continuing curious idea that there are "too many" hospitals and beds, the governments' next method of triage, both now and back in the mid-nineties, was to select hospitals for closure according to performance. This was sometimes understandable in terms of some of the institutions that were cut but not for those such as the Calgary General and the Queen E. George Subak, the ex-head of the Queen's Department of Psychiatry, says that one reason they all kept hoping that closure wouldn't really happen "is because we were performing so well in every sense. Teaching, for example – the Queen E was arguably the best primary and secondary care teaching hospital in the city or the province." The Queen E handled about 10 percent of the teaching for McGill – the premiere medical school in the country – and so was performing a service that could hardly be duplicated by either government or private clinics.

If poor performance as an institution was not supported by the facts, the province's next obvious criteria for axing a particular hospital would have been fiscal mismanagement. And it's here where, in the case of the Queen E, they could at least point to a few moles and freckles, although the government's charges of fiscal mismanagement mostly bewildered the people trying to save the hospital. Subak says, "It was being very well administered, with no major deficit or area of inefficiency, and everyone knew that. One way the province attacked us there was simply to doubt the veracity of Larivière's numbers. The Minister of Health, Yves Rochon, and the head of the Regie, M. Villeneuve, made him spend a lot of time documenting and supporting them. But there was no way they could deny the healthy state of our finances, even after innumerable meetings with different accountants and so on who were looking for supposed deficits between 1993–95. Finally, in August of 1996, despite all our efforts and despite the fact that they no longer had any reasons for it, we were closed."

Subak sighs before attempting to dispassionately analyze some forgotten detail that would explain why all this happened; he's still looking for the flaws in what he still considers to be the finest hospital the city ever had. "There was a period of fiscal difficulty, prior to 1991. That crisis at the Queen E, you could say, started with Director General Albert Nixon, who, because of government strictures and a culture that put the patients' and hospitals' professional needs above budgetary concerns, was constantly getting loans from the Royal Bank for different items; the Regie regionale didn't like that. They also didn't like him closing beds in the summer – they would've liked to have the hospital perform better by cutting jobs, not beds. The ER had to deviate ambulances sometimes because there were no beds due to such seasonal closings and that set off red lights at the Regie. 'How come the QE has such healthy performance records, yet is clogged up with chronic patients using up its beds?' they asked."

The reasons for the high level of chronic patients in the place had to do with what the hospital saw as its primary mandate to the community. "The population in our catchment area was aging and as they became affected with the diseases of age, they wanted to be in their normal, neighbourhood hospital, not some strange place far away," Subak explains. Then, as now, there were far too few chronic-care beds in the province, largely as a result of government policies based on theories about "returning patients to the community." They had closed many chronic-care facilities without providing adequate substitutions. When older relatives got to be too much to handle, people often took them to a hospital Emergency Room and left them there. They'd then become the hospital's problem and would either be kept in a hospital bed or gradually moved out to cronic-care facilities or old folks' homes as spaces slowly opened up. Today, this remains a serious problem in all public care facilities – in Europe and Mexico as well as here.

Back in the early 1990s, the Queen E had a 20 to 30 percent higher rate of this sort of "granny-dumping" than other city hospitals because of its perceived soft heart. Families knew that the Queen E would take good care of Grandpa while he was in limbo, and some staff colluded. Subak says, "Well, a few of the doctors ... 'stored' their patients at the Queen E. I guess they figured, 'I've worked here for 40 years, and if I want to park my nice old patient Joe, who has no place else to go, I should be able to!'" Considering that at the time the headlines were full of cases of scaldings, neglect, and abuse in the province's over-loaded and under-monitored elderly and cronic-care facilities, this was an understandable and compassionate thing to do.

As always in the history of a small and eccentric hospital, there were other anomalies at the Queen E that displeased the government bureaucrats. Subak says, "There were also problems with ORs getting clogged up with plastic surgery cases, just like today. But the big thing was orthopedics; there are so many of those procedures desired at any time, and the Queen E wouldn't turn its population away. So their OR bills were about 20 percent higher until the one-day surgery clinic, Dr Lincoln's initiative, was opened in 1989–90, and that helped a good deal. The chief surgeon at that time, Dr Coglin, was a media star, known for being the doctor to the Expos at the height of their popularity. Nobody could push him around, so his patients got their knee and hip replacements regardless of the budget!" Owen Ness, who headed the hospital board during this period, also mentions the same higher OR costs that brought unwanted Regie attention. "There was a clear explanation for that," he says. "The Queen E was the only hospital that would accept so many orthopedic patients. The surgery and especially the prostheses are very expensive so in order to stay under budget, most places simply refuse to do these procedures. These conditions are debilitating, very painful, and the joints deteriorate. The Queen E realized that and because they cared, got people into their ORs. The other hospitals made them wait."

THE LANGUAGE CARD AND OTHER VILLAINS

Responding to complaints that English-language hospitals have been hit
particularly hard, Executive Director Marcel Villeneuve of the regional
board said the closings were spread equitably across the network.

Graeme Hamilton, Montreal Gazette, 1995[22]

Stymied in their efforts to understand how poor performance, either
fiscal or professional, could possibly have been the reason for closure,
the people fighting for an English institution in Quebec naturally
jumped to the conclusion that their hospital was being closed because
it was English. This time-honoured Quebec excuse for indignation
turns out to be mostly untrue. In fact, four of the hospitals that were
eventually closed were French – a majority – and from a purely political
point of view, closing one more French institution would understandably have been too much for the predominately French electorate to
tolerate. In that sense, being English was definitely a disadvantage. But
when draconian demands to save specific amounts of money come
down from banks or rating agencies to a government, there's naturally
a point at which weak or marginal institutions are no longer available.
That means that strong, viable, fiscally responsible, innovative, and
invaluable public resources, such as the Calgary General, the Wellesley
in Toronto, and the Queen Elizabeth in Montreal, will be closed down
too. It's like selling off your valuables to meet your debts. You start with
the boat or the couch you never use, but eventually, if the debt is big
enough, you sell your bed or the bathtub.

During this period of the mid-1990s, the bureaucratic bodies that
mediated between the provincial government and its hospitals were
the sixteen "Regies regionales," or Quebec Regional Health Boards,
across the province. The Regies regionales were created on the theory
of decentralizing control so that hospitals could be more responsive to
their localities. But in practice, Ness says, "They were incapable of and
not empowered, in any case, to make any decisions." Surgeon Fred
Weigan says, "A government that micro-manages health care delivery
does not expedite communications; things just keep getting worse that
way. The Ministere de Sante decided to decentralize the top-heavy
Regie nationale de sante with sixteen or eighteen Regies regionales –
and of course ended up with sixteen top-heavy systems instead of just
one. I'm not saying their intentions weren't good. CLSC walk-in clinics
had a lot of merit, too, in theory. But the rot set in almost at once." For-

mer Director General Albert Nixon is still able to describe the immediate effect of multi-leveled government bureaucracies on patient care. "Back in the 1970s, if one of our X-ray machines broke, we'd tell Mr. Ouillette in Quebec, and he'd say, 'Order a new one.' Now, if it's not on your priority list at the beginning of the fiscal year – and why would it be if it hasn't broken yet? – then you can't get one. I think the Regional Councils were a big mistake. There are so many of them – it was just another level of bureaucracy."

That time-period for the Queen E was especially unlucky. The Hospital wasn't allowed to deal directly with the higher levels of government that must have known just what was going on. Instead, administrators descended into a Kafkaesque world where they were only allowed to talk to the Regies regionales, which had no power to respond and therefore almost no interest in the hospitals' ideas and demands. Owen Ness says, "The Regie, for example, didn't even bother to read the documentation we had done by an outside firm explaining why the Queen E shouldn't be closed. Their chief at the time, Marcel Villeneuve, just kept repeating his famous statement to any objections we had, however reasonable and well documented: '*J'ai fait mon lit et il faut que je dors dedans.*' ('I made my bed and I'll have to lie in it.')" Ness says sadly, "He was a very willing accomplice to the government, which had unilaterally decided to close the both the Queen E and the Catherine Booth, another old Montreal hospital. They figured they could get rid of 400 beds if they closed the Catherine Booth, even though it was a cronic-care hospital, not at all the type they were supposed to be closing, which just illustrates how the Regie refused to discuss or investigate anything, however basic. Later in the process, the Regie was horrified to discover that the Catherine Booth was in fact a rehab or cronic-care hospital, the very kind that they needed to keep open. They hadn't taken note of what it was when they slated it for closure, and they were too rigid to go back on anything they'd already declared."

In a democracy, when a government decree concerns a community institution that was built up over generations, largely with that community's funds, there is always supposed to be an appeal process. The Regie gave the doomed hospitals in Quebec only 30 days to come up with an *avis ecrit*, a written appeal, explaining in detail why they shouldn't be closed. "But that," says Larivière, "was a farce. Instead of explaining their extraordinarily arbitrary decision, they put all the onus on us to defend ourselves. It simply gave the appearance of democracy.

Owen Ness was the vice president of the board and at Alcan was VP of Human Resources. This exceptional person very actively negotiated with the Regies regionales on our behalf, but it was hopeless. They attacked our number of beds, the fact we had no long-term care facilities; they claimed they wanted to have ambulatory care service. So we tried a partnership with a CLSC – you could write a whole book about that. But it didn't work. We tried to become everything they wanted and posited a community health care center with private clinics, long-term care, day surgery, everything they claimed we lacked. Our doctors put up $1 million from their own pockets for this center! But the Regies paid no attention. It was like they didn't even read it."

Owen Ness lays out how inexpensively the Queen E supporters could have saved what was really vital about their hospital. "For only sixteen to thirty-seven million," he says, "we could have freed up the hospital not only for the clinic's uses as cronic-care, walk-ins, and radiology while retaining the best ER in the city. Fundamentally, I think this was about shutting down an English institution, however efficient, over any more French ones." There was, as mentioned, a great deal of political maneuvering around the province's exhaustingly famous language issue. Three French hospitals were being closed too; but St. Mary's was English, like the Queen E. Why did it, although considerably less-beloved, survive? Ness thinks its size was a factor. "It was slightly bigger, so it didn't fit their numbers so well. Also, like Santa Cabrina in the East End, there was a very powerful community behind it. There was no cohesive group of business leaders like that helping us. Our influential supporters had divided loyalties. They were also on the boards of the Royal Victoria, the General, and so on. They were afraid for these institutions too. So they backed off on defending the Queen E."

Owen Ness also spent energy trying to get the Queen E named a trauma centre and blames the people closest to the controversy. "Why in heaven's name not? The location, the expertise, equipment, it was perfect! We had the right institution, but no political pull." The hospital resorted to a lawsuit at the end to challenge the government's right to close them. "We spent $80,000 on it," he says. "We thought we'd be good on appeal; our lawyer was ready to prove the law had been broken by the closure. But Jean Lapostolle, the head of our board, I guess decided to back off." Even if local officials were not the root cause of closure, they seem to have done little to help the community heal. Ness says that after losing their appeal, "we tried to get possession of the building – one the government was desperate to get rid of it. The lawsuit would have given it to us for a dollar. Not only did we not get the building, we didn't even get to keep our name! That was given away to a private clinic, the Centre Queen Elizabeth, which set up in the same building."

This last blow was devastating to Queen E alumni, and Ness states, with some heat, "I want to be very clear about this. The 'Centre Queen Elizabeth' has *absolutely nothing to do with our hospital* and is not a hospital itself. It's just private doctors' offices, a radiology department, and a completely unrelated cronic-care unit." There is a good deal of anger still about the fact that the revered old building, built so gallantly by the founding Griffith family and other pioneers, still bears the Queen E name. Not only did the government refuse to let the survivors use it in ways more useful to the public, Ness and many others feel that the name was kept on their building largely to confuse voters about the drastic nature of the closures. Indeed, many Montrealers still believe that some part of the original hospital was retained in the private clinic that has been permitted to bear its name. Moreover, the chronic-care unit that occupies the Queen E's old nursing school does not have the highest reputation for patient care so the old Hospital's reputation is being diminished even after it has ceased to exist.

Mario Larivière has honestly tried to see the whole situation from the government's point of view. "Maybe, as they claimed, a few of the community hospitals in Montreal really were duplicating some services. So, how can you tell how many you need exactly? Should there be one on every corner? Should they be twenty minutes apart, or thirty? It's fine to design a system taking such things into consideration, but *it has to be part of a plan.* There was no plan like that in our hospital closures. For example, one major reason they gave for closing the Queen E and the others was that they were supposed to be 'outdated and superseded by the new Ambulatory Care Centres' that were being advocated at the time." These were to be highly specialized outpatient centers that handled airway management, that is, operations, as well as treatments that required local anesthetic, such as chemo, dialysis, and day surgery. There were no plans in the other Canadian cities and towns affected by closure, either, as well as no new ACCs. Larivière says, "They were right, that system would have taken up much of the slack left by the closures. But they were never built! Sacre Coeur, I wrote up the protocol for theirs. Notre Dame – they still don't have one ... we never got them ... The provincial budget just swallowed them!"

DEATH AND DESPAIR

Around here, people felt they had lost this one place we knew and
trusted. We wanted to go there, and even though they've been adequate
for our needs, [the remaining hospitals are] just not the same. We
wanted the Queen E. And now it's gone.

Elizabeth Tsuk, former patient

When secret financial deals are made between governments and
banks, the ripples affect the target population in myriad ways. In all the
cities affected, bitterness and blame estranged individuals and institutions, although in reality they each had very little to do with the tragedy. Many Queen Elizabeth doctors, nurses, and administrators remain
truly hurt and disillusioned about the lack of support they got from the
McGill teaching hospitals, so much so that a good many of them left
the province. Surgeon Ron Lewis is among many to have blamed his
alma mater. He says, "I became disgusted with the McGill hospitals
because of their bureaucracies. Of course, McGill still has the reputation and a strong, strong academic base; it's still superior to any other
medical school in Canada, except for the University of Toronto. So it's
very hard for me not to think that had they supported the Queen E, it
might have survived. If McGill had insisted, if they'd said, 'No, don't
close it! We need this hospital.' But they didn't. I think they had their
eye on the area for the proposed super-hospital already. To have saved
the hospitals that are still open and let the Queen E go ... but that's
that. It's done."

Lewis still believes, along with many others, that McGill didn't take a
stand for the Queen because "their first priority was their own professional and academic interest, which they had invested in the idea of a
new super-hospital. They also thought – and this is how even experienced people can badly misread governments – that they would somehow benefit from our loss, that the 'extra' money would end up in their
coffers. But it's like saying to a government, 'Oh, you can take that part
of our function away, the institution that does 10 percent of our teaching.' To the government, saying that doesn't inspire them to put that
10 percent into your other programs. To them, that means you'll do
fine on 10 percent less overall!" Lewis also believes ministers destroy
institutions because of their own pet projects. "Rochon's [pet project]
was this super-hospital, an amalgamation of all the McGill teaching
hospitals to be located not that far from the Queen E, in the Glen Rail-

road Yards. Some other minister might want to cover up the Decarie expressway or enlarge the Arboretum. But closing the Queen E didn't liberate money for the super-hospital or anything else, even though the reports were manipulated to imply it would."

Pat Titterton, whose bright career as a head ER nurse was destroyed, is also bitter and illustrates how the closures poisoned relationships within the professional community. Old wounds are remembered and in their frustration, people strike out at their own local groups rather than at those who were probably the real culprits. Titterton feels that, "McGill always resented us ... even though we weren't part of their teaching hospital program, we got more daycare surgeries than they did. Prior to closing, we were still getting traumas, which they resented because they were supposed to be the 'trauma center.' We were also popular because our surgical cases weren't left in the ER for three days. Ours were upstairs within 24 hrs. Dr John Harold used to say, 'They're either sick enough to send upstairs or well enough to send home.' We always kept seven to ten beds free for emergencies." Professional communities right across Canada are still fragmented by the feelings of betrayal and loss these closures engendered. It would be naive to think that quality of service is not affected to a degree by such deep gashes in professional trust and morale.

For the sake of argument, let's say that the bodies responsible for closing hospitals across Canada in the mid-1990s and that still threaten them today had little choice. After all, in the kind of economy people have created in the 21st century, balanced budgets are very important. This may be partially so because human relationships to economics can be expressed in numbers, which are very convenient tools of measurement. It's much more difficult to quantify what these closures did to the patients and the communities each hospital served. It's nonetheless clear how damaging such sweeping programs can be to morale, professional networks, care delivery, and methodology. Ex-ER Nurse Pat Titterton still gets depressed talking about what followed the act of giving up.

"It had looked pretty good for awhile. It became so awful when we realized all our work to save the hospital was of no use. The ER had to close first because that's where your patients come from. That was like a stab in the heart; you try to keep your staff's morale up and arrange courses and transfers. It took about eight to ten weeks to clear out the wards." George Subak of the psychiatry department explains that, "Whenever you close or amalgamate services, it's the transition period

that's hardest on every one. We had only four months to do it. I met
with Dr Beaudry at the Allen Memorial and transferred ninety heavy
cases to the Royal Vic. And, of course, I went over every single case with
nurses, doctors, social workers. Did it go OK? No. We tried everything
in the small amount of time we were given, but it's a simple fact that
you can't raise anxieties in people who are barely able to control their
anxieties as it is and expect a good outcome. Was it safe? No. The figures speak for themselves. And to this day, a majority of those ninety
patients still don't have good connections for help. To this day, they
don't have the autonomy they did."

As well, Ness says that in the dizzying last days of closure, the board
and the staff fought to save anything that could be used elsewhere or
would keep some part of the old institution alive in another form.
"Economic studies showed our viability to the very end. So I worked
with our consultant, Chris Cooper, trying to save whatever we could.
For example, the Department of Ophthalmology at McGill knew that
we could do cataract surgery for $650 an eye instead of their cost of
$1250, almost twice as much. We saw the Regie regionale about saving
the equipment that made that possible. They were such a mess; there
was no one we could find there with the authority to even talk to us
about it! So that didn't happen. At the very end, after we'd completely
given up, we met with St. Mary's to transfer our most expensive equipment. A priest had just taken over as head there. He and Lapostolle
talked about their personal activities and interests. I had to interrupt to
remind them, 'What about this radiation equipment? We have real
decisions to make here.' They were barely interested." Some good
equipment was saved, but much was trashed, put into storage, or lost.
Subak says, "It was all such a rush, such a waste."

The Queen Elizabeth's head of Ear, Nose and Throat, the late Eli
Katz, noted, "My department was better equipped than either the
Royal Vic or the General because over the years, if I wanted to buy
something, we found always found a way to get it. I used to go to every
convention of ENT and bring things back myself. And Albert Nixon was
a good man – if I got after him for a needed item, he'd try to get it from
the government or raise the money privately." At closure, this top-flight
equipment was seized, pending all the negotiations and new arrangements. "I wanted to buy it myself," Katz says, "but they said no, it
belonged to the government, even though I'd actually bought a lot of it
for the hospital myself! Then they locked it in a basement so long that

it became junk. No one ever got to use it." This kind of waste, of course, is a natural side-effect of the dissolution of any institution.

These stories illustrate that it's not just the obviously vulnerable patients who suffer when there are fewer hospital beds available in a country. The people who staffed the Queen Elizabeth and other once excellent, flourishing, small hospitals, whether their hospitals were closed or merely vastly diminished, have experienced considerably more trauma and stress during this downslide than the public can possibly realize. Like many others, Fred Weigan tries to laugh about how he and so many of the former staff and patients of the Queen Elizabeth hospital went through the five steps of grief established by researcher Elizabeth Kubler-Ross in the 1970s – five steps that she created to try to describe the most devastating experience faced by humans: their own deaths. They are: denial, anger, fear, bargaining, and finally, acceptance. He says it's taken most of his colleagues almost ten years to get to the fifth. "We still meet every November since it happened and try to support each other – at least 120 of us meet at the Squash Club on Atwater. It's a great evening. We have a very good time!"

Despite the brave words, intense anger is never far away from any discussion of the closed hospitals; some alumni find it so upsetting they can no longer speak about their lost institutions. The people who worked in these hospitals have, in fact, sustained fairly permanent psychological wounds. The physical health of the population is not doing so well either.

Larry Lincoln points out that, "These days, every year in January the ERs across the city are packed and the system is in crisis. For example, in 2004, the minister of health was bragging how they'd managed, for the first time in nine years, to avoid absolute meltdown – well, those are the nine years since they closed all those ERs, all those beds. Nobody is keeping track of what that decision has done to health care in our city, but if you look back, you can see so clearly that there's more stress on the system. It's not as good a system as it was then, to be sure." Lincoln concedes that there are many other factors responsible for the deterioration of Quebec and Canada's hospitals besides the mass closures of the mid- and late 1990s. "Hospital care has become more hit-and-miss, more haphazard. And of course, one reason is that it takes a lot more money these days to run a hospital because of the continuous leaps in expensive technologies. If you can't keep up, people suffer, and we don't seem to be able to keep up. You have to be very well-organized, and I don't think we

are. It's not just the technology. Nobody is looking at the health system
as a whole, taking time to try to figure this stuff out. Dealing with health
care is all putting out fires; it's crisis-management."

WHO SUFFERS

A battle to keep the Queen E as is may be hopeless, but they are right to
fight for what it does so well. Its emergency service is a model of care
and efficiency found nowhere else on the island ... This hospital has
revived the house call. Family medicine, social-service and geriatric units
treat the community at home.

Greta Chambers, *Montreal Gazette*, 1995[23]

Who suffers most when a hospital closes? Obviously, the mass closures
of hospital beds across Canada truncated careers and eliminated jobs.
But, of course, that's not all they did. Elizabeth Tsuk, quoted earlier,
was an occupational therapist at the Montreal Children's Hospital who
had several surgeries at the Queen E. She still misses the little hospital
and remembers, "We were so upset! I had Peter, my husband, making
green flags for our demonstrations. We marched several times. We felt
sure we'd save it; it was logical that it would be saved. Why would they
close such a place?"

When all the closures became a reality, extremely ill and vulnerable
patients suffered even more than families like the Tsuks. The Queen
Elizabeth's exemplary psychiatric unit, the one that had offered self-
immolation in the effort to save the hospital, had to abandon their
charges. "We were unique in the city," says Subak. "We had between
800 to 900 outpatients a month from the late 1970s on –thirty inpatients, rotating every ten days. There were *always* two beds kept open
for emergencies and we kept four or five chronic patients at a time, all
of whom had to be shipped to the Douglas [the nearest remaining psychiatric hospital]. Our unique position in the city lay in the fact that we
had psychiatric services available 24 hours a day, seven days a week,
despite having few interns and few residents. Moreover, we had people
on the staff like John Hughes who was arguing that mental problems
are a part of the human condition and can't be neatly separated from
physical ones. Of course, many of our patients had both."

Dr Subak still feels that the hospital that was closed was better at dealing with mental illness than anything that's come along since, and they
had the statistics to prove it. "We had a real community approach. I

mean, we made house calls, we saw these people in their natural habitat, we knew how and where they lived, in their rooming houses and so on. We knew when their conditions were worsening and they might lose their homes and be out on the street, so we'd be able to react. We also had, I think, an extraordinarily personal and humane approach to our clientele. They were mostly heavily bipolar and schizophrenic cases, but the incidence of the primary danger in those illnesses – suicide – was much lower in our out-patients than in other Montreal hospitals. The reason was close follow-up. The other hospitals had figures double or triple ours, per capita. We highlighted suicide prevention and really looked out for it."

Although today drugs are the primary weapon in the effort to keep the mentally ill out of enclosed institutions, George Subak claims that his department relied less on pharmacology than others. "We spent a lot of time talking to people, getting to know them. We had twelve psychiatrists at our height; only five at the end. We had lost our child and adolescent psychiatry section in 1994. It was closed in 1994 because the government decided to centralize everything in St. Justine and the Children's. We were helping children that were hyperactive, dyslexic, with drug prevention and so on. I can't tell you how those people are being served now. When the clients go into those big mega-hospitals they become anonymous – a number. They get lost, they give up more easily. Whereas, we were on first-name basis here and we followed up to make sure they didn't give up. Even though our department was small, it was beautiful – a real local service."

Owen Ness believes that since small community hospitals like the Queen E were lost, there have been many tragedies that people don't recognize. No Canadian studies have ever been undertaken to measure the effects when such services disappear so suddenly. Shortly before closure, he says, "In a single six-month period, two ambulance drivers reported that if they hadn't had the Queen E ER to go to, that is, if they'd had to go to the Royal Victoria, the General, or somewhere else, their patients would have died. The Bonaventure Autoroute was backed up with traffic, and they would never have been able to get anywhere else in time. That means that some patients in critical conditions from NDG, Montreal West, western downtown, and Westmount are undoubtedly dying before they get to a hospital now."

Ness suspects tragedies, but George Subak can name the dead. Even at the time, the media reported four psychiatric patients who killed themselves because they were losing their hospital. "The four suicides,"

Subak remembers sadly, "were the most vulnerable and sensitive patients who were very attached to us and our hospital. They felt they were doomed by closure. This was based on their previous experience elsewhere. We could help them hold on because we were so available, and in their experience, other places had failed them. They decided to give up rather than go through that again. Three were directly due to the closure of the hospital. One more I'd put in as well, a man in his early 40s with a major disorder, affective schizophrenia. He was very bright, sensitive, from a good family. When he found out we weren't going to be there for him any more, he jumped onto the expressway. Robert Prater, a university student. Another was a woman, very attached to us. She jumped off an eight-story building.

"They never would have killed themselves, I believe, if we had stayed open. We had such close follow-up. The Queen E was a safe place for them. They could call us and we'd come to their houses. And 24 hours a day, they could come in. Even if they'd been admitted twenty-five times before, they knew we wouldn't turn them away. That gave them the security and support to carry on. They knew they would always be cared for or could go into hospital when they couldn't cope. They also knew that wasn't true elsewhere. Suicide is impulsive behaviour. It can be changed – it comes from feeling abandoned." In the old days, George Subak would see people from the unit around his neighbourhood while doing errands. "I'd see my old patients at places like Dunkin Donuts. I'd say, 'why don't you come in and see me? You're not doing well.' And they would." Dr Subak hastens to temper some of his emotion over these very human costs of losing a hospital. "This is not to say that elsewhere, everyone doesn't do their best for their patients! I'm convinced there's no actual negligence going on. But in a big, big hospital with four units of 30 beds each, it's very difficult to have an overview and be aware of how everyone is doing. If the ward is small, the rumour-mill works; you hear when things are going wrong. You know where the crises are and how to handle them. And the fact that closure was a major crisis is reflected in the statistics. Between 1991 and 1993, before there was any hint of closure, we had zero suicides. In the two years up to and until closure, we had four."

Today, there's an ad-hoc group of former Queen E psychiatric patients that still meet at a local NDG coffee shop. They've never found any other hospital or any other doctors like they once had, so these Queen E alumni, whose bond is the care they once had, meet several times a week and try to help each other.

BIG VERSUS SMALL

When I was young and foolish I thought bigger is better. It's all phallic (laughs). I'm no longer impressed.

Surgeon Fred Weigan

Many people believe the Queen Elizabeth was chosen for closure precisely because of one of the things that made it so successful: a highly accessible, central location in the heart of the western part of the city. That location turns out to be only a few blocks from the site Montreal has chosen for its much-discussed, highly controversial "super-hospital." This ambitious amalgamation of five McGill teaching hospitals was supposed to break ground almost ten years ago but had yet to begin construction at press time. The location for the proposed "centre of excellence" is the Glen Railway Yards on the southwest side of the city, just below the Queen Elizabeth's NDG site and not far from the St. Lawrence River. Unlike the Queen E, which was accessible to autoroutes and city arteries alike, the new site is cut off by the railway tracks and the expressway and contaminated by years of industrial use. Hospital alumni figure that early plans for this massive amalgamation are one reason their institution wasn't considered as vital to the area as it actually was. Proponents of centralization originally tried to put nearly all the city's hospitals, French as well as English, in this area, but the project keeps being downsized, partially because of costs, but also because it's becoming more and more clear from international studies that this kind of health care centralization is a bad idea.

As Elizabeth Tsuk says, "Of course, I know that governments do a lot of crazy things, and closing the Queen E was a crazy thing. Now the super-hospital is an absolutely ridiculous idea. People from McGill believe in it. I suppose that's why it's going ahead. I think it's stupid and short-sighted because if there's some terrible catastrophe, you need more than one hospital! You need small hospitals that real people can get to – not just people with cars who can go anywhere easily. That was one of the great things about the QE, it was at a crossroads of buses and subways – the Children's too. To close the Children's and the Queen E both! How will people get there? Most of our patients, so worried about their children, came by bus!"

Whether or not the Queen E was a victim of the ambition of the super-hospital supporters back in the mid-nineties is to some extent just an adjunct of a larger problem. In fact, all community hospitals began suffering from pressures to centralize as early as the 1980s. The money needed for simple day-to-day operations in the smaller institutions – housekeeping, salaries for a sufficient number of employees, decent food services for the patients, basic equipment like beds and sheets – started being considered better spent if diverted to brand-new and much larger institutions. These were intended to garner world attention for various medical specialties, provide "cutting-edge" care for the most obscure diseases, give prestige and status to the profession, and attract investment from pharmacological and hospital equipment companies.

Elizabeth Tsuk has spent her life working with sick children. She points out, "When I worked at the Rehabilitation Institute, it was very chaotic, in a basement. It was just fantastic. Then it moved into a big place built by architects and everything got worse. The architects were horrible, nothing was made the way it needed to be for day-to day work. It's all a kind of monument to the architect, isn't it, instead of tailored to real needs? I'm sure that's what these super-hospitals will be like."

It's important to define the basic differences between hospitals. Medical professionals understand the differences much better than the general public but haven't clearly communicated them. Small hospitals aren't normally set up to handle rare or extremely complex cases. Consequently, the public has gradually internalized the opinion that the care it does dispense is somehow of lower quality than what might be available at a "world-class" institution, like the Toronto General, Mt. Sinai in New York, or a McGill teaching hospital in Montreal. What doctors know but the public seldom realizes is that the teaching hospitals' concentration on the medical profession's interest in innovation and career advancement may mean that the average person's hospital stay for the kinds of diseases that strike most of the country's population – gallstones, hip replacements, appendectomies, broken bones, or diabetes – will be less comfortable and more stressful in a big institution than in their community hospital, which is set up for these normal illnesses. Always granted, of course, that each hospital is decently funded to provide that care.

Derek Marpole is the very definition of what's called a "tertiary-care specialist." He does cardiac catharization, and he can only do it at a big teaching hospital, a "centre of excellence" or a "super-hospital." But even he points out that, "There's a very important place for good secondary care hospitals, which are so needed to take care of everyday diseases and accidents. It used to be they could take care of heart attack cases – the Queen E used to when I was there, before the technology advanced. Today, there's more specialist work and machines, so cardiac problems require tertiary care, but with other problems, most work can be done in small hospitals, and the patient care and contact is better. At the Queen, the care was very personalized, everyone talking to everyone." He pauses to remember. "I loved working there."

The main reason our society is so enamoured of the big and fancy in medical care is the technology that tertiary hospitals can afford to maintain. "Community hospitals can't handle the interaortic balloon pumps, access to ER surgery, cardiac catharization," continues Marpole. "But they can look after a certain scale of very common heart problems – acute coronary syndromes, rhythm problems. They can do resuscitations, of course. And one very important thing to remember is, the more technological a hospital becomes, the less hands-on and personal it is." The other important thing to remember is that good community hospitals know when they're out-gunned by a disease or injury and specialize in stabilizing patients and whipping them over to tertiary-care hospitals in the event that their condition is beyond their expertise.

Larry Lincoln, an orthopedic surgeon and the son of Quebec's former environment minister, Clifford Lincoln, is a lean-faced, dark, handsome man in his forties. As he puts it, "A community hospital's mission is to serve their community's day-to-day medical needs in a humane way. That means that only special problems, rare conditions, should be sent to a tertiary-care hospital like the General or the Royal Victoria. And yet, that's not the way it works; they end up doing the work that community hospitals are best at." Surgeon Fred Weigan says, "You can't be everything to everyone. At the Queen E, we didn't attempt brain or heart work. We knew our mandate. We sent anything suspicious off to the specialists. We had a direct line to the Neuro, only fifteen to thirty minutes by ambulance, and any time, day or night, I'd call them. Something wrong with the heart, we'd expedite that very quickly. That's the proper use of a community facility. You need a place for complex cases, but you also need a place for the every-day, the gallstones and appendicitis, the influenzas and broken arms."

Judith Levitan, a family medicine specialist now doing administrative work, is blunt about the differences between community and tertiary-care hospitals. She says that at most large teaching hospitals, "doctors place their highest values on research, fame, and glory. You just have to look at their requirements for promotion and tenure: publication, teaching, administration – nothing whatsoever about caring for the patient, nothing about the community, about experience, about practical expertise. I don't think it's appropriate for your professional teaching body to say nothing about actually practicing medicine when pursuing your medical career! I blame our university/government system as it now stands. What good is it, having specialists who know all about MRIs and how they can be used and so forth, if the line is too long for the patients in your institution to get one when they need it?"

Levitan says the competitive atmosphere in which our current system trains young doctors, pushing them into specializing by not encouraging general family practice or allowing them time to try the many kinds of medicine that would give them expertise in the most common ills of humanity, "has made specializations in weird and rare disorders the biggest prize you can pursue." She believes that because of the way teaching institutions bestow grants, status, and support, taking care of all the everyday ills that will beset the largest proportion of the population is now being left to the worst-funded or so-called 'least ambitious' doctors and institutions. "The greater and more complex the complications in a given disease, the higher your expertise in it lifts you in the hierarchy. That means that the stranger the disease is, the cooler the specialist, the more status he or she has. This is *so twisted* in terms of the public interest, so detrimental to what really happens in everyday treatment and diagnosis, because these very complex, serious diseases that they have elevated to such importance are by definition extremely rare! They don't afflict more than a tiny minority of the population. So work on the conditions that people are much more likely to get over the course of their lifetimes becomes orphaned and neglected in such a system."

Ottawa surgeon Ron Lewis understands why governments are looking in this direction. They think it will save money. "In Alberta," he says, "they say the medical budget is increasing by ten percent every year. Fifty percent of their budget is already going to health care. In a very few years, obviously, it will be their entire budget. What escapes people is that one supposed panacea for all this, to integrate hospitals into super-hospitals, like we've amalgamated cities into mega-cities, *only increases the cost of the health or municipal system.* It's supposed to be done in order to avoid duplication of services and whatnot, but if you look at the figures, it always increases expenditures. We've known this for a very long time with hospitals; there are many papers on the optimum efficiency of 300-bed hospitals. Say, for example, you look at gall bladder operations; that's much more efficiently done in a small rather than a large hospital. When you close or starve these smaller places, you create a system where all the care goes through the remaining big teaching hospitals. So it's not surprising that costs go up. This is exactly what's happened in Nova Scotia, Alberta, Quebec, Ontario, everywhere they've closed the smaller, community institutions."

Fred Weigan mentions reading an article by a group that builds hospitals. "These experts said the ideal size is 300 beds, give or take 75." He goes on to say, "we had 272 at the Queen Elizabeth. Having trained at big hospitals, the Royal Victoria and General, I was aware how top-heavy they were in comparison. Plus the egos were huge. The pure efficiency at the Queen E always took my breath away." Like others, he rhapsodizes about his small hospital's triage methods that had emergency patients in beds or on their way in minutes. "You'd walk in, were screened by an experienced nurse, seen by an experienced intern or resident, then the attending, and were on your way to a bed or x-ray within twenty minutes. The Tzar of Russia didn't get such care! That article by builders on size explains it in part. Just compare two hospitals with a small railroad station and Grand Central. How long does it take to get your ticket and find your train on each one? That's the degree of difference."

These stories hold true across the country. Ron Lewis, in Ottawa, cites the Riverside hospital, "which was very efficient and the same size as the Queen E." Then it was deemed too small and amalgamated with all the city's hospitals. "Back in 1995," he says, "government generated-statistics, released a month after they announced the Queen E would be closed, named it *the most efficient hospital in Quebec.* You'll see why this looks familiar to me. I mentioned that to the people at Riverside, and they said, 'Oh, yeah. Just before we lost control over our management, the government stats in Ontario said the same thing about us.'" This seems crazy, but it doesn't mean that there isn't, as Lewis explains, "a certain logic to amalgamation. It just doesn't happen in reality. The city of Ottawa amalgamated to save money. Immediately, everybody's taxes went up. Mine are 20 percent above what they were when I bought my house six months ago! The same thing has happened in Toronto and Montreal with amalgamation. All this expensive stuff we read about – kickbacks, waste, those kinds of problems – are most rampant in large, not small institutions. The bigger the institution, the easier it is to scam, the easier to lose statistics in the pile. It's the anonymity of the big city versus the small town. There is also no truth to the idea that amalgamation is better for the delivery of services."

Lewis and most of the other critics of the current move to mammoth institutions acknowledge that, "We can't go back to having all the little community hospitals we used to have – not because that isn't desirable anymore, just because it's not going to happen in the current atmosphere. But the value they had can be regained in facilities that are small and have control over their own management. Now that it's under the management of the Greater Hospitals of Ottawa, in effect amalgamated into a virtual super-hospital, Riverdale is all screwed up. It's hard to get local anesthetics, hard to take care of the outpatients. This has happened because it's been folded into the management of all the Ottawa Hospitals. They have to have their say in how everything is done. So you get delays in implementation, in supplies, a lack of personal input, and the lowest common denominator in care."

John Alexander Clark is the great-grandson of A.R. Griffith, the doctor whose life is reviewed ahead and who is generally considered the person most instrumental in helping found the Queen Elizabeth. Clark had little to do with the old hospital, but he did follow the family trade by becoming a doctor. He's a radiology specialist in Toronto and has worked in every size of institution. He says, "From a professional point of view, the biggest hospitals can be very, very frustrating." He points out that the current tendency to favour big hospitals or to consolidate smaller ones, "has no basis in medical science, reason, or even economics; it's purely politically driven. It's been proven time and again that there's no financial benefit once these mega-hospitals are established. Wellesley Hospital, for example, where I used to practice in Toronto, was well run with superb service to the clientele. But keeping it open didn't cut it politically."

Clark says that, "I've lived through several mergers in my career and frankly, I find large institutions don't function as well, especially administratively. You can get things done in a small place; the lines of authority are very clear. But big ones carry immense inertia, with all their levels of bureaucracy that have to be hurtled every time you want to do anything, from special to absolutely normal procedures. Access is not as good; waiting lists, typically, are much longer. What happens when you enfold several institutions into one big one are terrible upheavals in referral patterns and in the flow of services, which take years to settle. So there's not as much or maybe *any* care for some people in the short term because those referral patterns have been torn apart." Moreover, the most recent international studies show no indications that such actions make medical care cheaper or in any way better over the long term.

John Alexander Clark is, like Marpole, a very highly trained specialist, but he has made a conscious decision to "work in small institutions
now, and I'm much happier. My subspecialty is intervention radiology.
We do therapeutic work as well as diagnosis. Putting in tubes, wires,
catheters, and fiber optics has to be guided by radiology. Angioplasty is
generally done by cardiologists, but work on other blood vessels would
be done by people like me. X-rays guide the therapy, place the tubes
for drainage, so my specialty crosses a variety of fields. There are a lot
of popular procedures that require an intervention radiologist, like
uterine fibroid embolization. This sounds fancy, but it can all be done
in small institutions; you don't need big teaching hospitals for this kind
of normal care."

Intervention radiology is not alone; much of modern hospital care
doesn't require super-hospitals. How about the all-important budget?
Clark contends that although it seems counter-intuitive, you don't save
money by making two or three hospitals into one. "The public doesn't
realize the extent to which hospitals already band together on purchase agreements when buying supplies, machines, sheets, and even
doing laundry. Budgets are so tight that they've had to work together
economically for some time. Putting several community hospitals into
one building just introduces new construction costs and usually a net
loss of beds. Of course, the training aspect cannot be forgotten, and
that's supposed to be better. It's a major excuse for mergers and super-
hospitals. But as we make hospitals bigger, the training we give in them
becomes more esoteric. Politicians, professionals, and the various
funding bodies call for 'centres of excellence' and so forth in particular areas like trauma, neurology, or cardio, and they concentrate their
teaching on the really difficult cases that require all the bells and whistles of modern drugs and technology. That brings them international
status professionally, private investment from the drug and equipment
companies, that kind of thing. That would be OK to a point, but today
we're doing this to the extent that we're getting trainees who have
never seen a *normal* disease – never had to deal with appendicitis or gall
stones! What does that mean to the average person's medical care?"

Mario Larivière, who has administered scores of hospitals, says, "Yes,
we do need long-term care facilities, polyclinics, and yes, a CLSC or
other community clinic can provide home care, community foster
care, vaccinations, and so on. But you still need hospitals, that is, airway
management, for those constant, banal, but still life-threatening
events: gall bladder, appendix, airway obstruction, accidents. Sacre

Coeur and the Neuro in Montreal are not for those everyday things; they're for heart angioplasties, brain surgery, very complex cancer treatments, and difficult diagnoses. These big teaching hospitals help us go further medically. But you have to remember that at a small, community hospital, the cost of treating such a common episode is *half* of, say, Sacre Coeur's! That's because you don't need all those bells and whistles and specialists and fancy machines in the building to do most things."

La Riviere's profession requires a very clear grasp of economic issues, above all things, but he also understands how economic issues affect patient care. He says, "A community hospital is there to take care of the normal illnesses of the population. It has a different mission than a centre of excellence, and the two don't work well together. For example, MRIs and complex diagnoses should be located in the big hospitals, but oncology and radio and chemotherapy, on the other hand, should NOT be centralized. That's a tremendous burden on the patient. I've tried so hard to get it here in St. Eustace. Certainly, we have enough cancer here! Imagine how many people out of 250,000 have it! But they have to drive ninety minutes, when they're so sick, for treatment. What if they have no car? What if their spouse cannot leave work or the children? What does that cost them, or the system? The bureaucrats who've created a world focused on having super-hospitals, to the detriment of community ones, are like Drapeau with his dream for an Olympic Stadium; it's that kind of grandiose view in Quebec. The bureaucrats and ambitious physicians will make their reputation out of it. But they're not thinking about the realities of health care for the real people they're supposed to be serving."

The thing that no one steps back and admits, Larivière says, is that, "we're talking about mixing very different cultures – the super- and the community-care hospital – and you know, forced marriages never turn out. It just won't work. The cost will be enormous, even though they'll hide it from us. There's a staggering cost already we're bearing from the closure of those seven hospitals just here in Montreal. Unbelievable, irreplaceable professional experience, the slow development of institutions and protocols – all lost. And we never even did any kind of assessment after it happened and before jumping into these new fast-fixes." This kind of discussion about really looking at historical experience, about real costs and the differences in the types of care people actually receive, almost never makes it into the news when allocations of our health care tax money are announced. Instead, the discussion usually centres on prestige, attraction of specialists, and advancement of the profession. The community hospital advocates wonder what has happened to the central purpose: patient care.

Both Larivière and John Hughes point out that, "Fortunately or unfortunately, most of the people working on these decisions haven't been terribly ill; they don't know what it means to be in either a large or a small hospital or how that daily care plays out." On paper, big, fancy institutions with new equipment and so on seem inarguably better. "They also claim," Larivière says, "that we need new institutions because the old ones are in terrible shape. And that's true – the Royal Victoria is literally falling apart; it's dangerous. But if we'd put money into maintenance, that need never have happened! Will we build a super-hospital and then just let it fall apart? If we spend money on buildings and machines and rare disorders, will we still be able to pay for enough nurses and orderlies so they aren't overworked and exhausted? Will we be able to make the patients comfortable?" Pat Titterton, the Queen E's head ER nurse who is now living in Ontario, says, "Ontario just did a patient-input survey of all their hospitals – access to care, community services, financial performance, technical expertise – all rated on a scale of one to five. The two small, community hospitals, Armprior, which serves 7 or 8,000, and Renfrew, which serves 9,000, each got five stars. The huge one in Ottawa got only one or two."

LITTLE BITTY CENTRES OF EXCELLENCE

> The job of a community hospital worker is to serve the patient. You're not trying to become a famous, innovative physician. You're trying to serve the everyday health needs of a particular community. The irony is, that often also leads to innovative work.
>
> Dr John Hughes

Besides supposed economic savings, one reason that's given for centralization and super-hospitals is that such centres will attract top-quality doctors who produce innovations that will advance medical care and bring prestige and financial benefits to both the institution and the whole urban area. That seems logical, although many of the people actually responsible for medical innovations will argue the entire idea. Ron Lewis is credited with several important, life-saving surgical innovations beyond pre-operatative use of antibiotics – retroparital aortic surgery was just one of them. Lewis pioneered repairing the aorta from the patient's side rather than from the front. "The reason for doing it that way is that you can reach higher to do your work with less disturbance to the organs. I did it at the Queen E before closure, and I was the only one doing it at the Royal Victoria. But it never caught on there like it should have." Lewis thinks he knows why.

"When I moved to the Royal Victoria and the General after the Queen E, I was astounded to see that, in terms of carotid and vascular surgery, it was like a time-warp. I found that so many things I had learned there long ago as a resident, things that I had used and discarded as better things came up, were still being taught in the big hospitals as gospel. Twenty years later, they still had many of the same procedures and protocols. I thought, 'My God; time has stood still.'" He hastens to add, "This is not to say that in some areas they weren't further advanced; but a surprising number of old treatments were still in place at the big teaching hospital. The methods they were using for varicose vein stripping, for example, were exactly the same ones that I was taught as a resident. It took me five long years to get that hospital to buy a cheap piece of equipment, costing only $1,000, which made varicose treatment so much better for the patient. I believe that the reason for this isn't stupidity or lack of funding. It's purely size, which creates bureaucratic inertia."

Many hospital history experts, as well as other small hospital alumni, agree. Larry Lincoln was anxious that an older colleague, Larry Coglin, be credited as that hospital's main pioneer in arthroscopy: joint surgery done with fibre-optics. What Larry developed was very pragmatic – a methodology for doing knee surgery with local anesthetic. "All aspects used to be done with general anesthetic," he explains, "but in the early 1990s there was a crisis in anesthesiologists in Quebec; many had been let go, so there was a long waiting list for joint repairs. We at the Queen E were the first to try certain knee operations with a local; we could do a procedure that cost the government at least $100 for only $42. But because we billed for the local anesthesia and weren't anesthesiologists, we got in trouble. The government looked into us for several years; we just kept doing it and eventually they stopped trying to block us."

It's a relatively minor procedure and not appropriate to all knee problems, but it can be done with only local anesthetic. Lincoln says, "We could cut a three-month wait for that particular operation to one month. That's a time reduction of 200 percent! It was the same operation as with the general anesthetic. The only drawback is getting a local in the knee joint, which hurts, so we give Verset to calm the patient first. The other advantage, besides speed and cost, is they can walk right out of there an hour later, whereas they'd have to spend several hours recovering in a hospital bed if they'd been given a general anesthetic. The local numbs the knee joint so patients can walk. As quickly as five to twelve hours after, they start to get the benefit." Lincoln does nine to eleven knees at a time; the greatest limits on the numbers he can do are hospital budgets. "Knee and hip replacement prostheses are very expensive – $3000 plus equipment. Arthroscopy is better. The equipment is the big expense; each piece costs me several thousand dollars but as time goes on, we use it more. The problem is there are constant technological advances and hence a need for new instruments. So the major way the government saves money is to limit OR time, that is, simply to control access to the surgery."

The average patient's access to surgical care in any health system translates to how quickly their surgeon can get access to the Operating Rooms (ORS). Because the number of operations each surgeon is allowed to do is limited by both demand and government budgets, it has become vitally important that ORs work at a high level of efficiency. We hear about not enough beds, doctors, or nurses, which also plays a strong role in long wait-times for surgery, but one of the most common reasons why a patient might have to wait days or weeks for needed surgery is a simple physical problem within each operating theatre, called "changeover time." Surgeon Fred Weigan says, "Changeover, that's the time between when Patient A leaves and Patient B comes into the OR. In that time, you have to change the linen, take away instruments, mop, change clothes, re-scrub, and make everything brand-new for the new arrival. At the Queen E, we felt ours needed improvement. Ron Lewis, who used to be surgeon in chief at the Queen E and then became peripheral vascular surgeon at the Montreal General and the Royal Victoria, told me that in 2002 and 2003, a one and a half-hour changeover time was nothing unusual at those hospitals. At closure back in 1995, the Queen Elizabeth had ours down to *twelve minutes*, which is simply unequalled anywhere in the world."

The Queen achieved this miracle through "group consensus and communication. We'd study the situation together at our meetings, talk about it over lunches, and we'd realize that the bottleneck was, say, anesthesia; everybody could be ready but them. Or another time, we'd speak to the superintendent of the OR, because we'd figured out everyone was ready but the scrub nurse. Maybe they'd say, 'Oh, that's because her union has a break then.' And we'd come back and say, 'Well, can we arrange things so the break is better timed?' Once we'd figured out *what* was slowing us down, we'd all get together and make compromises. That nurse would change her break. She'd be willing to because we all got along so well that she wanted to help. And a doctor or a surgeon would re-orient his entire schedule. People were willing to make sacrifices because everybody did, on every level; and then things would roll. It was just magic, watching the Queen get ready for surgery!"

Daily medical care is frequently better at small hospitals, too, because both the administration and the heads of the various departments are more conditioned to place the patients' needs above technological, professional, or bureaucratic considerations. Surgeon Ron Lewis, now working in a very large hospital similar to those envisioned by Montreal's "super-hospital" boosters, reiterates his experience that big institutions don't simply drain the coffers of the small ones. He says, "In many ways, they can smother the very innovation they claim they'll inspire. The [large] hospitals are beyond conservative." He goes on, "I was thinking of an innovating project I'm interested in. So I printed out the requirements for permission just to do a preliminary study here. On the first page, it stipulated that I submit eighteen copies. I gave up; what's the use? What are the chances that eighteen separate people or committees will all approve any idea in any decent amount of time? I understand how this happens – part of this is the satisfaction people get from the idea of protecting patients from experimentation, and that's a viable desire. But I tried to introduce a protocol for adopting the use of Heperin, a common drug that's already being used all over the world. Five years and a lot of work later, I still can't get it accepted. It's a very useful study, a protocol to help me get blood results so we can look down the list, see if that drug is working; but these large systems are too inert to respond even to the commonplace innovations, to say nothing of really exciting ones."

"At a little hospital like the Queen E," Lewis contends, "things were different." He was allowed to investigate protocols successfully for the simple reason that the chain of command was shorter. "I was the only person in Montreal, except one at St. Luc, using an angioscope to do bypass surgery, instead of operating blindly." He says, "I did that from 1990 on. When the Queen E closed and I went to the Vic, I took that equipment with me. But over six years, they never once let me use it. And after five years of fighting to get that varicose vein equipment I mentioned, I remained the only one operating on varicose veins that way. It clearly expedites treatment; there's less morbidity, trauma, time expended. How they dealt with my request was simply to cut varicose vein surgery completely off their list." Lewis says, "So now, Montreal patients either have to come to Ottawa and see me or head out to the one clinic in the area which does it, in the far East End." Varicose veins are not, of course, a rare condition. As Judith Levitan predicted, its plebian status may be one reason why caring for it is not being pursued at a teaching hospital, despite the public need.

Lewis goes on, "I came here to this big hospital in Ottawa and proposed the same thing and initially they promised to look into it. I even offered to buy the equipment myself. It's never happened yet." Lewis thinks he knows why. "The system at these big hospitals is simply not set up to respond to changes and innovations in either treatment or the delivery of services. It's the same thing with laparoscopic aortic surgery. I was on the verge of being able to deliver that at the Royal Vic; I'd had a year of experience in the lab, but when it came time to buy the equipment, the system just wouldn't accept it. And here our laparoscopic equipment is hopeless."

Small hospitals can not only support great innovations but also facilitate careers and the advancement of the profession. Oddly enough, they sometimes do this better than the big institutions that concentrate on such goals. Albert Nixon, the Queen E's director general in the 1980s, married into the family that had founded the Hospital. He says, "Even in the old days, Uncle Harold [Griffith] understood all the secrets of a small hospital – how you attract and hold onto someone of the caliber of Ron Lewis, for example. When we got Ron as a young resident, we sent him to St. Mary's to learn vascular surgery, hoping that afterwards he'd come back to us. When he did, we gave him the support he needed! We were small enough that we could raise the money we needed for the new departments and technologies that attracted such people without committee meetings and long delays." Nixon had large donors on top, like the MacConnell and Molson families, to say nothing of their hospital's Women's Auxillary. No committees were involved. The money they gave was immediately available for practical use. "We used it to make sure our staff had what they needed to do the best work." Small size meant economic simplicity. Nixon did all this almost single-handedly. "I had no assistants – no bureaucracy. We had volunteers. That's how you can keep things running smoothly and without any bottlenecks, either for the patients or the staff!"

SUPER-SIZING THE STUDENTS

Medicine today and when I learned in the 1970s is like the difference
between the old days of baseball and today. I wouldn't go into medicine
if I were starting out right now. It's no fun.

Joe Mamazza, MSI pioneer

Anyone old enough to have had an old-fashioned surgical appendectomy and who has since experienced a cystectomy or had one of the
many other kinds of formerly highly invasive surgeries that are now
achieved through the use of fibre-optics knows first hand how much we
all owe to the surgeons who developed the new, minimally-invasive
technique of laproscopy. Scarring, healing time, and physical trauma
have all been significantly reduced. An appendectomy that used to
leave an unsightly scar and keep people in the hospital for a week,
dazed by morphine and unable to work for at least another week or two
after that, now leaves an almost invisible little dimple. Patients are
home within 48 hours and back to their lives in a week. They don't
have the painful adhesions and weakness from trauma that so often
used to follow this type of surgery. Joe Mammazza feels he owes many
of the opportunities to develop this important surgical innovation to
the atmosphere prevalent at the Queen Elizabeth hospital. He also
feels he owes his ability to have advanced his field to his early training –
a training which, like the hospitals around it, has since been super-
sized.

"Medical training today," he says, "it's all so pegged in advance. You
have to specialize so early. There's so much rigidity regarding what
you can and can't do that you never have the opportunity to find out
what you're good at. Specialists used to have to do general work first,
which could be applied to their program. No more. For instance, my
fourth year elective at McGill was emergency medicine at the Queen
E. Then I did my internship there. After six months I enrolled in their
oby-gyn residency. I thought I'd like that but I discovered that operating is what I liked. So you did four straight clinical years, then practice
or a year of research as one more year of training to 'round you off.'
My third year at the Queen E was research, which I looked forward to
until I discovered I also hated that!" The current system would have
kept him in oby- gyn, to say nothing of research, and some very important innovations in laproscopic techniques might have been many
more years in coming.

Cardiac specialist Derek Marpole agrees. When the rotating internships that Joe mentions were abolished, it had a very deleterious effect on the profession and is much to blame for the serious shortage of general or "family medicine" practitioners in Quebec and many other places. "Now you have to decide on a specialty at nineteen or twenty," Marpole says, "before you can possibly know what any of them are like. Going out to different hospitals on rotating internships was an ideal way to make up your mind. Besides, there aren't good grants or positions for family medicine these days, so students end up choosing specialties for purely financial reasons. Of course, the level of knowledge required to practice most specialties is probably so great today that you might not have time to put off specializing any more. But I can still remember pearls from my outside practice, before I specialized. I got to deliver a baby – to take care of little children! I'd never have a chance to do that if I were a young doctor now. You get the opportunity to see the bazillion ways that chest and arm pain might not have anything to do with the heart, whereas in a specialty, those patients have been weeded out. You hardly ever see them, so you don't really understand the full expression of the symptoms, even in your own specialty."

Judith Levitan believes that, "cutting the rotating internships in the late 1970s was the biggest single educational error the medical schools in Canada have ever committed! When it existed, you had an eighteen-month rotation, doing different specialties, helping with babies being born, doing some pediatrics, assisting surgery. You could really get a feel for what you liked or hated. You could go out with one specialty, come back and take another. Not now. Now you have to make your choice before you actually experience any variety. As soon as you can, you have to choose a specialty or you won't get one of the very few slots the government has left open in it and the grants and loans and so forth you need. Later on, if you find you've made a mistake about your life's work, you can't go back. You're stuck in that specialty." Judith adds that, "McGill may be the worst that way. There was an exit poll done by the Association of Canadian Medical Colleges that showed they have the youngest age for specialization in the country."

This system, which results in too many specialists and far too few GPs – a crisis that is probably the most important medical problem in Canada at this time – also has serious effects on diagnoses and slows treatment. Judith Levitan points out that not only people with normal but nonetheless painful and potentially dangerous problems like asthma, gall bladder, bowel, or kidney conditions under-serviced because there are too few GPs but also that the current system "often doesn't even work on the level of helping the few people who do contract the rare diseases. For example, the belief at the Royal Victoria and the Montreal General is still that GPs don't have the slightest understanding of the difference between primary and tertiary care. But it's the specialists, I find, who have no conception of the enormous range of diseases that afflict people. I mean, GPs are seeing patients presenting with all kinds of things. They have to know a little about everything and that's the point – a little, not a lot. So if they send someone for a consult who hasn't really got that disorder after all, the specialist decides that the GP is an idiot. The specialist never notices all the times the GP was right in sending on the patient; he takes that part for granted. And he doesn't have the slightest idea what other diseases are out there that can mimic the symptoms of his specialty and raised the GP's suspicions in the first place. He never bothered to learn anything about them because those conditions are not part of his specialty."

"The result of this status war," Levitan continues, "is that there's no communication between these two groups. The GPs have hardly any access to a specialist who might help them keep up with changes in a particular disease or treatment, and there can be a three-month wait to just *see* a specialist. If the poor GP calls him to ask, 'Well, in the meantime, can I help my patient by doing this or that,' the specialist is irritated by his importunity. I've heard them say things like, 'Don't call me up with this shit. Don't bother me!' So the GP – and the patient – are on their own, trying to figure out if the problem they suspect is the real one and if the specialist they're waiting weeks to see really is the right one. Huge amounts of time and taxpayers' money get wasted, both with these kinds of faulty diagnoses and with lack of treatment while the patient waits to see a string of possibly useless specialists."

Not only are there critically insufficient numbers of GPs with little access to the specialists who have become the disease "experts" but they have simultaneously, with the restructuring of hospitals in the mid-1990s, been denied access to their patients in most hospitals. So hospital care, which was once superintended largely by medical generalists, has been turned over to government bureaucrats and, to a lesser degree, the medical specialists. The general or family practitioners don't fit in anywhere. Specialists never learn about day-to-day diseases because they aren't supposed to, which is bad enough. Even worse is the fact that the problem also works in the opposite direction: GPs no longer get exposed to the teaching opportunities that have been provided by hospitals for 150 years, since their very inception. This is a revolutionary change in hospital care and management that has been unilaterally imposed by governments, once again with no studies on its effects, and very little professional input.

Mario Larivière, as a government bureaucrat directing a hospital, has straddled this change. He points out that pushing GPs out of the hospital system has had serious effects that few people, including the specialists and the GPs themselves, have completely grasped. "Community hospitals can be and always were teaching institutions. Our GPs need to know about real life, about what happens to their cases when they hit the hospital system. In just this past decade, they've been suddenly isolated in their private offices, sending people here and there, never seeing what actually happens to them, never being allowed to go in and see them when their conditions become acute."

Judith Levitan explains, "This completely changes the role of the attending staff. The trouble with what's happened to medical care is that no one looks at the big picture. No one looks at how patient-flow *works*. The Quebec government implemented this 'effectif medicament' system that decides what resources you're allowed to use – including staff. We can't provide a GP to go onto an orthopedic ward to assess folks who have had surgery. These people are their family patients or might be having other medical problems, too. But they've been classified by the government as 'orthopedic patients' so it's supposed to be a waste of money to have any other kind of doctor but orthopedic surgeons see them. Even small rural hospitals can't get the money to have the bodies to do this. And it's ridiculous. That's not how the human body works, just having one thing go wrong at a time."

Because of its traditional respect for generalists, the Queen Elizabeth was particularly attentive to this problem. Its methods should not be lost but studied as useful methodology today. Levitan says that the Queen E staff "fought that kind of rigid classification actively. For example, we didn't allow anyone to work in the Emergency Room, whatever their specialty, if they didn't have a practice. We felt that they had to be exposed to a wide spectrum of illnesses or they'd never recognize the right one in the emergency setting. We had four on-call groups of twelve doctors. You could call the doctor who was either the patient's GP or her specialist and check about what you were doing for them in the ER. You didn't have to start from scratch, taking down all the information about the patient, figuring out if her asthma symptoms were masking coronary ones and so forth. We had a staff phone book. I'd call all the people during a shift, saying, 'your patient Mrs X is here presenting with so and so symptoms. Do you want her admitted?' And then I'd have the guidance and input from someone who had known the patient for years. Of course, that doesn't mean you do what they say slavishly, no matter what you think about the current crisis. But it's such important input into your final decision!"

At the hospital she was working for after the Queen E closed, Judith reports that she asked for the staff phone book and they said, "What for?" "I explained that before doing a procedure, I wanted to check on a new patient's status with his regular doctor, and I was told, 'Oh, you can't bother the doctors about that. Just figure it out yourself.' Imagine people with chronic asthma or palpitations having to go through the full rigamaroll every time they go into the ER – maybe being given the wrong drugs, ones that don't work or that they're sensitive to – rather than letting the attending hospital physicians just call their family doctors for quick advice on what usually works! The result is that the patient is treated rudely, kept unnecessarily long, and, chances are, the information about their latest crisis never gets passed on! It's a heartbreaking loss of opportunity and decline in quality of treatment, and it costs the system untold amounts of money."

This situation has become so acute that in 2003, the Ministere du Sante announced a program to provide patient information online so that ER doctors would have some background on these patients and there would be fewer overlapping prescriptions and treatments. One scheme was the "Carte aux Puces" or "Smart Card." The province's medicare cards were supposed to be encoded with some of the patients' basic medical information that was stored in a central data bank. The public, however, didn't have much confidence because of the possibilities for fraud and privacy invasion inherent in this idea, and there remain serious security and technical difficulties in managing medical health records online. This entire problem is one of those situations that worked fine when doctors simply had access to each other; it was destroyed by the new, budget-centred ideas about health care. Now more money will have to be spent on an untried new system to try to fix what wasn't broken in the first place.

Derek Marpole explains some of the recent history that has lead to such a yawning chasm in the profession. "Internists, that is to say, young doctors chosing to specialize into what was termed 'internal medicine' used to be considered real specialists. Now the category has been split off into 'internal medicine' and 'family medicine,' and the internist has simply become a glorified family doctor. When this first happened, they either retired or became sub-specialists." Fewer and fewer GPs are being trained to make up for this shortfall caused by such confusing changes in the categories. "The number of GPs is more and more inadequate because training is way down. The idea was that GPs or family medicine doctors would man the government clinics, the CLSCs, and specialists would take up the slack their departure left in the hospitals. But in the rural areas of the province, there aren't any specialists to do that in the first place, and in the cities, there aren't any generalists available."

Not enough GPs are trained any more to staff even urban CLSCs, let alone small-town ones, and most Canadians under the age of forty can't find one wherever they may live. All the government decisions in recent years have mitigated against the generalists. Hoping to save money on salaries, governments have pressed Colleges of Physicians and Surgeons to limit enrollments. Because they have a vested interest in making sure their graduates will be valued and able to command large salaries, Colleges have readily complied. Surgeon Fred Weigan says that to add insult to injury, GPs were also prevented by professional rules from intruding into specialties. Specialists, however, have not been prevented from invading family and general practice. "The big hospitals really muddied the waters when they got into family practice," he says. "The GPs were so pissed off! What the hell are guys in specialized hospitals with all those bells and whistles doing horning in on infected toenails and rashes? They were over-endowed, I guess, hadn't got enough of their fancy cases, so they started keeping themselves busy with what was really general and family practice. That really caused a lot of negative emotions." This lack of respect for the proper use of general practice and its mandate in the management of small hospitals has had serious repercussions throughout the medical profession, as we'll see in chapter 7. Serious repercussions eventually affect patient care.

Older doctors like Derek Marpole have happy memories of the weekly luncheon/meetings at the Queen E where "everybody sat together; it was very open, democratic." At the big Royal Victoria, on the other hand, Marpole remembers, "the specialists sat together; no GPs were allowed at that table. The chief of medicine, John Beck, had a prejudice against family medicine. He was a very patriarchal, patronizing specialist – not an unusual thing." Orthopedic specialist Larry Lincoln agrees and thinks a hierarchical arrangement is a serious mistake because possibly the one quality that "was most important to patient care at the Queen E was the position of the GPs, family medicine physicians. They were everywhere, and they were well-respected. They were heavily involved in the wards, in the ER, and it was all interdependent. I guess what I mean by that is the Queen E was more consistent in its care. A patient would generally have a good experience in the ER and then on the ward as well. At the other hospitals I've worked at, well, elsewhere I've seen that only about half the nurses or doctors on the ward are interested in taking care of you; to the other half it's just a job. I've had a lot of upset patients asking me to get them another nurse. Our arthroscopy department, mind you, is really good. But we don't have a huge amount of contact with other departments, and that's another thing that was different at the Queen E. In most hospitals today, you're isolated and you spend time with other people from your department: cardio, neuro, the ER, whatever, but not there. They had all these mechanisms – the meetings, the lunches, the games, the parties, the teaching seminars, the conferences – to bring everybody together."

What does it mean, when the generalists are cut off from the other parts of the health care system in every way, even socially, as they are in our current system? Larry Lincoln notes that having GPs around "helps enormously with continuity of care and diagnosis." Elderly or very ill patients frequently have multiple medical problems. Yet typically in the teaching hospitals, the only doctors they see are the specialists that preside over their most current, acute condition. These doctors know nothing about the chronic ailments that may have indirectly caused the current problem. "There's a different system at St. Mary's, for example," he says, "that tries to alleviate those problems. Other GPs, although not your own, come and cover the ward. So we do have medical coverage in orthopedics, but it's also true those doctors don't know these patients in any other context. At the Queen E, the involvement of family medicine was very noticeable, part of the whole egalitarian fabric of the place. They were involved because it really was a community hospital. Once you got used to working that way, you wanted to keep working there."

What these doctors are describing is a system in which the profession is directed from the bottom up rather than from the rarefied and unusual levels of experience down. Surgeon Ron Lewis explains that the former method not only empowers and supports general practice and the patients, it makes life easier for specialists. As we see in chapter

7, he is supported in this belief by all the latest international studies. "When I got to the Queen E as a resident, it had started a new era as an affiliate of McGill. Cam Darby was chief of surgery when I got there; he's a remarkable man, retired now and living in Kingston. Starting with Cam Darby, we got surgical residents in from the big teaching institutions – new blood, if you will. Wilfred Palmer did the same thing the same year for Internal Medicine at the Queen E with the same result. So there was superb specialist care tied in with great GPs and a whole team of rotating staff and residents that could contribute. This remarkably efficient set-up isn't seen anywhere any more. Where I am now and at the many other big hospitals I've worked at as a specialist, you have to make an extraordinary effort to link up the various people attending to a patient. At the Queen E, you were in a position to really direct patient care because there was such good communication and exchange at all levels."

PERFORMING THE POST-MORTEM

The closing of the Queen E. certainly revised the political leanings of doctors, nurses, and patients there. It was like reaching out to touch the face of God and finding out he needed a shave. It was literally unfathomable.

Fred Weigan, surgeon

It doesn't matter what current medical problem you bring up, people who used to work at the Queen E will claim that everything from ER and surgery crowding to long-term follow-up was done better at their lost hospital. Despite sharing in the loyalty, surgeon Ron Lewis, from his new life in Ontario, says, "It's important not to exaggerate the perfection of the Queen E. It was good, but things went wrong there, too, and they were on the downward slide because of the budget cuts which were escalating at that time." Mary Owen says the thing that keeps up her morale during the tough current period when she's not allowed to nurse up to her standards is that, "I've got a good family life; my husband is very supportive. I do get discouraged though. I know I'm not providing the same care as I was. How can you? Patients lying in hallways, two nurses taking care of seventeen people in an area built for six. You can't pretend that's good care. And the worst part is, the Queen E would probably be like that now. I'm sure it would, except there would still be some good things left as well."

Mario Larivière says that the most important point to consider when we assess the changed medical landscape today is that "there were no studies to back up these closure decisions. None. And there was no follow-up either." There are still almost no reliable studies on what community hospitals do or on what advantages or disadvantages closing so many beds brought to Montreal's or any other Canadian city's health system in terms of professionalism, patient care, or even financial efficiency. Even the World Health Organization's and other international inquiries into the high level of lost beds found it difficult to quantify the effects of such changes. Instead, as outlined above, there's now a new flurry of further and even more radical changes being suggested, notably building the "super-hospital," which would cut yet at least another 500 beds out of the system.

Heart surgeon Ron Lewis was asked if there are any studies, statistics, or papers that could help measure changes in medical practice over the last ten or fifteen years. This information is needed in order to have an objective way to assess whether or not this kind of institutional centralization and professional reorganization is the right direction for our Canadian system to proceed. For example, do we know if the loss of GPs on the wards has appreciably increased patients' problems or hospital costs? Does the closure of so many beds, the crowding of ERs, the long waits for surgery and consults cause clear, measurable increases in serious complications or deaths, as conversations with many doctors seem to imply? If so, by how much?

But Lewis echoed many other sources, including Statistics Canada, John Hughes, and the World Health Organization, when he replied, "There are no studies answering these questions. There are no studies even showing whether morbidity, the death rate, has increased. Why not? It does seem reasonable that we should know such things. But suppose I collected all these cases that I suspect are happening because of the problems you mention and then tried to publish them. Do you think I could keep working here? How about if I gave my necessarily secret study to the *Ottawa Citizen* when it was finally done; wouldn't I have to leave the entire province?" In any case," he said after thinking a bit, "when Flory published about the success of penicillin in 1941, he had only ten samples. Some things are so obvious they don't require absolute proof – the kind of suffering and downslide in care levels we're talking about happens over and over. It's more than obvious."

This downslide might be obvious to doctors and hospital staff who deal with medical issues every day, but most people interact with the medical system for only short periods, generally late in life. As a result, they are completely unaware of how much of our hospital system was unceremoniously destroyed a decade ago and how much that fact has affected the various issues that characterize the debate on how to maintain and fund hospital and health care in Canada today. Everything from the importance of generalists and institutional size to spiraling external costs and the issue of privatization needs to be reassessed in the context of our recent great loss. The birth, success, and then summary death of so many hospitals in Canada should leave our society with myriad questions. It's time to consider them.

One question is: Why were so many community hospitals and hospital beds sacrificed in the mid-1990s in Canada and why are the remaining ones still under pressure today? The answer to that question was not satisfactorily provided at the time and remains a mystery to the people who fought so hard to keep their institutions open. Another important question is: Why were some of the departed hospitals so loved by their staff and public? If we take the testimonies above to be even partly true, it would seem to be a good idea to seriously assess the practices that we so recently discarded. Posing the two larger questions precipitates a deluge of smaller ones: Where did all that health care money that closure was going to redistribute, really go? Has the disappearance of these "extra" beds proven to be a benefit to society? Were the policies that drove the closures and that continue to place community hospitals in danger really a necessary step in the evolution of modern health care – that is, should community hospitals be replaced by a combination of clinics and super-institutions? Or, on the other hand, could these closures have been a serious, even tragic, mistake? Most importantly, how can we learn from this experience what is really vital to the kind of health care most Canadians clearly want to receive?

All too frequently, societies spend generations carefully building up their institutions. Then, often with great rapidity, situations or even management styles change and they decide to destroy them and to replace them with something new. We've done this in recent years with agriculture, transportation, and a host of other industries and are today living in an era of declining health, prosperity, and stability across the planet. That may even be because, over the last century in particular, we have almost never taken the time to assess whether the institutions we closed or practices we abolished really were filling vital needs in a manner that was viable for the long term and whether their replacements represent true progress as opposed to mere novelty. This is a serious flaw in the way we structure both our institutions and our societies. The only positive action that can now be taken to salvage something from the loss of many highly functional health care units and from the systemic changes to the Canadian health care system of the mid-1990s is to finally stage a post-mortem. As in a human post-mortem, the goal of a careful historical dissection should be to give us the ability to identify healthy, vibrant institutions on the rare occasions when we do get them; and that will avoid death and decay in the future.

It most certainly isn't in the interests of either governments or individual hospitals to provide the empirical studies – especially death and disease rates – that would answer these questions. There are some fairly reliable, although general, international studies that address certain points as we'll see ahead, but to answer all these questions, we have to look carefully for some other way to assess what worked, what didn't, and what we all need to think about reviving, preserving, or changing in hospital care. We could continue to experiment blindly with our health care institutions, of course, but without any kind of analysis, their ultimate successes or failures would just add even more unintelligible episodes to our collective past. In attempting to understand that past from its very beginnings, we may be able to tease out the general management and funding decisions that really did work. With some serious historical analysis, our old and revered medical institutions, even the ones that are gone, could to persist in some measure as useful guides to future generations of Canadian policy makers, doctors, nurses, administrators, and patients.

2

Growing a Culture

MINISTERING HEALTH

It was all something special; something special requires special people.
They had a history stretching back a hundred years. All those doctors
who were second-generation at the hospital or who had brothers and
wives and so on there; all those things combined to form a culture.
Mario Larivière, former director general, Queen Elizabeth Hospital

The Queen Elizabeth Hospital, like so many other small, community
hospitals across the country, owes much of its existence to the energy of
one person – Alexander R. Griffith, a general practioner. He was a
small, bespectacled man – quiet, humorous, religious, unworldly and
untraveled, and oddly unambitious for someone who helped found a
hospital and a dynasty of doctors. He came from unremarkable people
who were farmers in central Ontario and later moved to North Dakota.
His education was average. If there was anything unusual about Alexander Griffith and Mary Milne, the girl he married in 1888, it was their
devotion to the concept of living a life of service to others. Even that
was less unusual at that time than it is now. Today, we think of medicine
as a profession that attracts people who are socially and economically
ambitious as well as scientifically and mathematically gifted. But only
two generations ago, none of the rewards associated with the profession today, except perhaps those that come to an inquiring, scientific
mind, could be expected to accrue to those who sought a career in
medicine. Like teaching, being a doctor did grant some social status;
but the dizzying heights to which the profession would ascend over the

course of his career were not at all obvious when A. R., as the oldest Dr Griffith is most commonly known, set off from North Dakota to the University of Michigan at Ann Arbor to begin his medical studies at the age of twenty.

As Charles E. Rosenberg puts it in *The Care of Strangers*, his excellent history of the American hospital system, "Aside from a handful of surgical procedures, there was little in the way of medical capability in the [early 1800s] that could not be made easily available outside the hospital's walls – at least in homes of the middle class and the wealthy. Physicians could ordinarily do little to alter the course of a patient's illness and almost as little to monitor quality of life on the ward ... The hospital in early national America," he sums up, and this also holds true for Canada and for the rest of the Western world, "was defined primarily by need and dependency, not by the existence of specialized technical resources."[1] Therefore, the profession did not attract upwardly mobile technicians or scientists as much as it attracted people who wished to devote themselves to a life of service to the dependent, the indigent, and the needy. This fact is illustrated by how common it was for 19th century doctors to have sprung from very religious families.

To minister to the sick and poor in the almshouses and workhouses of the day required the qualities of selflessness, patience, kindness, and courage. This gave medicine an aura of devoted service that still clings to the profession today, even though it has largely turned into something quite different. But in the 19th century, medicine and nursing both tended to attract the type of person who today might join Doctors Without Borders or volunteer for a Third World NGO in a particularly desperate country. Such people needed great physical stamina and an unshakable belief, often despite a good deal of evidence to the contrary, that their efforts were doing people good at least some of the time. They also needed to be able to face a personal life of constant interruptions, disgusting and risky physical conditions, and be willing to earn very little money while providing constant, uncomplaining services to others.

A.R. Griffith was, by all accounts, such a person. He had elected to go into what was a largely unrewarding and selfless profession, but by 1900, within a decade of his graduation from medical school, the situation had evolved. Hospitals were becoming far more centralized and accepted as viable institutions by the population. Rosenberg says, "the prosperous and respectable as well as the indigent were now treated in hospitals ... medical knowledge [became] increasingly specialized ...

The hospital had become easily recognizable to twentieth-century eyes."[2] By the time A.R. Griffith's career was over, antibiotics were in general use and surgery had evolved beyond the wildest dreams of early imagination. Wounds and diseases that were a death's sentence only a few years before were being successfully treated. A.R.'s life spanned the entire breadth of this dizzying change: hospitals began as settlement and almshouses where the poor and hopeless were sent to die, but emerged as shining centres of technical and professional excellence that were attended by the pillars of society, now representing the forefront of civilized values in the new century.

Of course, for a farm family, even becoming the humble doctor of mid-century was an exciting social step. Despite their simple and devout background, A.R.'s family was not entirely without ambition. When he was three days old – the sixth child out of a future twelve – he was introduced to a relative by his proud father as "the young doctor," a gentle push towards his fate that he never quite forgot. This family story combined with their admiration of their beloved town doctor, the handsome, confident Dr Schooley. "He lived in the largest house in the village," A.R. remembered later, "and we boys were always thrilled when we passed his home, especially when chance brought a friendly wave from his hand."[3]

The Griffith family was devoutly Baptist. This branch of Protestantism was common in the U.S. but less so in Canada. It was a strict denomination that forbade liquor and many types of amusements but strongly encouraged practitioners to serve their fellow man in hopes of gaining God's favour. Despite these lofty values, at only thirteen, after a school career he joked did not reflect well on his reputation, A.R. left school to apprentice as a printer's devil. His lifelong interest in writing, printing, and communication in general was passed on to his son Harold and had a vivid effect both on the hospital he was to found and on his and Harold's careers. After working for a variety of papers and telegraph companies as print-setter, compositor, and reporter in his early twenties, A.R. finally felt compelled to go back to school to become a doctor in homeopathy, a branch of medicine much more common and mainstream at the time than it is today.

His son Harold describes the situation succinctly. "In those days," he wrote in a 1969 monograph on the history of the Queen Elizabeth Hospital, "there was rivalry and sometimes animosity between homeopathists and traditional doctors (who were sometimes called 'Allopathists'). Homeopathy is a system of drug therapy which was founded by Samuel Hahnemann in Germany in the 18th century and is based on the principle of 'let likes be cured by likes.' In other words, if one administers a small (in fact, miniscule) dose of a drug which in a large dose would produce symptoms similar to those from which the sick person is suffering, a return to normal health may be expected."[4] It's easy to see how in the days when vaccines were just being discovered, homeopathy seemed fully as effective and scientific in stimulating the "natural protective forces in the body" as its competition. Homeopathic doctors were fully qualified physicians, or allopaths, as well; they simply supplemented their work of setting bones or removing appendixes with these mild drugs.

"The advent of vaccines and antibiotics, as well as advances in surgery, made homeopathy less important," Harold admits in his monograph, but even in the late 1960s, he wrote, "those who have carefully studied it are still convinced that it contains much valuable truth." He pointed out that homeopathic doctors certainly did no harm with their treatments and in fact, "were in the forefront of the advocates of modern hygiene and treatment of the patient as an individual."[5] In their book on the history of anesthesia, Richard Bodman and Dierdre Gillies mention that homeopathic doctors were especially successful in their handling of the widespread scourges of tuberculosis and pneumonia. "Their success in treating such infections ... with small doses of drugs and bed rest appears today more rational than the conventional treatment at that time, which entailed bloodletting, purgation and the administration of 'ardent spirits.'"[6] Moreover, "the avoidance of alcohol as a drug of choice also meant that homeopathy was embraced particularly by temperance movements and fundamentalist Christian sects" and hence would have been particularly attractive to the Baptist Griffiths. In his own monograph on the Queen Elizabeth, Harold Griffith's father A.R. also mentions that in Montreal, in the 19th century, "the patients of the few homeopathic doctors were fanatical believers, and it was these laymen who obtained the charter for the Montreal Homeopathic Association back in 1865."[7] This was the Association that would go on to found the Queen Elizabeth Hospital.

Today, of course, modern medicine is firmly in the camp not only of the "allopaths" but of a scientific reductionism that is very different from the holistic approach of early medical researchers like Hahnaman. Today, not only drugs and surgical methods but also treatments and therapeutic options are supposedly corroborated by hard scientific data, the famous "clinical trials" that apply the most stringent standards of research available to science. Such trials ideally employ double-blind studies where neither the participant nor the researcher is aware which subject was given a drug or which was given a placebo. Typically, studies of this type are applied to a statistically acceptable number of cases. Even if the results seem to be significant, researchers are expected to make certain that no side effects or unwonted variables make the drug or treatment more dangerous than salutary. Furthermore, five years must elapse after such trials before the treatment is finally approved for use.

Proper clinical trials were only established a generation ago, in the late 1940s. When responsibly carried out, they provide impressive evidence that a drug or a procedure is probably both safe and effective. They are, however, extremely difficult to construct, especially when they relate to human beings, because people are so individually variable and their lives and genetics cannot be equalized in a laboratory. These facts go far to explain the constantly changing nature of their findings. Whether mammography is a good – or bad – or good – diagnostic tool in the fight against breast cancer or whether margarine is safer or more dangerous for the heart than butter are controversies that spring directly from studies using this reductionist scientific method. Such fluctuating findings illustrate how slight alterations in the composition and construction of different trials, even on the same drug, food, or therapy, can result in conflicting evidence, especially over time. Of course, their concomitant, stable discoveries – such as the fact that vaccines can now protect most people against smallpox and typhoid or that aortic and bypass surgery increase the lifespan of people afflicted with heart disease – represent therapies whose efficacy has been measured and proven by these same reductionist methods to the satisfaction of most researchers.

This approach to science was born in 18th century thought but only came to be widely applied to medicine in the late 19th century. It is being ever more stringently applied today and is the basis for "evidence-based medicine," which is discussed in more detail in future chapters. But in Alexander Griffith's era, medicine had not yet made the leap into this world of cold, hard, scientific facts. It hadn't begun to work out the protocol for clinical trials or even recognize the need for them. In fact, Charles Rosenberg makes the case that early medical practice, before about 1860 or 1870, was actually what he terms "anti-reductionist." In these early medical systems, doctors and patients did not look at evidence and studies but rather a "return to the state of equilibrium" that they associated with health. Like many still existing alternative therapies, they sought balance in the body's activities and emulated natural tendencies in their emetics, purges, bleedings, and so forth.

Even today, alternative therapies such as homeopathy and naturopathy, exercise disciplines such as Tai Chi, or the healing practices employed by traditional peoples, continue to use complex combinations of treatment, diet, exercise, drugs, and even social interaction and spiritual intention. It was believed that "each patient possessed a unique physiological identity, and the experienced physician had to evaluate a bewildering variety of factors, ranging from climatic conditions to age and sex, in the compounding of any particular prescription. The same speculative mechanisms that explained recovery explained failure as well. One could not hope for a cure in every case; even the most competent physician could only do that which the limited resources of medicine allowed, and the natural course of some ills was toward death. For example, the treatment indicated for tuberculosis, as a 19th-century adage put it, was 'opium and lies.'"[8]

It sounds like a very different and ignorant world; but lest we think science has utterly triumphed, we need to remember that in the case of chronic diseases, even the most modern medicine has not made all that much headway. In the 19th and early 20th centuries, for example, addictive opiates like laudanum were the treatment of choice for the many sorts of rheumatism and arthritis that raged through a population that did too much heavy work in cold or damp surroundings. Until very recently, modern doctors prescribed Non-Steroidal Anti-Inflammatory Drugs (NSAIDs), such as the patented Celebrex and Vioxx, to treat the many people still afflicted with these problems. NSAIDs kill pain just like the old narcotics but have recently been found to have serious side-effects, including an increased incidence of heart attacks and strokes as well as the effects for which they were already known – perforation of the stomach lining and damage to the liver, kidney, and nervous system. Many doctors and patients are beginning to feel that these side effects are arguably much worse than the constipation and habituation of the opiates.

Since many NSAIDs now come with serious warnings or are being taken off the shelves, doctors are going back to the more old-fashioned, less dangerous drugs. These give no patent revenues to large corporations, of course. Other than the even more dangerous steroidal drugs, NSAIDs were the only mainstream medical treatment generally available for these widespread and chronic conditions. In A.R.'s day, one could argue that, at the very least, the placebo effect wrought in a fervent homeopathic believer by *Arnica montana* or *Arsenicum* could also stave off symptoms for quite awhile and spare the patient at least some of the problems that might have come if they had immediately began using an opiate, or these days, an NSAID.

The dramatic impact that the introduction of reductionist scientific medicine has had on acute disease is central to any discussion of hospital care. However, that impact has been feeble when it comes to chronic diseases. The proof is that the same old homeopathic remedies, as well as many other alternative therapies, still remain popular with a broad section of the public – so much so that it's a rare pharmacy, even in North America, that doesn't offer some of these remedies. As for other parts of the world, such as Europe, the loyalty to homeopathy is best exemplified by the long-lived royal family of Great Britain, who resort to it almost exclusively. In this context, it's important to remember that A.R. Griffith was not as far from the mainstream when he decided to attend a homeopathic medical college as he would be today. When the young Alexander left his job as a newspaperman in Grand Forks, North Dakota, and went off to study at the University of Michigan in Ann Arbor in 1887, he was going off to become as fine and progressive a doctor as his father could have imagined.

This was only two generations ago, but we have to remember that science and technology have moved very rapidly during this period – and not just in medicine. A.R. delights in mentioning how he and his fellow students would gather together of an evening to watch the new electric street lights turn on. As street lights went from wax torches to gas to electricity in less than fifty years, so did medical studies proceed through disciplines such as homeopathy on their way to the complex specialties of today. A.R.'s explanation for his deserting the *Grand Forks Herald* for medical school was simple: "but ever burned within me memories of my father's prophecy when three days old."[9] That admission sounds as much like a heed to a calling as a desire for career betterment.

THE BOWERY

They say strange things and they do strange things on the Bowery, the Bowery. I'll never go there anymore.

Harry Conor[10]

The year was 1889 when Alexander Griffith decided to finish his medical studies in the dauntingly huge and faraway city of New York. He and Mary Milne, whom he had been courting ever since they were teenagers, decided to marry, not only so A.R. would have company when facing the big city but also to "grow up together ... away from the atmosphere of small-town influences" in the "greatest of all cosmopolitan cities." "What visions we had," he reminisced, "of art, of literature, of progress toward the higher estate of life!"

Mary Milne had professional gifts of her own, having studied nursing in North Dakota. The starry-eyed newlyweds arrived at their humble digs in the biggest city they could imagine, where A.R. "was to work and work" among the poor squatters and new immigrants. Mary became matron of a children's hospital connected with the Five Points House of Industry on Worth Street and earned the relatively large amount of thirty dollars a month – twice what Alexander got as a student nurse and doctor. This hospital was a workhouse or almshouse, and its conditions would have rivaled those of a shantytown in Afghanistan or Ecuador today. In describing another such worker of a generation before, Ezra Stiles Ely, a Presbyterian minister who began to preach in New York City's almshouse hospital in 1810, Charles Rosenberg says, "The young hospital chaplain entered the almshouse with much the same bravado and anxiety as if he had been undertaking a ministry in Burma or the Gold Coast [because in fact] ... the internal logic of the almshouse allied it more closely to the hospice of the Middle Ages than to the 20th-century hospital"[11] Things were only slightly better by Mary's day.

"Grandma Mary," says her granddaughter Barbara Griffith Clark, "was a strong, determined woman. Besides her work as Matron at the Settlement House, she raised four sons and made sure the family always remained very religious." The experiences the young couple had in their first three years of marriage were traumatic as well as noble and instructive. They were to stay with them all their lives and become the stuff of family legend. Being "very religious" was almost a necessity for early doctors and their wives. Hospitals and almshouses were organized by and around religious groups, and doctors were expected, if not forced, to attend all services. As Rosenberg says, "[Many] aspiring physicians would, indeed, have chosen between medicine and the ministry; both would have been pursued with appropriate gravity." He mentions George Shattuck, founder of a Boston dynasty of doctors and researchers, who chose with difficulty between "divinity and physick," and was "by no means unique."[12] It was a good thing that the Griffiths' youthful desire for art, literature, and progressive sophistication was tempered with religious asceticism. During their three years in New York, they were kept too busy dealing with poverty, disease, and endless work to enjoy much of the "higher estate of life."[13]

A.R.'s college, the New York Homeoeopathic Medical College and Flower Hospital, "was all confusion" because it was still under construction when they arrived. The couple took the precaution of getting lunch at 50th street because the college, located at today's highly urban intersection of 63rd St. and Avenue A, was "almost in the country." As A.R. was to write later, "a little to the north, on the site now occupied by Cornell Hospital, goats scampered on rocky fields held by Irish squatters living in crude huts."[14] Although the training would seem very rudimentary by today's standards, A.R. was enrolled in the first college in America to demand three instead of two years for a medical degree. Less than a generation before, all that was required of a practicing physician was that he attend three or four months of lectures, the content of which did not vary from year to year. There was no clinical training whatsoever. This circumstance was under revolutionary upheaval by the time A.R. got to the Flower Hospital. He also got practical experience by working that first summer as a student nurse in Charity Hospital on the infamous Blackwell's Island.

"I had never seen anyone die, and my practical knowledge of disease or treatment was nil, but, believe me, I saw death and disease in plenty those five months," he wrote many years later.[15] A.R. was appalled even then by the way, for example, that TB patients on the Island were mixed in with the general population and especially by the heartless way they were treated. People failing from the disease had to watch others dying in a clear and apparently unavoidable rhythm. "As they progressed toward the grave, they were moved to a line of beds near the door – always filled up rapidly as the bodies were carried out." At Blackwell's Island, A.R. witnessed "food ... served up in the crudest possible manner. Many times well-cooked cockroaches were picked out of the large dishes before being served to patients." Griffith, like any other physician of that century, knew that a healthy and clean diet was one of the very few weapons that his profession possessed against the progression of disease. Diets in the general population were poor, and doctors had learned that everything from childbed fever to tuberculosis and diarrhea might respond spectacularly to improving them.

Charles Rosenberg points out that because surgery was in its infancy, it was dreaded and very often fatal. This was an era dominated by acute infectious diseases, whose victims most hospitals refused to accept. "A disproportionate number of hospital cases were thus chronic or lingering ills – rheumatism, dysentery, bronchitis, heart or kidney ailments. Sufferers ... did not ordinarily die, but neither did they get well. However, in many cases, even the crude meals and shelter provided by the hospital [of the first part of that century] were an improvement over the patient's normal environment."[16] In the 1860s, for example, Thomas King Chambers, the senior physician at St. Mary's Hospital in London, England, had observed in a published paper that a "delicate and puny maid" suffering from "purulent abscesses yielding two pints of pus daily," still retained her appetite, and so they fed her roasts, steaks and soups "like a gigantic gladiator." He felt her subsequent complete cure was due to this rich and sustained nourishment.[17]

A nineteen year-old servant girl in the same hospital recovered from menstrual problems and anemia in 1858 by being carefully provided with good "beef tea" and protein.[18] Witnessing the revival of difficult cases on healthy food was so striking to the doctors of A.R.'s day that it goes far to explain the wonderful kitchen kept at his own hospital, the Homeopathic, and the reason why food remained the largest single expenditure in the hospital's annual budget until well into the 1980s. Anyone who has eaten hospital food in Canada recently might long for a return to this aspect of early 20th century practice.

A.R. and Mary's experiences among New York's poor and disenfranchised left them shaken, but contemporary "proper" hospitals weren't much better. *The Care of Strangers* describes mid-century conditions in better places – conditions that undoubtedly were mirrored in the poor settlement houses and tenements that greeted A.R. and Mary in New York. "There were rarely places to wash or dry bedding even in the best-run hospitals ... Passersby were assailed not only with the stench from hospital privies, but the sight of tattered sheets and blankets waving from windows and makeshift clothes lines. "Sheets, as one complaint put it, "too filthy to be beheld by any one without loathing and disgust." And much as Alexander had witnessed with TB patients, "Operations would ordinarily be performed in the common ward ... [and the] dead bodies were often left in the wards or placed directly in coffins while surviving patients looked on."[19]

Besides all this, before the 1860s in many hospitals, "patients were always getting scurvy, despite their caregivers having known for a century how to avoid it." This may be shocking, but two other common complaints, that sick people had to sleep on the floors or in corridors and that there were inadequate supplies, "with nurses [being] forced to tear up threadbare sheets and blankets to serve as bandages,"[20] are reminiscent of the 21st century conditions brought on by budget-tightening. Today, patients also sleep in hallways and contract avoidable infections caused by the re-use of pieces of expensive surgical equipment, such as contaminated laparoscopes, which were designed to be thrown away.[21]

Of course, by and large, the 21st century hospital is still light-years ahead, if only because we now accept the germ theory. Before the 1870s, even in the prestigious halls of well-established hospitals, "Surgical education and practice ... was still primitive and limited ... surgeons operated in street clothes or in blood-stained frock coats left at the hospital; the hair and face were never covered. Instruments, patients and hands were rarely washed except after surgery to clean off the blood. The wooden operating table and floor were stained with years of blood, pus and discharges and were only cleaned to wipe them dry between operations."[22] In London in the 1870s, at St Mary's Hospital, even for operations such as mastectomies, colostomies, joint excisions, and amputations, there were "no preparations, not even washing of a limb before amputation ... The same instruments were used again and again, and the same bloody operating coat was worn by the surgeon, usually a threadbare frock coat. If the wound filled with pus, each ward had its own sponge to swab it out, the sponge being passed from wound to wound."[23] No wonder that infection was accepted as a normal outcome of any surgery, although by A.R.'s day, McGill surgeons were at least drenching themselves, their nurses, the patients, and the walls with continual sprays of carbolic acid, which "often caused dermatitis and occasionally nephritis from inhalation."[24]

The quality of the staff was almost as bad as the surgical methods. The normally forgiving and tolerant A.R. says that leaving the charity hospital Training School where he worked as a nurse enabled him to "pass forever from the companionship of some of the worst specimens of manhood you could imagine, who had entered that school to train as male nurses. No wonder this school ceased to exist."[25] His experience was far from unique. Because of the constant prevalence of infection and the poor standards of an underpaid staff charged with keeping them clean, contemporaries talk about the characteristic stench of all hospitals, "of stale pus. It was something which could be recognized hundreds of yards away from the institution."[26]

The untrained nursing and orderly staff might be drunken, thieving, or immoral, and A.R. had reason to dislike them, but they had their own point of view as well. One of the few of this uneducated and unremembered class to have left a written account is John Duffe, a ward nurse and ex-sailor who worked in New York Hospital's Marine House in 1844 and kept a diary of the experience. He recounts many cases of theft. Watches, valuables, even furniture and bedding were constantly disappearing into the pockets of the staff as well as being carried off by patients and visitors. His labours trying to nurse the patients were enough to turn anyone cynical and sad. "He was an experienced dresser of wounds and infections, and administered countless baths and enemas,"[27] but does not seem to have been appreciated or promoted for his skill. Like A.R., he had to contend with terrible food, but he also had to put up with abuse from his "betters." In a passage that conjures up *Oliver Twist*, Duffe writes, "If putrefied vituels (sic) be injurious to the stomac I am shure we will soon be all rotton for our butter is rotton and stinks worse than a Sconk. But it must be borne with, for like everything else if we complain our godly Superintendent will tell us you may consider yourself discharged. For the Lord sent it and you must eat it, you hireling." His duties included scrubbing the filthy floors, washing the sheets, fetching the "roton" dinner for the men on the ward, but mostly "carrying and luging (sic) of Slops and all kinds of filth and dirt." Duffe could only take a day off if he could find a patient willing and able to substitute for him. At the end of one diary entry, the poor man writes, "So ends this days work, for work we may call it without end."[28]

After his traumatic period as just such a nurse, A.R.'s next job was as junior physician at the children's hospital where his wife was matron. Conditions were not much better. In fact, the luck of the Griffiths' draw is either so bad as to be farcical or simply illustrates the norm of big city medical practice for beginning physicians at the time. "This district," he wrote, "was the worst in New York. Baxter Street – Jewish clothing houses – Mott Street and cheap Chinese eateries – Mulberry Street and Italian immigrants – Division Street and millinery (or what we would now call "sweat") shops – all closely connected with the Bowery in its palmyest days."[29] The Bowery in this era, of course, is now legendary for its poverty and Dickensian living conditions. Not only there, but even in wealthier areas, people were not generally treated in hospitals or almshouses "unless they had no relations or were beyond hope. So the hospitals were full of the dying or disenfranchised." Hospitals, for most if not all of the 19th century, did not admit either the contagious or chronically ill because, "The former endangered the hospital's staff and patients, the latter undermined its limited ability to provide beds for the potentially curable."[30] Both of these are medical facts true to this day. As we have noted, the Queen Elizabeth's continuing compassion for the chronically ill actually helped bring about its demise as an institution. More recently, many experts are becoming nervous about whether or not to admit victims of emerging pathogens to regular hospitals because the contagion decimates the very staff needed to combat it.[31]

Then, as now, there was an ideological battle between privately and publicly funded hospitals. "Private hospitals," as Rosenberg points out, "sought to admit only the morally worthy," in the same way they seek to admit only the economically worthy today. The "two-tier" medical system that many people fear may be the advance guard of a serious restructuring of human rights and equality in the 21st century was in full force back then. "The prostitute and alcoholic," he writes, "like the victim of typhus or smallpox (who were always assumed to be contagious) or cancer (acknowledged as incurable) would be excluded and left to the almshouse ... Lying-in (maternity) patients were often admitted to private charities if married, rebuffed if unwed." Of course, if such patients could pay very high prices, finding treatment was another matter. "The Pennsylvania Hospital would admit incurable cases if they paid their way, and even venereal, alcoholic, and contagious cases if they could afford care. The rate for smallpox victims was five dollars a week in the 1840s, for venereal and alcoholic cases four dollars."[32] In an era where ten cents would buy an excellent meal in a nice restaurant, the cost of five dollars a week was simply astronomical. Diamond Jim Brady could afford to get small pox or syphilis. Most anyone else could not.

Those able to pay for treatment at home might also be very poor, but even in A.R.'s day, they usually chose to be operated on there, in what he called "those awful tenement rooms." Rotting food, hoards of children, dirty laundry, and even rats accompanied the doctors' efforts. Nor was the physician as yet protected by widespread public confidence and veneration. In recounting the fate of an Italian woman who was operated on by a colleague, A.R. says graphically, "Results were not satisfactory and the husband searched for my friend, carrying with him a stiletto. Remember, in those days the surgeons always expected pus following an operation – if it were creamy and bland everything would be all right, but if the odor was objectionable and the tissues friable, then the surgeon sadly shook his head. In this case, the surgeon never reappeared – and there was plenty of pus."[33]

Even when occasionally efficacious, this doesn't sound like the opportunity to enjoy art, culture, and progress in the big city that the young Griffith couple had anticipated. But A.R. and Mary carried on through three tough years. As graduation approached, a Canadian school friend, Hugh Patton, urged Alexander to set up practice in Montreal. Doctors were cheap, plentiful, and not always sought after, so choosing the wrong city to begin a practice could end in financial ruin. A.R. paints quite a picture of himself coming up north in mid-winter to this "smart, French-Canadian city." "I wore a Prince Albert coat and a plug hat," he writes. "This seems laughable now, but every young doctor in New York at that time was so arrayed. It was tragic when I stepped off the train ... and found very cold weather with snow banked on both sides of the street. I borrowed a cap and warmer over-coat ... and remained a week, entertained by Dr Patton."[34]

COMING HOME

My father was an ideal family doctor because not only was he a skilled clinician, he was a genuinely friendly man and loved people. His patients became his friends; he was interested in all their activities ...

Harold Griffith[35]

Despite his discomfiture, the hopeful and stylish young doctor was entranced with the look of the place, especially after the filth and mis-eries of the Bowery. "Beautiful farms surrounded the city – there was no Westmount, Outremont, no Verdun. Horse-drawn street cars were replaced during the winter by large, closed sleighs with plenty of straw on the floor to keep the feet warm." So although he got invita-tions to set up practice in New York and Philadelphia, he and Mary chose to move to Montreal, in June of 1892, with the snow thankfully gone and "the birds singing and happy ... Montreal seemed slow and old-fashioned after the Bowery ... How could we ever make a living here?" And in fact, "People in the Point did not want to rent to us, thinking we would never be able to pay. Finally we secured a place of seven rooms at 535 Wellington St [in today's Point St Charles]. The first rent was $12 a month."[36]

Today, a young GP wouldn't be able to beat off new patients with a stick. But back in the 1890s, young doctors had to lure patients in and hope for luck. A.R. mentions that, "The Venerable Archdeacon Kerr of Grace Church called to welcome us. He was disappointed to find we were Baptists, but welcomed us all the same. He went home and told his wife that 'another doctor had arrived in the Point to starve!' We remained the best of friends as long as he lived." A.R.'s good humour, self-deprecation, and ability to mix with those who were considered exotic, as well as his ability to fully appreciate gifts that were not scientific but ethical and spiritual, were qualities he proved able to inculcate in his children and colleagues. "Another friend I found in those early days," he wrote in 1934, "was father Tom Heffernan, now of St. Augustine's; we have remained friends all these years ... [and] his interest in homeopathic medicine is well known. Last summer, when my medical friends were in despair over my fate, Father Tom came to see me. His little visit and his blessing as he was leaving turned the tide, and slowly I came back. God bless Father Tom."[37] In order to appreciate how unusual this kind of relationship was, it helps to remember that between the 1890s and 1930s, there was such an atmosphere of bigotry and even violence between Protestants and Catholics in North America that, all across the Midwest that A.R. had so recently vacated, Protestants regularly burned Ku Klux Klan crosses on property belonging to Catholics. Baptists, in particular, had great animosity towards Catholics or "the Papists," as the pejorative went, so that the idea of friendship between men who were such committed practitioners of these two faiths is worthy of some notice.

Griffith was also noticeably egalitarian and unthreatened in his relationship with what his generation would have termed "the ladies." Linda Mary Jacobson, A.R. and Mary's eldest granddaughter, remembers her Grandmother Mary and how "managing" she was. "That's the reason we didn't just share the big house up by Lac des Sept Iles in the Laurentians," she says. Various other family houses were quickly built nearby because "her son Jim's wife couldn't stand her and the other two daughter-in-laws couldn't either because she was always dominating them." Linda Mary said the terrible conditions Mary and A.R. had lived under when young and doing charity work in New York had left such an impression that even the grandchildren and great-grandchildren heard stories about them but, "I'm afraid I can't say much about Grandma's child and girlhood; she wasn't a talker that way.

But my father loved to talk about things like his childhood! And he loved to write."

A.R.'s many personal essays and speeches, including the slightly forced upbeat account of his time in New York, are all written in a humble, cheery style that his son Harold would reproduce almost exactly. In them, A.R. always refers to his wife in the most glowing terms, as his "best friend, wonderful companion, beloved wife," and so on. Yet their marriage does not seem to have been as happy as their children's would be. Linda Mary, the first grandchild, lived with them when very young; she thinks her grandmother's career desires, cut short by four little boys born one after another, were frustrated and that she took out a naturally dominating, organizational nature on family members. She remembers Linda, Harold Griffith's wife, saying that, "whenever she went to the Griffith's, they were always arguing! Of course, it may have been intellectual sparring, because she meant the whole family, the boys too. She was from a much quieter family, very gentle people, so the Griffiths' forthright ways may have been upsetting to her." Whatever outsiders make of their characters and relationships, in his writings A.R. never misses an opportunity to extol his wife and, in an era of absolute masculine supremacy in economic matters, he goes out of his way to publicly point out that Mary supported them in New York with a salary twice the size of his own. In general, his continuing attraction to such a competent, professional woman explains a good deal about his attitudes towards the women with whom he would work later in life.

A.R. was given the chance to share an office with two other doctors who already had their own practice. The chances of anybody stumbling in looking for a new medical man were slim, but during his very first week, "a patient came in with a badly lacerated hand. Dr England was not in, nor was Dr Hutchison to be found, and so they tried the new doctor. The office was scarce furnished but we had an oil stove – one burner – and plenty of hot water. Also I had some Calendula solution. A dozen stitches, a wet dressing on the dirty, oily fingers and hand – brought a 100 percent result and a boon to my medical reputation! To this day, I have patients who come to me as a direct result of this Calendula."[38] A.R. Griffith's granddaughter Barbara has saved his hand-written, yellowing medical records, beginning from that first patient in 1892. In the same year, he was paid the princely sum of three dollars for administering ether while his friend Dr Patton operated on a child's foot. He mended another hand and a foot for fifty cents each, and a Mrs Butter received a consultation for free.

Before he got a full practice, A.R. reports that he used his free time to both keep up his daily studies and insert himself into his new community. "We went to Church, to *all* the Churches. Within two years I joined the Oddfellows, Foresters, Masons, Royal Arcanum and Royal Guardians. It kept me poor paying fees and kept me out many nights, but I gained experience and friends." A.R.'s final advice to young doctors starting out includes "another ethical way of advertising. Have some member of the family come during evening office hours to report how a patient is progressing. The people waiting will immediately gossip on the large number flocking to the new doctor."[39]

The Griffiths stayed on in their flat on Wellington for twelve years; all their boys were born in that house, delivered by the man who brought them there in the first place, A.R.'s friend Hugh Patton. When the youngest of the brood was three and Harold, the second eldest, was ten, they finally were able to move to a nice house on Peel Street, which was both home and business. Their granddaughter Barbara remembers it well; she even lived there as a baby because her father, Harold, "was in Philadelphia for his second internship. I slept in a bureau for three weeks down there, then we moved in with Dad's parents on Peel. And after that year, mom and dad took an apartment on Grey and Sherbrooke for three years then moved, and my sister was born on Marlowe, near the Homeopathic's new building."

Barbara remembers the Peel Street house as being lovely. "In Grandpa's day, you'd come into the patients' waiting room, which was the parlour, and Grandpa's office was at the back. I remember a little room next to the office with beakers and test tubes that I thought was really fascinating." Besides being full of children and grandchildren, this was where most of the Homeopathic Hospital's early business was carried out, as well as A.R.'s practice. Barbara went there for years after school for her piano lessons and also remembers going on house calls with her grandpa. "I'd wait outside in the car while he went in."

Medicine is one of several modern professions where stopping well short of your limits is an important virtue. A.R. was, as his son said later, an "ideal family doctor," not only because of his genuine interest in all aspects of his patients' lives but because of his humility and loyalty to the gentle medical art of homeopathy. The late 19th century was still not removed from the often homicidal practices of bloodletting, purging, and other violent treatments like icy baths, intentional wounding and scarring, and large doses of poisonous chemicals such as arsenic. A.R. was proud of affecting cures that spared his patients both the knife and violent medications. "To cut and slash and delve into the human body never did appeal to me, and many a patient I kept from the surgeon by medical treatment," he says, "although, when the 'little pills' failed or the symptoms warned, I always summoned the surgeon." Despite his gentleness, early in his career, A.R., like every other doctor of the era, lost several mothers to complications of childbirth, which he never forgot. Decades later, he still publicly blamed himself for not recognizing certain symptoms. "With these two cases early in my practice," he wrote, "I became very anxious and gave greater care to pregnant women." That care often included homeopathic pills like "Mer Cor.6x," which he credits for saving a woman suffering from what we would now call toxemia, which even today is a dangerous condition of late pregnancy. "She still lives," he noted happily in 1934, "and is herself a grandmother."[40]

In many respects, A.R. was old-fashioned even for his era. The age of surgery had already arrived. Antiseptic methods and ether, introduced in the 1880s, heralded "an activist, intrusive style of practice and a decreasing emphasis on the conservative or expectant management of many syndromes." In *The Care of Strangers*, Charles Rosenberg points to another old-fashioned doctor of the age, James Knight, chief surgeon between 1863 and 1887 at a children's facility, the New York Hospital for the Ruptured and Crippled. To some degree, the description of Knight also fits Alexander and even Harold Griffith of the Homeopathic/Queen Elizabeth. Knight "was a physician who assumed a holistic – and paternalistic – attitude toward his patients and the hospital's work generally. He placed little emphasis on operative procedures and a great deal on diet, exercise, fresh air, bandages, and appliances."[41]

The Griffiths, father A.R. and sons Harold and Jim, were able to extend some of the more valuable aspects of Knight's approach by nearly a hundred years by fusing them with the coming, and to some extent, opposing reductionist scientism. But as for Knight himself, as Rosenberg says, "By 1887, he had become an anachronism. He was succeeded by Virgil Gibney, a youthful and energetic orthopedist. Numbers of operations increased rapidly and lengths of stay decreased; Gibney himself lived outside the hospital. The surgeon was no longer content to guide and monitor, to negotiate a multidimensional path to physical and social health." Today many people – especially those with little hospital experience – still romanticize the profession and think of doctors as being more like Griffith and Knight than Gibney. While it is true that, "Aseptic surgery had far more to offer many patients than the bandages, regimen and braces of mid-century," Rosenberg points out that the new-model surgery also "construed its responsibilities in increasingly narrow and [disease-centred and] procedure-oriented terms,"[42] a tendency which was to have very far-reaching consequences.

This fundamental change in philosophy and approach has seldom been properly analyzed and confronted by those taking the lead in moving medical and hospital care in the corporate and technological directions it is headed today. Any analysis has tended to assume that the move towards scientific reductionism was simply all to the good. But as we grow into maturity, we gradually realize that most events are comprised of both good and bad elements. The new approach brought much of undisputable use but obviously, a few things began to be lost on the way, most of them having to do with the nurturing and humane aspects of medicine. Rosenberg points out that as early as the 1920s, "almost all the criticisms of the hospital so familiar to us were already being articulated by critics ... Concerned observers of the hospital pointed toward a growing coldness and impersonality; they deprecated an increasing concern with acute ailments and a parallel neglect of the aged, of chronic illness, of the convalescent, of the simply routine. They warned of a socially insensitive and economically dysfunctional obsession with in-patient at the expense of out-patient and community-oriented care."[43] Over the years, many voices have sought what Rosenberg calls "an understanding of the patient's social and family environment," the more holistic caring epitomized by the old-fashioned family doctor, that would bring medicine out of the hospital and back into the community, increasing our understanding of the actual causes of disease as well as multiplying the possibilities for appropriate therapeutic treatment.

This kind of approach, although never far from more elevated medical discussions even today, "was not to prevail. Those aspects of institutional care not centred on hospital wards actually decreased in significance as the hospital and its [increasingly chemical and technological] inpatient services have grown ever more prominent in the culture of medicine."[44] Today, as Rosenberg points out, the hospital has become "an institution clothed with an almost mystical power, yet suffused with relentless impersonality and a forbidding aura of technical complexity."[45] Hospitals are created and supported by human beings for social and moral purposes, yet they increasingly seem oddly isolated from, one might say almost indifferent to, the real social needs of most humans. Current hospital care analysts can learn a great deal by studying the details of the successes and failures of people like Gibney, Knight, Griffith, and all the other pioneers of the surgical and chemical techniques that have enabled so many of us to stay alive today. It would be most helpful to investigate ways to break the hospital's social isolation, which set in so early in its short history, so as to determine which future directions will yield the most dividends for our societies and which directions are doomed to fail.

RESTRICTED ACCESS

Patients admitted to the wards on presentation of an order signed by a Life-Governor or member of the hospital staff.

Back cover of the Annual Report of the Homoeopathic
Hospital of Montreal[46]

A.R. Griffith died in 1936 at the age of seventy-two, before the full demise of homeopathy as a mainstream medical treatment, and was therefore able to use it throughout his long career. As a gentle, deliberate man, the gradualness and benign doses used in homeopathy continued to appeal to him, and he raised both his doctor sons to appreciate this branch of medicine, probably as much through his stories about its effects as by overt clinical lessons. Harold, who was to become one of the world's first specialists in anesthesiology and who remains the most famous figure in this field even today, remembers following his father in the Homeopathic Hospital of Montreal, "where he would lead me around the wards and introduce me to the patients and I would pretend to prescribe 'Bryonia' or 'Pulsatilla' or some other homeopathic remedy for them."[47]

But even in 1894, homeopathy felt itself becoming the poor relation of medical practice. As Harold Griffith puts it in his monograph celebrating the seventy-fifth anniversary of that hospital in 1969, "The Montreal General had been in operation since 1821 and was already famous as a teaching institution, but its facilities were crowded and the wards open only to doctors who were members of the Medical Board. The Hotel Dieu, founded by Jeanne Mance in 1642, welcomed the private patients of any qualified doctor, but it, too, was crowded, and the French language was an obstacle for many English-speaking Montrealers. In 1893, another great hospital was nearing completion, the Royal Victoria, gift of Lord Strathcona and Lord Mount Stephen. Why couldn't one ward of this new hospital be set aside for the patients of homeopathic doctors?"[48] This reasonable hope would not be the last time the McGill hospitals let down the humble outsider and the homeopaths were crushed. The reasons why the big teaching hospitals of Montreal refused doctors like A.R. and his friends, however, went well beyond any expression of disdain for homeopathy as such.

Rosemary and David Gagan, in their remarkable book on early Canadian hospital care, *For Patients of Moderate Means,* point out that, as in other cities, "The limited supply of private rooms in Montreal's Royal Victoria Hospital was so much in demand [that already] by the 1890s they had to be rationed among the attending medical staff and admission prioritized by medical urgency."[49] In general, the demand for hospitalization in Quebec alone led to a 22 percent increase in the number of new hospitals – a statistic that includes the new Homeopathic. Moreover, although hospitals were once built to care for the sick poor, with some small accommodation for the private patients whose fees would help to pay for the main work, "by 1914, these wards were shared equally by medical indigents and the new class of paying patients." In some places, the demand for private care was already outstripping charity work. For example, the Victoria Hospital in London, Ontario, in 1897 "at the last minute ... summarily redefined 20 percent of the 140 beds already planned for new construction" to respond to this new demand by the upper and upper middle classes.[50]

Despite a "valiant effort" by the Homeopathic Association, national and even global demographic developments were as much behind the denial of access for Montreal's homeopaths to the city's new facilities as were the differences in their approach to care. A.R. and his friends couldn't help taking this as a rebuff of their beloved Hahnamann's work, however. A.R. wrote philosophically that "these hospitals were necessarily closed institutions,"[51] but the denial of access was a serious blow. The bad news came down in January, 1894; in July of that same year, however, the Homeopathic Hospital of Montreal was founded. A patient of Dr Patton's, Mrs Geogiana Duff Phillips, unexpectedly presented the Association with a cheque for $10,000 with which they purchased a large house on McGill College Avenue.

When it was clear that a homeopathic hospital was going to become a reality, the very first act performed by the Association was to found a Women's Auxiliary. Its second act, before providing salaries or even a living remuneration for doctors and surgeons and before equipping a proper operating room or buying modern medical equipment, was to establish a Nursing School. The school was physically attached to the hospital so that the new house had young women professionals living inside it from the moment it opened. Although not universal, this was not an unusual practice.

The Homeopathic doctors who needed the hospital both to advance their profession and to achieve their goals for public health care understood, as Rosenberg puts it, that in terms of "the patient's experience of care ... the most important single element in reshaping the day-to-day texture of hospital life was the professionalization of nursing. In the 1800s, as today, nurses were the most important single factor determining ward and room environment. Nursing, like professional hospital administration and changed modes of financing, has played a key role in shaping the modern hospital."[52] Nurses of a high professional standard were an absolutely fundamental requirement to the survival of the clients in this new, tiny, and pretty rudimentary clinic. A.R. refers to the first patients in their fifteen-bed facility as "pioneers," admits that equipment was in short supply, and that, in their hope of attracting customers, he and Dr Hugh Patton "frequently ... did not charge any fee for professional care, and only $2 a day paid for the room."[53] But they had their Nursing School, and both he and his son, Harold, would never abandon it.

In this new world of professionalism, nurses were important for actual care but doctors themselves would become involved in the administration of the institution far more than they had ever been before. Rosenberg explains that prior to the middle of the 19th century, the hospital "was not directed by a bureaucracy of credentialed administrators; it was certainly not dominated by the medical profession and its needs. Lay trustees still felt it their duty to oversee every aspect of hospital routine. The hospital was very much a mirror of the society that populated and supported it, a society rooted in deference and hierarchy, a society in which traditional attitudes toward the responsibility of wealth were very much alive. Medical men needed and used the hospital; they could not control it."[54]

"Laymen," that is, important community figures as well as the financial donors who were drawn from the religious and business communities, administered these early institutions. Despite having no medical knowledge, they also decided who should be treated, what therapy they should receive, and even how long they should stay. In the United States especially, where private hospitals were more common than the public religious hospitals founded in Canada, people were let in not just on the basis of medical diagnoses, "but to a significant extent on the basis of social standing." Rosenberg explains that, "In almshouses, salaried agents of the governing board pretty much admitted everyone. But in private hospitals, physicians could not guarantee admission to their patients, even to beds they attended, but only recommend them to the committee."[55] Even out-patients had to get a signed certificate from a contributor to the hospital.

So the people who donated to the hospital had the privilege of recommending patients – usually two – but more according to the amount subscribed. "No patient was to be treated without a certificate from one such subscriber," Rosenberg says. "And even when individual philanthropists supported free inpatient beds, they often retained the right to approve the beds' occupants." This control was never absolute, at least. Patients still had to have a medical examination to make sure they weren't incurable, contagious, and so forth, and these kinds of necessarily medical evaluations naturally became ever more important. By mid-century, just before A.R.'s day, "control over the number of available free beds [rather than social restrictions], served as the most significant everyday constraint within which physicians decided to admit or reject a particular applicant."[56] Nonetheless, with such non-medical decisions being taken every day, it is understandable why, from the turn of the century through the 1970s when governments in Canada finally took over, physicians fought so very hard not only to work in hospitals but also to hold on to the right to administer them and to decide who needed what type of care.

Because poorer people needed a special recommendation from well-placed subscribers to get into a hospital, most did not even attempt it. They did their best at home. Private, that is, paying patients, might go in for a particular reason – caught sick while traveling, or needing emergency surgery – but they had ways of softening the experience, often significantly. The other patients were "public." That is, they either paid what little they could or their costs were absorbed, more or less, by the various charitable and religious groups affiliated with the hospital. "Most prospective [lower middle-class and middle-class] patients," Rosenberg notes, believed that, "accepting any kind of charity was humiliating." So generally, "only the destitute and friendless would look for relief from pain and want."[57] Entering any hospital was also a major commitment of time; until the middle of the century, the average stay was counted in weeks or months, not days. Women in the 'lying-in' or maternity ward of the Pennsylvania Hospital between 1807 and 1831 stayed, on average, for a whopping fifty-two days; "indigence, not difficult pregnancies or deliveries, dictated such extended hospital care."[58]

The really poor and destitute, including people such as sailors and prostitutes, were sent to separate institutions and treated more like convicts than patients. In such institutions, patients who were at all functional had to take care of themselves and help with housekeeping; they often ended up with most of the work of nursing the others. In short, the lunatics ran the asylum to the extent that a large part of a typical institution's efforts was control of their patients. This explains the obsession with rules that has dominated the hospital experience almost ever since. There were many: against smoking, for example, or spitting and loud talking. "Inmates" were also required, "without exception," to attend religious services on Sundays, and actual punishment cells were often maintained where patients could be incarcerated for drinking, fighting, and "eloping," that is, attempting to escape hospital care! In 1846, the Hospital Committee of Philadelphia's municipal hospital agreed to put a patient who tried to escape, a sick man, on bread and water for forty-eight hours "and as soon as the Physician in Chief says his health will permit, he is to receive one (cold) shower bath a day for one week." The New York Hospital limited difficult patients to a "low diet" or locked them up. Rosenberg points out that these institutions were "as much boarding house and convalescent home as [sites] for treating the acutely ill." Besides eloping, being obstreperous – "a black market in whiskey and tobacco flourished in every hospital despite the best efforts of superintendents and governing boards to end it," – and refusing medication, Rosenberg notes that, "a passive but final mode of resistance was suicide, a problem that plagued large urban hospitals well into the twentieth century."[59]

As for the staff, a similar chaos and brutality often prevailed. It is important to understand that, as Rosenberg says, "Nurses and attendants were not professional in the sense we have come to understand the term." They were drawn from recovered patients or from people who had had some outside nursing or housekeeping experience, somewhat like the people who were recruited to man emergency drug rehabilitation centres in the 1960s and 70s. Until A.R.'s day, they were also separated from the lay trustees and physicians who controlled the institution by a very wide social gulf. Moreover, nearly all the servants, nursing attendants, washerwomen, and coachmen lived *inside* the hospital or workhouse. Often entire servant families made these fearsome institutions their only home and therefore, to a considerable degree, were in a position to govern it. Despite the trustees' and physicians' complaints of lack of order and control, as Rosenberg says, "we can only assume that there was a well-defined order in the hospital, but one for which the ambitious young physician felt neither empathy nor understanding."[60]

Many, including A.R. Griffith, complained bitterly of staff theft, "drunkenness, elopement and fornication, and the perfectly systematized ... understanding which exists between the persons concerned." Private patients could escape some of the dangers and inconveniences by bringing in their own servants, who might comfort them but cause further disruptions by disobeying or causing envy among the regular staff. These patients were able to supplement their diets, rooms, and bedding with comforts and even luxuries, unlike the poor or "free" patients, and they didn't have to perform the cleaning and nursing duties demanded of free inmates, "nor were they exposed to the eyes and hands of medical students as 'clinical material.'"[61] So the "two-tier system" we hear about so much today was in full force early in hospital history and must have caused a good deal of envy, fear, and anger in both directions.

In most respects, early hospitals were social microcosms of the outside world. "Education, piety, genteel dress and diction brought appropriate respect; venereal disease, alcoholism and low ethnic status brought a parallel disdain." At the Philadelphia almshouse in 1846, for example, when more space was needed for lunatics, the entire black, male, medical ward was appropriated and its inhabitants moved to the attic.[62] At a meeting to comment on proposed building plans, Philadelphia's Episcopal Hospital medical staff urged that rooms for 'colored persons' should be in rooms smaller than those suggested and separated from the main building.[63] Venereal patients, from the earliest days, had to pay disproportionately more for their treatment than other patients; female venereal patients were often not able to get treatment at all, because it was assumed they were always prostitutes. "Attending physicians at the New York Hospital were chronically unwilling to visit certain wards, particularly the black and the venereal."[64] So there was rampant prejudice and social injustice as well as a lack of rudimentary hygiene and professional control.

Of course, social change was in the air; these tendencies would not persist into the 20th century. As the middle class expanded, more doctors insisted on admitting patients who were not rich enough to pay full amounts but who could pay something towards their care. The process took time, however, and at St. Mary's in London, England, where the governors continued to fight their doctors' wishes to admit patients on medical and not social grounds, changes in attitudes towards greater equity in care were not to triumph until after the end of the 19th century. In 1899 and 1900 at St. Mary's, the pressure became intense from various doctors and surgeons to admit not only people such as respectable middleclass widows, retired doctors, and clergymen but even, in one famous case, an alcoholic publican, on grounds that placed both the severity of the disease and its scientific interest to the doctors on a plane well above social class.[65]

This expansion of hospital access to all walks of society almost immediately led to increasing demands for state intervention in the provision of medical care. As early as 1905, hospitals in Germany were already under public authority and maintained out of public funds – a condition that was praised in many quarters in England. This tendency was to increase, of course. Despite the doctors' triumph in getting people admitted for medical reasons by at least 1900, however, doctors' influence on the hospital ward was surprisingly weak in the years when A.R. was in training. The house physicians, who were now called "residents," lacked the clinical experience or status necessary to control the rest of the staff. The much more prestigious attending physicians "appeared infrequently – to admit patients, oversee an occasional difficult case, or to teach during the brief medical school year." Throughout the 19th century, attendings and surgeons rotated their responsibilities, "with three- and four-month periods of duty diluting still further the attending physician's potential influence." To sum up, Rosenberg states that it was not any of these various classes of doctors, but the ward nurses, who were often tough, old women who had once been patients and by whose names the wards were known, who "endured."[66] It was their influence, whether brutal or kindly, which shaped life on the ward, then as now. And the new administrators of the new hospitals realized that the professionalization of these nurses would solve many of their problems in running the wards day-to-day.

As for what was expected from doctors at the time, "The house physician's contacts with his ward patients might often be characterized by a casual brutality, but its casualness was as significant as the brutality."[67] North Americans, at least, were repelled by the prevailing European style of patient-doctor interactions and a Bostonian wrote of one of Paris' leading clinicians in 1832: "If his orders are not immediately obeyed, he makes nothing of striking his patient and abusing him harshly."[68] As one British surgeon observed as late as 1897, three years after the Homeopathic had opened, "Formerly it was fashionable to treat [patients] roughly, to disregard their feelings, even to swear at them."[69]

The physicians and laymen and women on the board who managed the earliest hospitals were also very far away, both socially and spiritually, from both patients and staff in the 19th century when the push to modernization first began. But the superintendent, the person who would today be called the CEO or general director, was very close to the patients physically and remained so for some time, especially at hospitals like the Homeopathic/Queen Elizabeth. In nearly every hospital in the earliest days, this person had similar duties to those that government-appointed bureaucrats have today. "The trustees exerted their legal authority through him. He was responsible for purchasing, for discipline, for hiring and firing within the 'house' he administered."[70]

The terms "house" and "family," often employed in the old documents, were not just metaphorical. As Rosenberg and other historians note, "The residents and apothecary ate at the Superintendent's table while his wife normally served as matron in particular charge of the women's wards and such 'female departments' as cleaning and laundry." The qualities desired in a hospital manager of the early period, Rosenberg notes, "were neither hospital experience nor medical training, but rather ... prudence, responsibility and piety ... It was expected throughout the century that the Superintendent would live, with his wife and children, if any, in the hospital, and eat every meal with his house staff and apothecary. When the trustees sought to fill vacant superintendentships, recommendations of wife as well as husband were solicited, for she bore an appropriate responsibility for maintaining the institution's moral health."[71]

All this is to say that when founding their new hospitals, the pioneers – who in Canada included those opening the Royal Victoria or expanding the Calgary General just as much as the small band creating the Homeopathic – had a vision of a great deal more fairness and professionalism than they had seen in their careers thus far. And the Homeopathic was more advanced than most, even at the time. From its foundation, as Harold Griffith says, "the policy of the Hospital was to have an 'open door.' That meant that not only was its door open to penniless patients, but also that it was permitted for any reputable doctor to admit his private patients and treat them there,"[72] an implicit invitation to the middle- and lower middle-class. Quite a few years

before this power was granted in England, doctors had come to domi-
nate the hospital board of the Homeopathic and were deciding who
should be admitted. This board retained the egalitarian desire to serve
the poor that had motivated A.R. and Mary Griffith from the first, and
they had also chosen not to treat other doctors the way they had been
treated; they did not bar them from access to a hospital when their
patients needed such care. Of course, it should be noted that the
Homeopathic also needed both kinds of clients – not only to preserve
their mandate of protecting the general public health but in order to
survive economically – a fact that gradually became clear to more hospitals around the world.

ROOMS FOR ALL

> The removal of the nurses to their new home has provided two excellent
> wards where semi-private patients are admitted at the low rate of $1.00 a
> day. This is a great advantage to many who are unable to pay the higher
> fee required for single rooms.
>   A.R. Griffith, Medical Superintendent's Annual Report, 1900[73]

A.R. Griffith was a devoted homeopathic doctor, but this approach,
which seemed to work best on the chronic ailments like arthritis, bronchitis, or digestive problems that filled the hospital wards of the 1870s
and 80s, was to fade against the onslaught of the large number of infectious diseases that would decimate urban populations at the end of the
nineteenth century. In *For Patients of Moderate Means,* Rosemary and
David Gagan have noted that just as the Homeopathic and many other
Canadian community hospitals were opening their doors, "Canada was
experiencing both a health and a health-care crisis."[74]

This health crisis was a direct product of industrialization, urbaniza-
tion, population growth – especially through immigration – and the
unsanitary conditions that prevailed "as the result of inadequate and
overcrowded housing; non-existent or ineffective sewage and garbage
disposal; untreated, unprotected, and regularly contaminated municipal water systems and private wells; insufficient regulation of food and
milk supplies; unsafe and overcrowded workplaces; and large concentrations of seasonally impoverished and malnourished working
poor."[74] This last description sums up the kinds of illnesses that A.R.
Griffith and his fellow doctors commonly saw both in the streets and in
the older health care institutions of Montreal at this point in their

careers. Typhoid fever, tuberculosis, sepsis, complications of child-birth, and avoidable accidents in the workplace constituted their main patient load, as it does in the third world today, and the high levels of this kind of misery, then as now, were not very susceptible to changes in medical technique because their primary causes were due to social and economic circumstances.

Added to the problems of an imperfect medical comprehension of the action of germs and the spread of disease was the fact that most cities were being overwhelmed by a population explosion of new arrivals, nearly all of them poor – the mass exodus of people from farm to city brought by industrialization or the people fleeing impoverished countries abroad to come to Canada. For example, Winnipeg grew from a small town of 8,000 in 1881 to a large city of 163,000 by 1916 because of its position as a "focus of westward immigration, the western hub of a transcontinental transportation system, and the commercial center of the new wheat economy of the prairies."[75] Winnipeg was not alone. Along with such demographic pressures "came public health problems that produced annual epidemics of environmentally induced contagion. One observer likened living conditions in Winnipeg's immigrant North End to those of a European village in the Middle Ages, but he might have been describing the working-class districts of any Canadian city, among which Montreal's east end was the most notorious."[76]

However, for the first time in history, hospitals, rather than the traditional arenas of homecare or neighbours' help, shouldered the burden of trying to heal these new masses of sick people. "Caring for the perennial victims of seasonal epidemics of air- and water-borne contagion became a major responsibility of community hospitals after 1890, and was one of the reasons for their rapid expansion."[77] Historian Terry Copp, in his book *The Anatomy of Poverty: The Condition of the Working Class in Montreal, 1897–1929*, points out that such care was more difficult and lasted for a longer time in Montreal than in other North American cities. Even in A.R.'s day, "The connection between inadequate wages, poor housing conditions, and a mortality rate which marked Montreal as one of the unhealthiest cities in the western world was perfectly clear to many contemporary observers." Copp says the main reason for Montreal's lag in the areas of hygiene and housing was a highly "defective piece of legislation," Quebec's Public Health Act of 1886.[78]

This was the period of the "burst of scientific creativity associated with the names of Pasteur ... and Koch" who not only pioneered the

germ theory of infectious diseases but also discovered sepsis or steril-
ization as a way of combating them. Montreal was not left out of this
"truly revolutionary change in the history of mankind," as Copp puts it.
The city boasted two institutions that were "very conversant both with
the new discoveries and their implications for public health," the
McGill Medical School and the Laval Faculty of Medicine. However,
this local knowledge was not translated into political action. Although
the Quebec Board of Health suggested entirely modern methods such
as "compulsory smallpox and diphtheria inoculation, the medical
inspection of school children, adequate controls over the purity of
milk, treatment centers for tuberculosis, and water purification programs," it had no political power. In a situation that may sound familiar
today, the municipalities, which had to find the tax dollars to pay for
such initiatives, did not prioritize investing in public health "except in
time of epidemics," so the Health Act was almost completely ineffective.[79]

The figures for this period really are shocking and outstrip anything
but an active war zone today. In Montreal, "between 1897 and 1911,
approximately *one out of three babies died before reaching the age of twelve
months*. As late as 1926, the rate was still 14 percent, a figure almost
double the average for New York or Toronto" at the time. [80] Although
the early records of the Montreal Homeopathic show the numbers of
infant deaths as coming close to the combined loss of patients to tuberculosis, typhoid, and pneumonia,[81] this problem was partly masked at
the Homeopathic by its location in the prosperous center of the city as
well as by the special focus of its doctors and its board. Montreal's
infant deaths were mostly due to diarrhea and enteritis caused by poor
water supplies but were greatly exacerbated by the general level of
health and education of the parents and the family's housing, so they
varied from only 43.9 per 1000 live births in St. George, where the
Homeopathic was, all the way up to between 212.9 and 213.8 in St.
Henri and Ste. Marie, where the poor French working class and immigrant slums were found.

The Homeopathic had its share of such patients but because it was a
homeopathic hospital, part of its clientele at least had to be relatively
discerning. Deciding to use a homeopathic doctor involved information gathering and informed choice. Additionally, the discipline itself
relied heavily on treating "the whole person," that is, paying attention
to diet, housing, mental and emotional health, and general family living conditions – the very causes of most of the ills of the day – which

explains much of its success at the time. This attention to patients and their larger needs is philosophically quite different from the emerging interest in learning about and treating diseases themselves. It is also one reason why the Homeopathic/Queen Elizabeth extended an unusually enthusiastic welcome to psychiatry in the 1980s and 90s. The Hospital's long history had trained the board to see the mental and emotional state of the patient as a natural adjunct of daily patient care. Looking at the whole patient became so engrained at the Homeo-pathic/Queen Elizabeth that in 1972, almost eighty years after its founding, a proud grandfather asked the Hospital's cook to fry a freshly caught trout for his youngest daughter who had just given birth. "The kitchen did so," says the sister of the patient, "without batting an eye! They even served it with a flower and a bottle of wine."[82]

Fresh trout would have come under the umbrella of patient morale and illustrates a continuing administrative concern with surroundings, diet, and mental well-being that was deep enough to have survived most of the 20th century. Back in the 1890s, it must have been one of the key factors that helped bring down the Homeopathic's child mor-tality statistics to a level four times lower than found in the rest of Montreal. Another contributor, of course, was the parents' education. The predominately French-Canadian working class people of the nearby east end were underpaid, living in often deplorable housing, and had been taught that babies needed "very quick weaning to bottles filled with *la bouille traditionelle*," a mixture of beef extract, cereal, and, of course, the local water. This cultural tradition was probably based on the mother's poor health and the very close pregnancies common at the time, which even in 1900 were blamed for adding to this group's high infant mortality.[83] Despite gradually getting more control over water and milk sanitation, Montreal was to continue to suffer regular health-care crises well into the 20th century because of political lassi-tude. Nonetheless, by the time the early epidemics of typhoid and tuberculosis were abating, around 1900, Montreal's hospitals – not its homes – had become the first line of defense of public health, partially because hospitals were the only defense left.

Individual hospitals at the turn of the 19th century liked to think that their sudden popularity was due to their own high standards of care, but in fact that care was not to significantly affect death rates until the advent of good surgical procedures and antibiotics almost fifty years later. The factors that really made a difference at the time were the basic demographic and social changes wrought by the Industrial

Revolution that made the earlier practice of caring for one's family at home simply impossible. "Among working-class families, neither urban living conditions nor family economies were amenable to the prolonged nursing of the sick at home. Families of six or eight, sometimes augmented by unmarried boarders, crowded into one or two- room tenement flats, were incapable of segregating the sick, especially the contagious sick, from the healthy, or of ministering to their needs. [As well,] material survival depended on the collective contribution of all who could work to sustain the household's precarious income. A family quarantined by public health officials for six or eight weeks was effectively impoverished for [at least] the duration of the illness."[84]

So hospitals became the only option for the working poor and the lower middle classes when they became really ill. Even the upper middle classes, who had formerly been able "to afford surgeons, physicians and special duty nurses for private medical care at home," fell victim to the financial panic of the mid 1890s, one of Canada's most severe economic depressions. At this point, they, too, were forced to "economize with hospitalization, which included a private room, board, nursing and attendance by the best medical practitioners available, all for eight to twelve dollars a week, and without the stigma of being identified as, or having contact with, a charity patient." At the same period, these hospitals were trying very hard to become cleaner, quieter, more professional and more worthy of peoples' trust. "With the return of better times, these individuals became an important new clientele of users who were able [and willing] to pay ... because they were no longer terrified by the prospect of hospitalization, which from experience they now knew would do them no harm." [85]

All these tendencies were reflected in the Homeopathic Hospital of Montreal's earliest years, although as usual there were some individual aberrations. Because of its earnest desire to become the most accessible hospital possible, the Homeopathic was one of the first hospitals in the world to make arrangements for affordable care for the lower middle classes instead of catering just to the highest and lowest ends of the economic scale. There was a real danger then, as now, for such people as clerks, farmers, factory workers, or even nurses to fall between the cracks of a system that rewarded penury and destitution with free care – care that was seen as too humiliating for straightened but respectable families to face. There are no statistics from the period to give us an idea of the number of people who may have deferred medical care or surgery for reasons of shame or the fear of pauperizing their families with home-care costs, but it's obvious from anecdotal evidence as well as rapidly changing public policy that this number must have been significant. In any event, as early as 1900 and well ahead of general practice, the Homeopathic began offering "semi-private" rooms at the astonishingly inexpensive rate of a dollar a day. "This is a great advantage to many who are unable to pay the higher fee required for single rooms," A.R. wrote proudly.[86]

At the same time that other hospitals, and the Homeopathic itself, were wooing paying patients in their ten dollar-a-day rooms with luxurious furnishings and special diets that included wine served in crystal goblets, A.R.'s friend and fellow founder, Arthur Patton, lamented in the *Annual Report* of 1906 that between September and December of that year, "over 100 paying patients were refused admittance for lack of room, for the same reason a large number of public cases were refused."[87] Like other hospitals, the Homeopathic subsidized its non-paying patients by attracting about twice as many paying patients. Patton noted the fact that the public cases still totaled 100, "by far the largest number we have ever cared for ... it may not be amiss to draw your attention to the amount of work we are doing and the smallness of the Provincial government aid we receive, viz. $100.00 per annum, which is less than half the sum received by institutions in our city which do not aid the poor to anything like a proportionate extent."

At this time, Canadian hospitals that were open to the public still had to depend to a large extent on the fluctuating and unpredictable philanthropy of private donors. But as early as 1900, the numbers of patients and their demands for medical attention were making the idea of increased government funding for medical care a viable consideration, even for hospital administrators as independent and conservative as Dr Patton. This simultaneous burgeoning demand for and need of health care in the 1890s, as David and Rosemary Gagan note, also coincided with "several interrelated developments in medicine and health care, [all of which] converged ... to stimulate the re-invention of the hospital as a health-care facility for the whole population."[88] These revolutionary changes in the hospital as an institution came from three quarters: investigative laboratory science; the birth of the science of public health; and the "ascent of a skilled workforce of medical assistants, professional nurses, and more importantly, their sisters in training, the student nurses of Canada's newly founded schools of nursing," with the first and the third developments supporting the birth of the second.

A RISING PROFESSION

> For five years the nurses of the training school slept in the hospital
> building, and were most uncomfortably crowded. The inconveniences
> and discomforts were numerous, but the nurses were always patient,
> cheerful and uncomplaining, doing their work with credit to themselves
> and honor to the Hospital ... much praise is due Miss Moodie and the
> ladies of the Auxiliary for the new Home leased and furnished in the
> adjoining building.
>
> A.R. Griffith, Medical Superintendent's Report, 1900[89]

The discoveries of Joseph Lister, Louis Pasteur, and Robert Koch completely revolutionized surgery. That same revolution – the discovery of
the importance of an antiseptic environment – cut down not only on
the rate of post-operative infections but also the other great killers in
hospital wards: puerperal fever, typhoid, and various hospital-borne
infections. Eventually even tuberculosis declined, although it took the
discovery of antibiotics before it was fully under control. The simple act
of washing hands and surfaces as well as scrupulously boiling bedding
and disinfecting instruments made a staggering difference in the rate
of infectious diseases. As their friends and relatives went in for small
surgeries and infections such as typhoid and pneumonia – and then
walked out again, actually healthier – people were encouraged to look
upon the hospital door as a portal not leading to death but as an opening to hope. And the newly trained doctors and nurses working within
were the most hopeful of all.

These people, as well as early hospital administrators, saw this new
understanding of the spread of disease as their chance to finally make a
real difference. What they wanted were new standards of order and
cleanliness, based on a professional understanding of the behaviour
and spread of germs. The dirt, chaos, and disorder were being
replaced with an ideal environment of antiseptic perfection that could
only be achieved by trained staff that understood its purpose and
importance. Hospital workers and administrators realized that this new
era of clinical order and professional cleanliness could only come from
new forms of education tailored to inculcate real professionalism.

Almost every new hospital with high standards also felt that "their"
new standards of professional health care could not be entrusted to the
outside world but would have to be created within their own, attached,
educational institutions. From a purely economic standpoint, these

institutions would not only train the truly professional nurses they would need, they would also provide a constant pool of extremely cheap, yet professionally trained labour. Dreary physical work still abounded. The bandages still had to be wound, the medicines measured, the brass polished, and the patients fed. But now that germ theory was understood, the floors had to be scrubbed even more rigourously and the instruments, beds, and linens had to be not just scrupulously clean but also medically sterile. This required a staff doing what is really scut-work with a professional understanding of why and how.

By the end of the 19th century, hospitals were realizing that what they needed were "medical assistants with [at least] a rudimentary background in anatomy, physiology, *material medica*, hygiene and toxicology." *Canada Lancet*, among other medical journals of the era, "reported compelling evidence that professional nursing reduced patient mortality rates."[90] Given the financial restraints in every hospital, however, how could such educated, carefully trained people possibly be paid? The apprenticeship side of teaching nursing solved the problem. If the school was "in house," each student would be at the disposal of the Hospital between eighteen months to three years, on hand twenty-four hours a day to clean, serve meals, and do laundry, all in the name of "training." And at first, there was a great deal more of this kind of "training" than there was course work and medical theory. Nonetheless, there was resistance from many doctors to the whole idea of medical assistants. They feared their professional status, still so new and precarious, would be infringed upon by less highly-trained workers. As David and Rosemary Gagan put it, "the debate over the appropriate medical role of the professional nurse, once launched, was never entirely resolved, and is still resurrected from time to time." However, hospital administrators clearly understood that it wasn't entirely the fully-trained graduate nurses who were so sorely needed by the patients. The free labour given by the pupils, "who flocked to the often hastily-conceived training schools," was "the life-blood of cash-strapped hospitals trying to cope with a rapidly expanding population of patients."[91] This is one reason why many hospitals instituted their in-house schools so rapidly.

Life for the young women who did arrive in droves to these schools was so economically tight that it's hard for us to imagine. At the Homeopathic in 1895, they had to provide much of their own equipment, including dresses and aprons, catheters, thermometers, a hypodermic syringe, and more, all for a salary of three dollars a month at the beginning and going up to seven dollars during the last eight months of the eighteen-month training period. Their room and board were free. The rooms were often cold and crowded and the food at some hospitals was far from exemplary. The desirability of such work was heightened by strict rules of acceptance. The "girls" had to be unmarried and fairly old, between twenty-five and thirty-five at first, with "testimonials as to character." By 1907, hospitals such as the Vancouver General were paying a princely ten dollars a month on top of board, but besides the actual course work, the students' duties included twelve-hour shifts, six days a week, with a patient load of twenty per shift. Obviously, not much time was left for actual study, and young nurses slept as little as interns do today. The hospitals depended on this pool of cheap, daily labour and also brought in extra cash through it.

Like other hospitals, the Montreal Homeopathic made money on its student nurses by sending them out to take care of private patients; most of their pay for such services went to the hospital. Despite some exemplary attempts at equity between the sexes in this hospital, the Homeopathic's "Rules for Nurses on Outside Cases," which were very similar to their rules for in-house patients, are devastating by today's standards. These young women were "to attend the sick, both rich and poor, in hospitals, hotels or private houses, wherever the Superintendent may appoint." With typhoid, cholera, malaria, and TB still major problems in Montreal, to say nothing of the daily rout of lice; "bloody flux," or infectious intestinal ailments; gruesome abscesses, ringworm, and mange; and people frequently dying of sepsis or tumours, these assignments must often have been fairly horrific. And the nurse's responsibilities were total. "The nurse's time belongs to the family employing her. She is to take entire charge of the patient, and of the sick room, and of the closets and bathroom used in connection with it." In often highly infectious, dangerous conditions, she had to clean, disinfect, ventilate, make the fires, empty the bedpans, sweep and dust, prepare clothing and any special "invalid food," administer all medications, serve the meals, keep daily records for the physician, and keep track of all his orders. "If her attention be not of necessity wholly devoted to the patient, the nurse is expected to make herself generally useful," more or less as a servant. She also had to "maintain a dignified reticence in regard to the disease, its treatment, or the methods of other physicians, and ... to hold sacred the knowledge which to a certain extent she must obtain of the private affairs of such households."[92]

Harold Griffith later wrote that such a woman had to have "integrity, devotion ... and incredible endurance." Although by 1910 or 11, there was some outcry against such obvious exploitation and inequality – the Vancouver City Council found the situation "outrageous" and demanded an explanation from its hospital board – the exploitation has continued in some form even into the present day.[93] Nurses were, as Rosemary and David Gagan put it, "the hospital's principal domestic servants, with a broadly defined understanding of germ theory, aseptic procedures, patient care, medical record keeping and [especially] deference to their superiours."[94] This deference, a feminine delicacy and subservience born of the still very strong "gendered lines of authority" of the 19th century, was both the nurses' cross to bear and their most important professional shelter. Virtually all hospitals of the era exploited young women's eager desires to take advantage of the only respectable independent profession outside of teaching that had opened up for them. Some, however, did so in ways that would lead not only towards greater male-female equality in the future but also would give rise to far better professional care for the patients.

GENDER EQUITY

These are all honored names in the history of the Hospital, and the names of many more men and women should be added – particularly the names of women.

Harold Griffith[95]

Seen in its full historical context, the Montreal Homeopathic's infant Board of Directors' first act of establishing, or rather, officially recognizing an already functioning Women's Auxilliary, was far from unique. In Europe and North America, women had been the primary caregivers and healers for centuries and were also the driving force behind the establishment of work- and almshouses well before they began to help establish community hospitals in the late 19th century. However, the Homeopathic's willingness to credit women's work publicly and to accept women as professionals, important funding sources, and even administrative equals, is notable from its beginnings and was to grow throughout its history to become one of its most interesting and unusual characteristics. It's useful to compare its attitudes with those of a very similar institution, the Moncton Hospital in Moncton, New Brunswick, which was also a small, community venture with a comparable beginning. The Moncton Hospital was founded only four years after the Montreal Homeopathic and, like it, benefited enormously from the women who were deeply involved – it might be said almost entirely responsible for – organizing, funding, and supporting the institution in its fledgling stages.

W.G. Godfrey, the author of a history of this hospital, *A Struggle to Serve: A History of the Moncton Hospital*, records that throughout the 1890s, a local group called "the King's Daughters" was already busy helping poor families. This association of women organized the first meetings to discuss starting a small hospital in the city and brought together the requisite clergymen, doctors, aldermen, and society figures. Initial meetings went so well that the King's Daughters decided to "amalgamate with all those women in the town who feel an interest in the matter."[96] This community outreach enabled them to form a Ladies' Aid society similar to the Homeopathic's Women's Auxiliary. Within a week, it was raising funds and organizing a mass public meeting.

The core of well-educated and well-trained physicians already in Moncton was quick to get involved in such a venture. On 11 January 1895, the first public meeting was held and women attendees still outnumbered the men. Annie Purdy, wife of Dr Clinton Purdy, was particularly active and emphasized the need for their own nurse's teaching school. Like all medical care reformers of the era, she assumed that the hospital would primarily cater to the destitute, but she pointed out that "those in our city who are away from home ... will gladly avail themselves of the opportunity which the private wards will afford of giving them board and excellent nursing for very little more than they would pay for board alone."[97] It was Ann Purdy's speech on this occasion, with shrewd suggestions as to where and how to raise funds, which was credited with gaining support from the audience, including the city's mayor. A supportive editorial in the local press admitted that "the Ladies" had taken the initiative in founding a city hospital. But now that the ball was rolling, the editor felt this enterprise should pass "largely out of the hands" of its initiators, who nonetheless "should feel gratified with the result."[98]

Subsequent fund-raising was successful largely through the efforts of the Ladies' Aid. On 5 March 1895, the Moncton Hospital was incorporated, complete with its own training school for nurses. Twelve local men were named as trustees with a further two trustees to be appointed from the ranks of the city's physicians – all of whom were male. Finding operating budgets to make the new building a functioning reality, however, was again bounced back to "the initiators," the Ladies' Aid.[99] The old city almshouse was refurbished and triumphantly opened as the Moncton Hospital in June of 1898. Of the 437 visitors on Open House day, 250 were women. But as Godfrey notes, every person singled out for public honours and congratulations was a man. Very deserving of such praise they were, having also tirelessly worked for the hospital; but, as Godfrey points out, "Amidst all the congratulations there was only a brief mention that the trustees and the matron were 'assisted by some of the ladies.' At the hospital's birth, they were forgotten."[100]

In this, the Moncton Hospital was neither unusually unfair nor ungrateful. It was only typical of its times. Nearly all these charitable institutions, including the earlier almshouses, either refused or downplayed public recognition of the "anonymous and overlooked" women who shared and shaped their early history.[101] So it's interesting to see that when the first Medical Board was proclaimed at the Homeopathic Hospital of Montreal, a year before the fourteen all-male trustees were named in Moncton, its vice president was a woman, Mrs Charles Morton. Eight women served in professional or managerial capacities on this board composed of sixteen people. The administrators of the new Homeopathic not only remembered who had originally provided much of the funding to make its existence a reality they also gave them full administrative parity, way back in 1894 – something few hospitals have achieved to this day.

The nursing school founded by Homeopathic reflected the same very modern, almost nonchalant recognition of the women that continued to make its functioning possible. This institution, the Phillips School of Nursing, was named for the woman whose small but completely unexpected gift of $10,000 had enabled the hospital to open in the first place. Her face graced many of the hospital's early Annual Reports, and even after the institution had far out-grown its initial building, she was still referred to as its "benefactress" for many decades. Georgiana Duff Phillips was never on the board, but A.R. Griffith and Arthur Patton were. For reasons attributable both to their personal characters and their homeopathic training, they did not take what she had done lightly.

Despite such admirable attitudes, their tenuous financial position meant that the Homeopathic exploited the student nurses in the Phillips School as strenuously as did other hospitals of the time, albeit with better perks, such as free medical care and excellent food. However, they also took steps to make sure that their nurses could become outstanding professionals and able to move on to independent work. They were one of the first hospitals in Canada to pay them an increasingly decent wage. In 1894, as soon as it was created, the board had voted to import their first lady superintendent of nursing from Edinburgh, Scotland, a city then seen as the epicenter of modern medical practice. Miss Jessie Thomson, despite a quite large salary of $400 a year, left only two years later when her own theological bent asserted itself. "She felt called to become a missionary in China," Harold Griffith wrote in his hospital history, and she died there in 1899. The choice of a top-level professional woman set the tone, however, and from her era forward, training was both rigorous and demanding. The position of lady superintendent was also one of the highest paid and most influential positions in the institution.

The same quality that enabled A.R. and his staff to accept as equals those people who were disenfranchised in other environments may also have been responsible for their openness to innovation. As John Hughes put it over a hundred years later, "the misfits always found a home at the Queen E. People who wouldn't toe the party line elsewhere could practice and flourish there." For example, the same year it was founded, the Homeopathic's new medical staff of nine physicians grew by two more young doctors: Arthur D. Patton, Hugh Patton's brother, and Dr E.M. Morgan. The Patton family had neatly divided itself into doctors of medicine and divinity, the common tendency of the period already noted. But Dr Morgan, having specialized at the New York Ophthalmic Hospital and who had previously worked in Queens and Philadelphia, was an unusual breed for the period. He set himself up as something rather rare and exciting for the 1890s: an ear, nose, and throat specialist as well as an osteopath, "and was one of the first Montreal doctors to dabble in electrotherapy ... [keeping] an X-ray machine in his office from around 1900."[102]

In 1920, Morgan established the first X-ray department in the Homeopathic, a very early date for such a department in such a small institution. Radiology became his new specialty until his retirement in 1941. The hospital rapidly became a haven for this kind of innovator in medicine and technology; this quality would lead to its spectacular advances in anesthetics, laproscopics, and other therapies and techniques mentioned in the first chapter. As for Alexander Griffith, he was appointed medical superintendent in 1898, "and was re-elected annually to this office until his death in 1936." His son Harold noted many years later that despite the inevitable quarrels between the "strongly opinionated" doctors of the day, "on the whole things went along harmoniously." This was in large part due to a becoming humility that no doubt helped get A.R. re-elected every year. "He was never jealous, and realized there was plenty of work for everyone ... and he delighted in helping younger doctors get established."[103]

This blend of a burning ambition to attain the highest medical standards, coupled with an open access to all sorts of doctors and patients and an egalitarian, family atmosphere is the best way to describe the culture of the Montreal Homeopathic Hospital. Such an understanding an institution's underlying culture makes some of the arrangements at the Homeopathic/Queen Elizabeth described in the beginning of this book more comprehensible. What may have seemed so singular and quaint – the old Queen E's exceptionally fine kitchen, its medical superintendents and general directors taking meals with their whole staff and walking the halls at all hours, always available, takes on another sheen when seen in the light of general hospital history. The brother- or father-son teams, the status of wives, the intermarriages between nurses and doctors, are all expressions of the idealistic and familial nature of early community hospitals.

The goal of these early institutions was, of course, to elevate and perfect the medical profession to some degree. But that elevation was set firmly in the context of a greater goal: the general improvement of the health of the entire general public. The rich and influential men and women who founded these institutions were beginning to understand very clearly that individual health, including the health of their own families, was dependent on the health of the public at large, including the poorest of the poor. So in this sense, increased funding was a goal only to be sought insofar as it either improved the medical profession or the standards of care. What we expect in the health care field today, actual profit, was unimaginable in this early concentration of efforts that centred on containing epidemics and avoiding needless deaths.

Health care during this period was therefore not seen as it is today, as a money-making industry, but the exact opposite, a debit from the collective good that could only be staunched or partially repaired through charity, government subsidization, and much selfless and often unpaid labour. Early hospital founders and managers did not dream of gaining large amounts of monetary profit from their work of caring for the sick. Everything beyond operating expenses – that is, after very modest living wages for doctors, nurses, and support staff had been paid – was immediately invested into expanding the institution's ability to provide more and better care. Hospital administrators, who were generally community leaders as well, used the funding that came from their paying patients, the contributions from private benefactors and state authorities, and the voluntary help of the community at large to increase the number of beds, the availability of medicines, the modernity of the equipment, and the quality of medical research. That's why they never got ahead in an economic sense. In order to pursue the ever-advancing standards of care in the last years of the 19th and the entire 20th centuries, they were always spending up to or beyond their limits.

An emphasis on good nursing and a pattern of suddenly finding funds in the community just as the institution's resources became stretched to their limits characterized the rhythm of growth of the Homeopathic/Queen Elizabeth throughout its existence. It was not alone in this tendency, of course. Nearly every community hospital and most of the larger teaching hospitals expanded this way. As medicine was steadily becoming more effective, the old almshouses and charity wards were being seen as inadequate and undesirable. "Proper" hospitals with surgical departments and in-house care delivered by trained professionals were increasingly seen as a necessary adjunct to the new techniques and equipment that were proving so efficacious to the public good.

Fundamental to this change was the growing understanding that if a part of the population, the poor, was allowed to remain in chronic ill health, all the population, including the rich, would eventually suffer. Money was therefore never seen as the end goal of a hospital, but as its means. The real "end" was a safer, longer life for everyone in the population. Today's intense interest in hospital bottom-lines, the massive profits available in pharmacological and health care services, and especially an insistence on showing a profit while caring for the most helpless, depleted, and debilitated members of society, would have been utterly alien concepts to the founders of early hospital care.

As we go deeper into the 21st century, we will see that many of the health care institutions that were so idealistically built up in the past are either gone, like the Homeopathic, or are now crumbling. Many of the medical, governmental, and business experts analyzing this decline are suggesting draconian remedies that involve cutbacks in daily funding on the one hand. On the other, they are pushing for new constructions to house state-of-the-art machines and equipment designed to treat the most rare and dramatic conditions. So far, these plans have done little to reassure the Canadian population. That's because, as most analysts agree, this approach seems to be doing violence to those old ideals of patient equity – that is, of taking care of the whole population, not just part of it. As for the concept of humane care that attempts to treat the person and not just the disease, that too, as 2004's *C. difficile* crisis in Quebec made clear, has become a rare quality.

The public is repeatedly told that the paternalistic family-doctor days are long gone and that may be true. But very few of the people suggesting public/private partnerships and private clinics, increasing corporate and pharmacological control over public health, increased consolidation of community facilities into super-hospitals and centres of excellence – in fact, any of the other medical buzzwords of our day that will be discussed in chapters 5, 6 and 7 – seem to be interested in gaining any detailed understanding of the means by which so much astonishing progress was made in the early development of hospital care.

In the future, if we want to have recourse to anything similar to what A.R. Griffith and his staff were trying to achieve, that is, if we want to serve the health needs of the largest number of people as professionally, humanely, and equitably as possible, the biggest question in our minds ought to be a very simple one: How in heaven's name did those largely ineffective doctors go so very rapidly from the chaos, misery, and blatant inequality of the 1860s and 70s to the levels of professional control and real social advancement that were reached by 1900 or 1920, only a few decades later? When entire social systems are being overhauled, as they are at present, it's useful to be aware of what may have held them together in the first place. If we step back and do some serious analysis, we may find that while there's little doubt that the surfaces of such formerly functional systems have often become eroded beyond service, the skeletal foundations that ultimately support all such human endeavours are not so subject to the pressures of history – or even of economics – as we might think.

3

Family Medicine

THE GOOD LIFE

Menu:

Oyster Patties		Whitebait a la Boyer
Spuds	Peas	Pommes douces
Banana Salad		Grape Juice a la Griffith
Hokey Pokey		Shivering Jimmy
Pumpkin Pie with Mother's Special – Crab Apple Jelly		
Fruit	Cake	Candy

Selections from the annual dinner menus of
The Griffith Boys' Club, 1908–1911

No history featuring the Montreal Homeopathic/Queen Elizabeth Hospital would be complete without a trip to see a beautiful, turn-of-the-century cottage in the Laurentians, the lake and mountain country north of the city. The old pine building is tall and narrow with a deep gallery wrapped around two sides; it's a perfect example of turn-of-the-century rustic style. It has a native stone fireplace in the living room and a peeled-bark rustic stairway to the uninsulated sleeping rooms upstairs. The wide, shady porch is lavishly furnished with swings, hammocks, and tables capable of seating twelve or more. Smelling of balsam and wood smoke and strewn with the old camp pillows, photographs, toys, and the nursery school and professional award plaques of four generations, it is still the focal point of family life among A.R. and Harold Griffith's descendents.

The Griffith family cottage faces a long, undeveloped chain of three islands across a mirror-calm and sparsely inhabited lake. Although it remains almost unchanged over the last one hundred years, the house is in perfect repair, with old boats and furniture waiting attention in a nearby shed. From the time he was eight, this was Harold Griffith's younger brother Jim's favourite place. His eldest daughter, Betty Griffith Jennings, is short like her uncle and possessed of the Griffith friendliness and physical energy. Her own, modern summer home is just a few steps away, but she says that A.R.'s cottage is still the place where the old folks reunite every summer and all the grandchildren, nieces, nephews, and in-laws get to know one another.

The area was a wilderness in the late 19th century, populated only by Indian guides, trappers, and loggers. A lumber baron named George Ross "discovered" their lake, Lac des Iles, and built the first summer house. Two other early families were the Bridges and the Motts, the latter deeply involved in turn-of-the-century missionary movements. By this time, Mary Griffith had given birth to the youngest of their four boys and A.R. had built up a thriving practice in Montreal. In 1901, one of his more distinguished patients – Betty doesn't remember if it was a Bridge or a Mott – invited him to come up and join their new cottage community. It wasn't entirely a disinterested act, Betty says. "They really needed a doctor near by; there wasn't anyone in those days. So Grandpa would work all week in town and again, most of the weekend here. You never knew when someone would come over for stitches, a broken arm, or because his wife was having a baby." The working weekend spread horizontally into the second generation. Betty's father Jim, her mother Florence, who had been a nurse at the Queen E, and her uncle Harold continued this tradition of working from their vacation cottage. "I'm sure Grandpa had the same experience," Betty says. "Mother said she'd never delivered so many babies as up here. 'I think they plan it for our arrival!' she'd joke. 'I have to go out every day and deliver babies!'"

In those days, the only way to get so far was by train. "A.R. would come to St. Jerome on a train that took all day. He or Grandma had to bring all the provisions with them. There weren't really any stores and of course no power for the first 50 years they were there." They used gas lamps and wood stoves. Moreover, Grandma Mary left her maid and driver back in Montreal. It doesn't sound like much of a vacation from a hard-working life, but the Griffiths not only thrived on these energetic holidays, they passed on a taste for them. Betty says that her father's many duties even fifty years later meant that, "We didn't see Daddy (Jim) a lot. That was our life. Mother understood; it was the same with Linda and Harold and with Grandma and Grandpa. No, we didn't resent it! People were in trouble – you'd go."

Linda Mary Jacobson, the elder of Harold and Linda's two daughters, remembers that within a couple of summers after they had moved into the cottage, A.R. organized a "Griffith Boy's Club" as a way of both entertaining and instructing his four lively boys, then aged between twelve and six. "They would meet every week; I think there were a maximum of thirteen members besides the Griffith boys," she says. A.R. himself was listed as one of the members, not the president or founder of this "boy's" club, so a democratic atmosphere clearly prevailed. It went on for about four or five years. Linda Mary says, "They had debates especially, discussions, and a big, exciting dinner at the end of the year. They all had to learn how to conduct meetings and make speeches. We have some of the minutes of the meetings – they're very funny. The big, formal dinner was given in the winter and Grandma did all the food. She was a fabulous cook."

The sumptuous menus included fried chicken with bacon-tanglefoot sauce; oyster patties, jarred wild strawberries, Lac des Iles trout, cakes, candies, and a family staple: pumpkin pie with, of all things, crabapple jelly. Pumpkin pie was always served this way at the Griffiths' and each person has an opinion about the success of the dish. Linda Mary really liked it, but her sister's husband, Dave, to much laughter, finally admitted that he "never got used to it." There were exotic desserts the family has now lost the recipes for, like "Hokey-poky" and "Shivering Jimmy." Grape juice, variously named "a la Griffith" or "a la Bon Repose," the house's name, is always listed on the menu in a place of honour, in larger, bold type, presumably because it stood in for wine in the teetotaling Baptist house. These were two-colour menus of blue and red type on elegant, parchment-coloured paper with two gothic fonts; they look like wedding invitations. For most families of their modest means, the cost of having them printed would have been prohibitive. But although A.R.'s income was quite modest, his granddaughters assume he had connections in the printing business. After all, "he used to be a journalist and a printer's devil!" Linda Mary says.

The menus list the current members and the evening's speakers, who most often were doctors from the Homeopathic up for a fun family weekend. Other dignitaries or neighbours did these honours, too.

Harold wrote later that the Boys' Club meetings "were every Friday evening and consisted of speeches, both prepared and impromptu, debates, recitations, an annual minstrel show, and so on. Officers were elected every month to give everyone a turn; the secretary kept minutes, and my mother and baby brother Arthur were the permanent refreshment committee. We had frequent open meetings to invite friends and, at the annual banquet, we were able to invite girl friends, including Linda, to come and help serve as waitresses." There were formal toasts: to the lakes, their guests, "the ladies." As the years went on and membership grew, the toasts became more elaborate and the guest speakers more distinguished. In 1910 and 11, they included toasts to McGill and the Medical Profession as well as King and "The Dominion Government," and speakers included A.R.'s medical board colleagues and McGill professors. Harold wrote, "I am sure this Griffith Boys Club had a great influence on our lives, and is just one example of the wise ideas of my father on bringing up boys."[1]

Besides this club, Betty says A.R. encouraged his boys, at least the two eldest, to go into business in order to make their own pocket-money. There are pictures of Harold and Jim with their row boat. They went around the lake selling snacks and sundries from cottage to cottage. Betty says, "It was a very elaborate business for young boys. I can't remember how much money their account books showed they made, but it was in the hundreds of dollars! It taught them all about handling money and running a business, being responsible, keeping track of stock and change, and being clear about credit and so forth. And, it was physical work. They had to row the boat and carry the supplies in and out by themselves."

Linda Mary remembers some of the things her generation would do at the cottage. "A.R. and Daddy (Harold) liked to organize fishing contests. Grandpa wrote funny stories about the fishing contests and concocted awards. He also used to have us kids and the grandkids see how many kinds of trees or shrub leaves we could gather and identify; he loved to go on long walks in the woods. He'd organize a sailing regatta for the kids every summer; they still have the same regatta he started on this lake!" It seems incredible that busy doctors like A.R. and Harold found time on their brief "vacations" to organize contests and regattas for their children. "I guess parents are so much more lazy now," Linda Mary says. "There weren't easy ways to keep children busy then. Everything, from softball to boating, required organization. And Daddy would organize chores too. Every summer he'd have a list ready on the fridge for the "Cook's Assistants." It listed who would chop, fetch things, wash dishes, and so on, on what days. Everyone just did it; there were no arguments or malingerers like there might be today."

Family joys were to change little over the generations. At the cottage, the Griffith boys learned how to have fun while being responsible and productive. Today, the cottage teems with great- and great-great-grand-children helping to weed the gardens, tidy the dock, and set the table between swarming up and down the hill carrying floats and fishing tackle. The late Ken Jacobson, Linda Mary's son and father of two of A.R.'s smallest great-great-grandchildren, spoke with obvious feeling about the cottage property as being "sacred" to their family. He was eloquent about how much it meant to him as a child, what a joy it always was to go there, and "how important it is that children grow up surrounded by nature and with people who have the time to play with them and really teach them."

SECOND GENERATION

Love God and serve your fellow man.

Harold Griffith's advice to his children

Harold and Linda Griffith had five grandchildren. One of them, Tom Jacobson, a massage therapist who works with very ill people, says, "I think it's entirely possible that Harold had an influence on my entire life and especially my choice of profession. He was nothing short of heroic in my estimation. I have an early memory of being down at the wharf here at the cottage, playing and enjoying our usual summer activities, when a big motor boat came roaring up. There was a frantic man inside, speaking French. 'Où est le médecin?' Then a flurry of activity as my grandfather was whisked off, practically in his swimsuit, clutching his bag. And then later, he's back, with a story of how it all went well. That element of heroism was combined with the family stories about his fame as an anesthesiologist and researcher. He and my grandmother exuded a very strong sense of service, and both my mother and father were in service as well. So our family culture was oriented around service, not business."

Tom's twin brother, Ken, worked with disturbed children at the Michael Reese hospital in Chicago before his death in 2006. He remembered, "Harold and Linda never said things like, 'Oh, those people bothered us when we were on vacation.' I think they accepted that as just what they did. Harold had a wonderful attitude about work and play ... he would escape to what we called his 'office' to write – really that old workshed over there, and that work was integrated in the family life. It wasn't a big deal, like his work was so important. We were allowed to bother him if we wanted. But I thought of that shed as a spiritual place. He had his desk upstairs, but down it was the workshed, and he'd make chairs in there, do all the repairs for the house, fix broken wheelbarrows and windows and so on. When we were small he'd help us make little boats, and then we'd sail them in the water. These kinds of activities in that simple little shed created for me an idea of a kind of holy workspace, where you can have it all. These are very powerful memories."

Harold and Linda's daughter, Linda Mary, has another memory of what the cottage represents to the family. She says, "Grandpa died in 1936. It was up here. I remember saying good-by – they were taking him to the hospital. He never came back. There were five carloads of flowers at his funeral. Those were the days when people expressed their feelings like that." Harold, in the Homeopathic Hospital's annual report the very next year, wrote:, "No one knows better than I how much my father's long service as Medical Superintendent meant in personal sacrifice of time and comfort and money. I can only say that we, to whom you have now entrusted the medical administration of the Hospital, will try to carry on with something of the same spirit which animated our predecessors." Harold meant these words, and A.R. and Mary Griffith's legacy continued at the hospital and in their own family – most likely because the institution and the family were so intertwined. The late Dave Clark, who married Harold and Linda's daughter Barbara, threw light on professional nurse and doctor relations at the Queen Elizabeth Hospital when he mentioned how perfectly Harold and his young colleague, Dr Dierdre Gillies, "who was Barbara's best friend and like a member of this family," worked together in the operating theatre at the Homeopathic. "Dierdre was also up at the cottage every summer and almost every weekend."

If Homeopathic colleagues were treated as family, family often rated professional respect. "Harold absolutely never told his daughters to do things because they were women, and both had careers – Linda as a social worker and Barbara as an architect, back in the fifties. He treated people as people," Dave Clark said. When asked if becoming a social worker was a kind of religious vocation, as it was for Harold, Linda Mary says simply, "I always wanted to do that," and adds, "actually, Dad became less religious, in an organized sense, as he got older. For one thing, Sundays were the only time he could sleep in a little! Linda continued to be very involved in the Baptist organizations. My father said he just wanted us to know one thing: '*to love God and serve your fellow man.*' I always remembered that. The family had a big emphasis on doing service."

Because her father "loved nothing more than to be with his grandkids when he was older, and he knew them very well," her son Ken was always relating life experiences to things he learned from Harold. Ken said that working at Michael Reese, a famous "world-class" hospital, "was a bit of a deception. I remember thinking, 'These people don't seem to have it right about their own interests and connections with their patients.' They didn't ever have the same kind of warmth and human interest as my granddad. It was more a technical thing at Reese." When asked about how he dealt with the harrowing work of trying to heal the terrible psychic wounds he saw every day, he said gently, "Remember, my own father is a social worker and so is Mom. It's how I grew up. I learned how to deal with these things around the dinner table. Mother marrying a social worker in the first place, I realize now that I'm an adult, was not a coincidence. Harold was very happy about that, you know. And why did she fall in love with my dad? I think it was her expectation that good people should be like her father. She might have imagined we'd all become like Harold."

Many children in the Griffith family did not go into service professions, although a large number did. Of those that didn't, Harold's eldest daughter Barbara, an architect, says, "We were encouraged to be whatever we wanted. And we try to do the same for the next generation." Tom, the massage therapist, says, "All through high school, I thought I'd become a doctor. I was pre-med in college too, when I started getting interested in other things. I remember having conversations with Grandpa about my decision not to go to Med school. You'd think he'd have been all for my continuing, but he totally agreed with me. He said 'Medicine isn't going in the direction it should.' He felt that instead of concentrating on helping people, 'it had attracted people obsessed with money and power.' You know, the most he ever made was about $30,000 a year, despite running a hospital and coming up with all those innovations. But that was never an issue. We always felt like we had enough. And when I did get into massage therapy, he was really supportive. He found it very interesting, as a therapy ... He knew it was really, to some extent, very close to what he had tried to do as a doctor."

Despite having helped invent an entire specialty and defending it all his life, Harold remained a generalist at home as well as work. Tom says, "My grandfather was equally responsible for my love of history. He read to us a lot. I got that love of reading and that marvelous, jovial attitude towards life that showed us that reading was a powerful, even magical activity. He was also a huge baseball fan. We'd play family softball here and when he came to visit in Chicago, we'd go out to professional ball games at Wrigley field; our own dad really wasn't into baseball. There were many other things. He had a very broad spectrum of influence on me."

John Griffith Clark, the one grandchild who did become a doctor, a radiology specialist, agrees that there was no pressure on him one way or another even though, "When I was younger, I wanted to be just like Grandpa. We were the second generation, of course; he was mostly retired in our memories. We didn't see that he was never home like Mom and Linda Mary did. He was just a great grandpa. He was always there for us kids. We'd eat lunch and then he'd say, 'Let's go for a trek in the woods!' and off we'd go. We'd do tons of activities, tinker with machines, build stuff, make toys, go sailing. He was always the one reading us stories at bedtime, especially the family favourite, Seuss's *Thidwick the Big-Hearted Moose.* Or at least he's the one I remember the best; he read so vividly!"

John continues, "So when I was young, I guess I was torn between a service or science career. I was looking for something open, challenging, varied. I wasn't heading into a standard medical career, ever. I wasn't really interested in that primary patient contact. In my physics days I was into medical imaging research and that led to medicine simply because I thought doctors wouldn't listen to my research without an MD degree. Grandpa and I talked very little about my professional choices. It wasn't his style to take me aside and give advice, influence me one way or another, and anyway, I think I was only in second year med school when he died. Of course, I think it definitely pleased him that I was becoming a doctor." John's cousin Ken noted, "Harold was truly a non-judgmental person. He just had a glow to him. He wouldn't push you, he'd kind of steer you in the direction of the things that are undeniably important in life, like honesty or kindness, nature or reading. But he wouldn't interfere. As for us all 'following in his footsteps' in some literal way, he wasn't like that," and his brother Tom adds, "He had a lot of heart. He was a very loving grandfather. We got nothing but love and acceptance from him."

Neither Linda Mary nor Barbara feels they were raised in the clichéd doctor's home where the little woman tirelessly keeps house for and serves the busy physician. Linda Mary says, "At home, in a way, both Linda and Harold dominated. Linda had authority; she taught kindergarten but quit when she got married. That's simply what women were expected to do in those days. Her family was a big part of our lives, too. We did a lot of visiting with her parents and siblings, back and forth. Her dad was a doctor, too, leading the same kind of service life, working very hard with new immigrants. Their grandfather had been a doctor as well, and all her sisters were teachers. Daddy told us that when he proposed to Mom, she made him wait until the end of the summer for an answer, and then they didn't get married for three years! Those where the days when people took their time getting to know each other. But they were very happy, and he was proud of how beautiful Mom was. Once he said to me that, 'It's hard being married to a beautiful woman." I never figured out quite what he meant!"

Harold was amusingly relaxed about subjects like sex and wrote with obvious good cheer at the end of his life that he and his wife had been enjoying it well into their eighties. He also said publicly that he thought masturbation was quite good for people and admitted to practicing it himself. Despite having a reputation as a strict teetotaler in the hospital, he had a cocktail brought to him in his workshed at the cottage every night. When he was younger and his mother Mary, the true teetotaler, was alive, he and Linda met at his brother Jim's property down the lake, ostensibly a destination for a regular evening boat-ride, really a private meeting for a before-dinner nip.

Harold's younger brother Jim, head of surgery from 1935 until his retirement in 1961, was known with amusement at work as "a very different article," as the late Eli Katz, the hospital's ear, nose, and throat specialist, put it. "I knew them from 1951 to 1992, when Harold died. Jim was much more talkative – someone who made no secret of having a drink now and then. He was nice, he was capable, but rougher; there was a real contrast between them, like North and South. For instance, Jim was outgoing and he used to swear sometimes, and I'm sure I never heard Dr Harold swear. Jim didn't go to church much; he'd say something like, 'What the hell for?' He actually ran as a Progressive Conservative candidate in Westmount in the late fifties, and Duplessis was so pleased he promised him money for the hospital. He gave it; the stone was laid in 1960 by the man himself and is still there. But Harold was the opposite of that kind of political animal. He was very reserved and polite and didn't smoke or drink. At the annual banquet, maybe he'd have one glass of beer. And he never insulted anyone or spoke harshly, very good qualities in a hospital administrator!"

Dorothy Mapes, another survivor from the days when the Griffith brothers ran both medicine and surgery, says with some amusement that, "In the days between the 1930s and the 1950s, the chief of surgery was God. So those two brothers had a lot of say about how that hospital was run. But at the same time, when we had problems we could turn to both of them, to Jim as well as to Dr Harold. Jim was more hale, more outgoing; Dr Harold more gentlemanly. But anybody could take their professional and their personal problems to them." From the days when they rowed across a choppy lake together to deliver potato chips and candy to far-flung cottages or wolfed down cranberry jelly and pumpkin pie before trying to emulate grown-up debates, Harold and his younger brother Jim were never very far apart. Jim Griffith's professional life was to be as intimately tied to the Homeopathic/Queen Elizabeth as Harold's and A.R.'s – none of them ever worked anywhere else.

Ken Jacobson analyzed the connection between his grandfather's life at the cottage and his role as a medical administrator and innovator by saying, "Harold had vision as well as energy. I think his secret was that he had confidence that he could materialize his ideas, whether a child's boat or a new way to administer anesthetic. He was also very practical. Whether he was working on a wheelbarrow or organizing a convention of experts from around the world, he could manage all those very pragmatic things that have to be done. He could also explain anything to you, in very basic terms. He didn't use that physician's jargon. He didn't think that these matters needed to be made more complicated than they already were."

Harold's late son-in-law, Dave Clark, volunteered an example. "Harold was the main person who formed a cooperative to save the three islands you see from the house by buying them and holding them in trust. Only these three of the lake's sixteen islands are protected by virtue of our owning shares in the corporation. Of course there was a real push to develop them, like the thirteen others on this lake, and the municipality even tried to tax them as if they were developed. We got good politicians to help and we eventually got the approval of Quebec and the municipality to form a holding company without any development." Dave was standing near one of the cottage's big front windows on a cloudy, breezy July day, with its view of the still-untouched island chain. "Today," he said, "there's so much emphasis on making money. Harold didn't throw money away, but he wasn't looking for it. He worked for the love of this place to protect it. I remember him, at the age of eighty-nine. He stood on this porch and said, 'I came here as a boy of nine, and that view hasn't changed.'"

Although the three Griffith men, Jim, A.R., and Harold, were commendably effective, devoted, and focused, the gifts and talents the Griffith family brought to their hospital are far from unimaginable. All three doctors were real people, with many different facets and normal human faults. Much of what enabled them to become so productive, admired, and emulated by their families and colleagues was the strong set of values developed within their families. These are the common human values still held by many people today, but what was unusual was that the Griffiths' values were not compartmentalized. It's obvious that Harold, for example, was the same person at work and with his family. His core beliefs were apparent in every facet of his life, whether he was reacting as doctor, researcher, administrator, local citizen, nature-lover, baseball fan, husband, father, or grandfather. In that sense they are unusually obvious and help explain the effectiveness of the hospital he ran.

WAR STORIES

The harbour is full of ships, [one] with African troops in their native dress, a sort of flowing gown wrapped around them like a big white bath towel, and on their heads high red fezzes, as gaudy as roosters.

Harold Griffith, *Diary*[2]

Harold and his brothers attended a variety of Montreal High Schools and did tolerably well. Harold was especially involved in local church activities – several different denominations, actually – and also worked for the YMCA. This sounds slightly prissy today, but both the Boy Scouts and the YMCA movements were a new experiment. They were volunteer secular organizations that were heroically trying to civilize a young, urban, male population all too prone to violence, gambling, and drink. The Y's remarkable achievements in providing healthy and safe temporary housing, help for the poor and distressed, and hobbies and recreation for young people in rough environments were so successful that today we take their many improvements in urban social life for granted. But during Harold's era, many enthusiastic young men were helping build these organizations from scratch. They were the kind of clean-cut, middle-class boys who today play sports and get elected class president, both of which Harold also did. In his early years at McGill, Harold worked as a writer and editor, like his father before him, admitting later that he was more interested in his work for the brand-new *McGill Daily*, Canada's first college daily newspaper, and as editor-in-chief of the 1914 *McGill Annual* than he was in his first medical courses.

Like so many before him, Harold Griffith felt torn between two keen interests: medicine and religious service. In the earliest years of the 20th century, thirty years after his father's experiences, medicine as a profession still depended as much on ideals of charity and service as upon the new goals of science and technology. As an adolescent, Harold was passionately interested in missionary work. "I was wrapped up in the work of the YMCA and was convinced that with my help the whole world was about to be converted to Christianity," he wrote with self-deprecating good humour many years later. His major ambition was to combine the two and become a medical missionary. This interest was partially formed in his boys' club days at Lac des Iles where neighbours such as Dr Mott and a Mr Turner, famous for their involvement in the world missionary movement, must have made stirring speeches at the various banquets and while sitting around his parents' table.

Harold was also keenly sociable and excelled at organizing dances and parties for the various churches and service organizations to which he belonged. Although his future wife, Linda Aylen, was a high school companion for a while, he had several other girl friends, one of whom he proposed to in 1915. He was undoubtedly feeling vulnerable just before shipping out for war at the tender age of 19 but was declined in a classic "Dear John" letter he got at the front. The three eldest Griffith boys all volunteered for service in World War I. Harold explained that they enlisted largely because they thought the war "would be a grand adventure that would only last a few months." Four long years later, all three miraculously returned home physically unscathed, although he later wrote, "I have often thought what an ordeal the war years must have been for my parents, with three of their boys in dangerous positions. While friends of ours were falling on all sides, not one of us was ever wounded or suffered serious illness."[3]

Harold was at Vimy Ridge as a stretcher-bearer and on the lines in several other harrowing battles. A year passed after Vimy before he finally wrote his mother, Mary, about trying to get the wounded out of trenches knee-deep with mud and under fire. He admitted candidly that, "We expected every minute to be our last. I remember looking at Jack Rooney while we were all working for dear life and he smiled so cheerily in his bright Irish way. A few minutes later, he was blown into the air."[4] Like everyone else at the time, Harold refers to the Germans as "Fritz" and "the Hun." But despite this, he was already the calm, fair, objectively compassionate person his colleagues describe in decades to come. "The rest of the day is a hazy, confused memory," he wrote, still about Vimy. "Prisoners were coming in, either carrying our wounded or helping each other. They provided us with invaluable help all day long." And this was a battle in which Canadian troops were known for their ferocity and bravery as well as for very rough treatment of German prisoners. Although still very young, Harold always saw the human side of the situation. "I remember," he wrote, "finding four Germans doing their best to drag along one of our men whose arm had been shot off almost at the elbow. I got him onto a stretcher, tied up the raw stump, stopped the bleeding, but put him aside [figuring he would] die. Half an hour later when I had a minute's breathing spell, I went to look at him and found him alive and conscious and with returning pulse. I sent him off by the next squad and I've often wondered how he got on. All this time, the German shells were falling close to us...I was dressing a wounded man when a flying piece of shell struck the poor chap again and broke his leg."

The worst part of the day was still to come. Harold's mother was steeped in the medical profession, so she didn't need to be spared realistic detail. "Shortly before dusk," Harold wrote, "it started to snow, just enough to whiten the ground and add freezing to the many forms of death men could meet that day." Harold had a minor breather in the dug-out, so he decided to go see if he could help with transporting the wounded. "At the railhead I found a great congestion. Those responsible for the clearing of the wounded along the railway had simply disappeared, leaving fifty or sixty poor fellows lying in the snow. I saw the officer in charge of the prisoners and arranged to have all those cases carried out at once by the Germans, and then took thirty Germans back to our dugout with me where I still had twelve or fourteen stretcher cases. They were tired and hungry and sullen. I was unarmed and alone with them."

In the dugout, the nervous young soldier found, to his joy, "two dozen tins of bully beef, some bread and biscuits and most precious of all, a long drink of water each!" These transformed his frightening charges into "the most grateful, good-humoured group imaginable." Harold remembered some high school German and a few prisoners could speak French, "so we got on quite well. After our meal, a rest and a smoke, everyone turned to with a will and we cleared all the cases." Harold managed to find someone to take the prisoners away to a suitable shelter and then went back to the railhead, only to find "a poor, half-frozen, snow-covered wounded German lying motioning for help." Harold managed to get the man onto a miraculously passing truck. After that, he lost his way getting back to the dugout "and stumbled over ground which the night before had been Hunland. But at last about midnight I flopped down in the mud and blood of our dugout and fell asleep."

Harold had the good fortune to be saved from a situation that would likely have led to his death. Thanks to some McGill connections working on his behalf, he was transferred to safer Navy duty, patrolling for subs in the Mediterranean. Although young and not formally trained, Harold had obtained his transfer through a former McGill professor, who was now an admiral, on the strength of his still very slight medical knowledge. He was regularly called upon for first aid duties, stitching up or dressing wounds, and helping give ether to sailors injured on board ship. There were many more people nearby whom Harold could do nothing to help, however, including sailors within his convoy who drowned before his eyes after a submarine attack and a few miserable survivors of the Armenian genocide whom he soberly reported seeing in camps during shore duty.

Later, near Jaffa, which is a centre of fighting and suffering to this day, the only good thing that happened was that "the retreat of the enemy was so hasty they didn't take time to poison or fill in the wells." Harold describes the population as being "in a wretched condition – starving and they are so used to oppression they don't yet realize that they are now free. Many are still starving, either too dejected or too frightened to apply for help." In November of 1917, he wrote that, "The Turks had been maintaining a sort of 'Red Cross' hospital in Jaffa for children, but it had become utterly neglected. The poor children are now without clothes or food or supplies of any kind, lying sick and dying on the bare stone floor." Although his Admiral was sending for aid, their own supplies were inadequate and even their own wounded were being evacuated overland by car and train because, Harold wrote, "Disease is rampant all through Palestine. We have not entered Jerusalem yet as it is a hotbed of plague."[5]

This period pretty much marked the end of Harold's enthusiasm for saving humanity through missionary work. He would concentrate on physical and emotional healing from then on. It's a shock to be reminded that Harold Griffith was really only a college boy throughout this period – at the back of his 1917 war diary, he proudly recorded having read thirty-two books in six months, including classics like *Lorna Doone*, *Quo Vadis*, and *Les Miserables*. He wrote with unsparing realism about the horrors he saw but with equal skill and more enthusiasm about interesting officers and their mechanical talents and games and jaunts with friends to the exotic sights nearby. His discussion of world events, however, sounds more like the ruminations of a man of 40. On 3 January 1918, he wrote, "I suppose in history the Russian Revolution will go down as one of the most far-reaching events of this period. The news we get from Russia is very scant. Apparently, the ultra-radical 'Bolshevics' are now in control of the government, but how sincerely they are supported by the nation it is hard to say...Lloyd George has weathered a severe political storm arising from a speech he made in Paris in November...[And here] the submarine continues to be our most serious menace. But I suppose we'll pull through somehow."[6]

THE HOME FRONT

We were lucky we had no serious accidents as I often worked under conditions I would hesitate to risk now.
                                        Harold Griffith speaking of the early 1920s[7]

When they returned from war, this generation of "boys" did not receive any money to help them with post-war training, as veterans did after World War II. However, other considerations were extended to them. For example, Harold's younger brother Jim had enlisted a year after Harold, at the age of seventeen, and hadn't yet taken his final high school exams. "After the war," Harold wrote, "it was decided to give such young soldiers their matriculation without any exams and Jim entered with the class of 1924, only two years behind me." After a single year's internship in New York, Jim Griffith returned to Montreal. "He never really served a residency in surgery," Harold wrote, "but he liked that line of work, and joined the surgical staff at the Homeopathic in 1925. He set up a general practice in Verdun that became really busy, but he had a real aptitude for surgery. When Dr Novinger, the chief surgeon, died suddenly in 1936,

Jim succeeded to the post of chief surgeon and was very successful at that post for the rest of his life."[8]

Casually falling into a demanding specialty like surgery, particularly in a hospital where his father was the medical supervisor, makes it sound as if standards at the Homeopathic were pretty elastic. In fact, they were stricter than most at that time. Few people today realize how young the entire concept of a medical specialty is, now that generalists are rare. Although there were specially trained surgeons by the end of World War I, surgery had not developed into a profession with members with legally or even morally required courses and certificates. Jim was behaving as almost every other young surgeon did at the time. He was good at surgery and he liked it, so he ended up doing it. Other specialties, from dermatology to anesthesiology, barely existed even as concepts. In fact, it would be Harold Griffith who was a primary force behind the professionalization of anesthesiology – a specialty he never took special courses to attain.

Harold's early professional life was shaped by experiences that are almost eerily similar to his father's thirty years earlier. "One of the standard requirements for a McGill M.D. was to serve several weeks' intern service at the Montreal Maternity Hospital during the final year," Harold wrote. "I got out of this obligation by going to New York for a three-week course at the New York Maternity Hospital, during which students had an opportunity to see deliveries in the hospital and of doing deliveries in the tenement district of the Lower East Side ... The students were sent out alone, without any nurse or other helper and with very little equipment, only a Kelly pad, scrubbing brush, bichlinde tablets, and a pair of scissors to cut the cord. No gloves and no anaesthetics." The patients benefiting from the attentions of these young interns were almost all recently arrived immigrants from Greece, Italy, or Poland who were living in five-story tenement houses below the Brooklyn Bridge.[9]

Harold later wrote, "It seemed as if all the babies were born on the fifth story, with one cold water tap serving four apartments, and one toilet. It was also the rule that all babies must be delivered with the mother lying on the kitchen table, not in her bed. All the other children were sent to neighbours or put out on the fire escape. The father was usually in a very emotional state. It was prohibition time in the U.S., but usually the father had a bottle of some homemade liquor and insisted on the doctor drinking the health of the new baby. [On one occasion, although] I tried to resist, the father felt quite insulted and I finally had to take a taste of some liquid fire made of raisins. I ended the week with severe diarrhea – very uncomfortable." Harold, like his father before him, finished this work with relief. "It was really very primitive obstetrics...and couldn't compare with what we were used to in Montreal."[10]

Even work back at home was fairly rough. Only a few months after he had been writing his mother from Europe about Vimy Ridge, Harold was back home and living in his father's hospital. "Before college resumed in 1919," he wrote, "I moved into the Homeopathic Hospital to start my career as a student intern. Ted Waugh had finished his term and Walter Scriver also joined me at the hospital. We made a good team, and never quarreled."[11] Resident doctors still lived in hospitals until the 1950s and even into the 60s.

As mentioned in chapter 2, all early hospitals were homes for most of the people who worked in them. By Harold's time, the orderlies and staff were no longer living under the institution's roof, but nurses and young doctors did live there. Two other young medical students, Gavin Miller and Archie Wilkie, both of whom later joined Harold on the faculty of medicine at McGill, were part of his live-in crew. The medical students who joined this struggling community hospital were doing work that ranged from nearly the highest to the very lowest, without most of the differentials in status granted to class, or even sex, that had characterized both earlier and later institutions. "We took night calls," Harold remembered, "attended to out-patients, did the routine lab work, catheterized male patients and prepared them for operation, assisted the surgeons and gave anesthetics. We even carried helpless patients to and from their rooms, pulled them upstairs in the old hand-operated elevator and...helped the nurses scrub the floors."

Harold wrote at length in early memoirs about the professors he was studying under during this period and, true to form, called attention to the people who were the most unusual. He made special mention of taking genetics from Dr Carrie Derrick, "one of McGill's pioneer women teachers." Harold goes out of his way to be inclusive, a habit that is strong today but was certainly not typical of his time. Of his McGill class, Medicine 1922, he wrote, "We were a fairly serious crowd, about half of us war veterans, but in one way we were really unique; it was the first medical class to which McGill had admitted women. We had five, all good students. Two of these first women graduates went on to become McGill teachers of distinction – Jessie Boyd Scriver in pediatrics, and Eleanor Percivall in obstetrics and gynaecology."[12] The closest colleagues in his personal career as an anesthesiologist, not surprisingly given his lack of chauvinism, were women: Enid Johnson and Dierdre Gillies.

Harold's career was shaped by both women. Enid Johnson was his partner during the 1940s and as a team, they experimented with and developed the revolutionary new anestheic techniques described ahead. Harold was upset when Enid left Montreal to marry and practice in the Maritimes, but a young physician named Dierdre Gillies arrived to do her residency at the hospital. Her father was a famed early anesthesiologist from Scotland. She became best friends with Harold's daughter Barbara and soon became Harold Griffith's protégé. For the rest of his life they would run the anesthesiology department side by side. After he retired and contracted Parkinson's Disease, like a third daughter, she took care of him.

NEW CURES FOR A POST-WAR WORLD

Two record years during the great war ... mean our Hospital has practically been filled to capacity all the time. A larger and more modern building is becoming a greater necessity every day ... There were times when we were hard pressed for emergency cases, and beds had to be speedily improvised.

A.R. Griffith, report of the Medical Superintendent, 1917–18[13]

The 1918 flu pandemic struck the world just as the war was finishing. "The epidemic which had been raging in various countries and which I had encountered months before at the Dardenelles struck Canada in full force," Griffith wrote. "In Montreal, schools and other activities were closed and people were dying in the hundreds. Doctors were of course overwhelmed with work. The deaths were mainly due to pneumonia following a few days' illness, which was marked by aching head and bones and total weakness. Father was fortunate in having homeopathic medicines to use. His patients simply did not acquire the pneumonia and almost all recovered. So many patients had the same symptoms that it was possible to use the same homeopathic remedies in many cases – *gelsemin, eupectorium, belladonna, aferiumphos*, etc."

Harold's observation of this crisis affected the way he used all types of chemical medicines later in life. "I became convinced that there was much truth in homeopathy, although I never believed that '*similia similius currentor*' is a universal truth. There is no doubt, however, that in many cases an infinitesimal dose of a drug will produce the opposite effect of that same drug given in a large dose. I made many calls on patients in that difficult autumn of 1918, but I only really lost one case." Harold's observations are born out by the morbidity statistics included in the annual reports. Despite a significant increase in patients and the number of days they spent in the hospital, the influenza epidemic caused no more than three or four deaths at the Homeopathic in 1918 and 1919, and even pneumonia deaths were no higher than in previous years.[14] In 2005, *Ode* magazine reported similar anecdotal evidence from homeopathic hospitals in Europe.

In 1918, when Harold was returning from the war, the hospital was facing an overcrowding crisis and urgently required an expansion. Only twelve years before, 1907, it had acquired two more houses adjacent to the first building on McGill College and completed its first major expansion. The Homeopathic could be proud of their excellent handling of the influenza crisis and their continuing decent results against tuberculosis, with an average of two deaths a year, as well as typhoid, with only one death out of the twenty cases that were the norm in such a hospital. But by 1919, a hard-pressed A.R. Griffith wrote, "Every month the Hospital has been filled to its utmost capacity and usually there is a long waiting list. Never has the need of a new hospital been more apparent ... We ought to have at least twenty-five public beds. Our present accommodation is constantly overtaxed."[15]

In this, they were typical of almost every hospital in the country. As previously mentioned, the general population was growing and increasing numbers of paying patients were beginning to trust these institutions. Most significantly, the non-private, that is, non-paying, patients were especially increasing in numbers because of immigration and industrialization. In the early years of the century, when one might expect more deaths in the presumably less carefully-treated public wards that were still so feared and avoided by the middle classes, the Homeopathic took care to compare figures. They found that most of the deaths in those years were among the private patients, a result that is perhaps less surprising in that they were the only members of the population with the means to afford to be hospitalized for long, fatal illnesses such as cancer. In 1906, for example, A.R. Griffith was careful to note that of that year's twenty-four deaths, "five only were public patients." He even gives circumstances of their deaths, noting that two were over seventy-eight and one died of a cerebral hemorrhage after having been brought to the hospital in a coma. That means the other nineteen were all private, paying, well-to-do patients.[16] In terms of public versus private deaths, this was a typical year.

This was still almost twenty years before the new building was secured on Marlowe Street and the little Homeopathic, for all its brave words, was then trying to cope with treating nearly 1,500 people a year. It must have been a difficult, even frightening place much of the time. Harold Griffith, in his own memoirs of the period, admits that at this point, little progress had been made in general hospital care since his father's youth. "Pneumonia was 'captain of the men of death,'" he wrote, "typhoid fever and tuberculosis were lurking everywhere, puerperal fever was a dreaded complication of childbirth, syphilis prevalent and hard to treat, pernicious anaemia was invariably fatal, diabetes incurable."[17] Harold continued with this grim picture, describing how, "Some diseases which are rarely seen now were then common. There were no sulfa drugs or antibiotics. In my senior year at McGill, Banting made his first announcement of insulin ... Juvenile diabetes, which had been almost invariably fatal, was brought under control. Pernicious anaemia was [still] common and almost always fatal. I remember giving my first transfusion to a patient with pernicious anaemia. I used a medical student in my class as a donor. We didn't know much about blood groups or incompatibility. And although the patient felt bucked up for awhile, he didn't last long."

Harold also mentions that in the 1920s and 30s, "the brain and chest were almost inaccessible to the surgeon's knife."[18] In terms of surgery in particular, although the profession was a step ahead of the 1850s' use of whisky and biting rags to kill the pain, chloroform and ether were still the only way to keep a patient alive while the surgeons attempted to hone their skills at appendectomies and amputations. Because of the harshness of these chemicals, many patients succumbed to the anesthetic rather than the disease. Besides, their effect on the respiratory system made many forms of basic surgery on the human throat and torso impossible.

This description of Harold's new profession, which had held fairly steady for at least thirty years, was about to change radically. A tidal wave of technological advancement, largely brought about by the continuing industrial revolution and greatly added to by the exigencies of the recent war, was about to strike. It hasn't receded yet. This advancement came in three crucial areas, two of which were already in place by the late 19th century. The first to bear practical fruit was the professionalization of nursing. The second was the discovery of microscopic pathogens and the consequent development of public health practices such as immunization, pasteurization, and food inspection. The last and most recent was the development of antibiotics in the 1930s and 40s, which was also accompanied by breakthroughs in anesthesiology and therefore in surgery.

Nursing, as soon as it was professionalized, was quick to bring lowered human mortality rates through attention to hygiene, nutrition, and general care. In public health, the initiatives that made an enormous difference included legislation to control the purity of food, water, and milk, along with official inspections and fines for infractions. Antibiotics allowed doctors to control many of the most virulent of infectious diseases and finally, better means of performing surgery meant a vast increase in successful operations. The combination of the new understandings of germs along with the new government oversight and regulations resulted in the control of some of the worst infectious diseases, such as typhoid, that had accompanied the industrial revolution when large numbers of people crowded into cities.

To this day, the simplest forms of public health care, that is, sanitation and inoculation, have had more to do with improving child mortality and general human longevity statistics than any other development in medical science, including our many high-tech drugs and technologies. The educational and preventative side of public health also remains the least expensive way to care for a population's health. The costs of preventing infectious and other diseases through taxes, education, and legislation – for example, lowering cancer and heart attack rates by discouraging smoking and junk food – are far less costly to a society than dealing with the acute illnesses that result from the lack of a vibrant public health sector. To put it more bluntly, apart from the development of diagnostic tools such as x-rays and MRIs, neither of which actually heals but both of which can catch a serious condition early in its development, very little that has come out of investigative laboratory science has increased human longevity or well-being at a rate that approaches what had been attained by the turn of the 20th century when the discovery of germs and subsequent emphasis on simple cleanliness, a good diet, and clean water made an enormous difference.

So, although the genius doctor in the lab coat has been the adored hero of the 20th century, in actual fact, only a few drugs, such as insulin and the antibiotics, have greatly increased the survival rate and longevity of the population in a statistical sense. The effectiveness of antibiotics, we are now learning, is severely limited by overuse and therefore only available for a set period of time. The majority of the other drugs prescribed today only alleviate symptoms. Steroids, the drugs that control blood pressure, and the long list of chemo-therapies may induce fairly long and very welcome periods of remission from certain diseases, although this relief is often accompanied by side-effects. All the same, these few drugs have made a big difference in everyone's perception of modern medicine.

There is one more highly important discovery in the realm of chemistry that changed survival rates forever: the perfection of drugs that induce anesthesia. Surgical advances required the ability to put people to sleep *long enough* so that doctors could hone their skills and techniques for hours at a stretch. Today, as we all know, surgery not only rebuilds shattered hands or skulls: it can also replace arteries, livers, and even hearts. It can be argued that the incredible, microscopic sewing dexterity of modern surgeons was a human talent that always lay within the realm of the possible. The big difficulty was developing drugs that would allow patients to sleep through invasions of their bodies that would otherwise have been too much of a shock. The deadly effects of shock, respiratory blockage, or chemical overdose, which had made major operations such a limited option when the Montreal Homeopathic was still young, magically vanished, almost overnight. And interestingly enough, the world-famous genius who developed the most effective anesthetic drugs of our age, the ones that made the entire surgical revolution possible, was a humble GP from the Montreal Homeopathic Hospital. His name is very familiar: Dr Harold Griffith.

GREED, CURSES, AND GETTING HIGH: THE HORRIBLE HISTORY OF ANESTHETICS

My husband's great gift, which he devoted to the service of mankind, proved a curse to himself and his family.

Mrs Elizabeth Morton, wife of the man credited with the first anesthetic use of ether[19]

One would think that a book titled *Essays on the First Hundred Years of Anesthesia* would bore the average reader. However, this book, written in the 1970s by an anesthetist named W. Wesley Sykes, is full of exciting descriptions of South American arrow poisons, operating room explosions, and the exploits of an early 19th-century English squire and bird enthusiast named Charles Waterton, who penetrated unknown jungles, rode on a live crocodile, and handled rattlesnakes with his bare hands – all because of his vivid interest in exotic poisons. It also includes bitter anecdotes about some of the most tragic-comic inanities ever perpetrated in the name of science and modern medicine, recorded with a sardonic wit that would do credit to a BBC satire. And yet it actually turns out to be relatively restrained and prosaic, considering the drama stuffed into every cranny of the history of anesthetics.

In discussing the 1890 account by a famous German surgeon of some anesthetic difficulties he suffered while performing a surgery, for example, Wesley Sykes quotes from the doctor's autobiography:

> "The operation (for a lung condition) was proceeding normally, when, through a cause we were never able to ascertain, the glowing cautery set light to the ether vapour being used as the anaesthetic. The violent explosion that followed was repeated almost immediately as an oxygen cylinder blew up. The patient was killed on the spot, the Sister and the assistant were injured, and I lost an eardrum."

"This," remarks the author, "is exactly like saying, 'I dropped a lighted match into the petrol tank, and then, through a cause we were never able to ascertain, the car caught fire.'"[20] Further on, he mentions a surgeon named Deloup who used a solution of "4 percent cocaine for spinal anaesthesia in the early days of the method. After 100 cases, he concluded that this was as safe or safer than general anaesthesia. His experiences of general anaesthesia must have been indeed unfortunate."[21] Even the mild and generally forgiving Harold Griffith, when discussing why he took a special interest in anesthesiology from the very outset of his medical career, stated that "from what I had seen of our use of ether and chloroform in the War, I knew there must be a better way of administering anesthesia." He was referring to slopping some ether on a handy rag, clapping it over a wounded soldier's mouth and nose, and holding him down while he choked, vomited, and then became either satisfactorily unconscious or dead.

One of the reasons that anesthesia remained primitive for so long is that from the beginning it seems to have attracted the interest of an assortment of what we would now call dilettantes, mountebanks, mystics, and magicians, rather than serious scientists. These early researchers imparted a carnival tone that didn't leave the subject until well into the 20th century. This tone probably came from the fact that the effects of a successful anesthetic really are nothing short of magical. Historically, the whole concept of the apparent cessation of consciousness and its subsequent miraculous return was viewed primarily as a spiritual event. From the Paleolithic on, virtually all traditional peoples consumed the narcotic or hallucinogenic plants native to their regions in order to achieve a state of delirium and semi-consciousness, which they universally associated with a heightened spiritual receptivity. Often this drugged state was believed to be identical with death, from which the users would miraculously return with enhanced powers. At the same time, the concept of using the same or similar magically powerful natural drugs to forestall the deadly effects of pain and shock, so that a sick or injured person could recover, is a practice nearly as ancient as the quest for spiritual delirium. There is evidence that the earliest societies understood many of the physical effects of the opium poppy and several other narcotic plants, especially *Mandragora autumnalis*, the fabled mandrake root that is a relative of deadly nightshade; *Hyoscyamus albus* and *H. niger*, white and black henbane, respectively; *Datura stromonium*, jimson weed; and *Cannibis sativa*, or marijuana. All of the plants mentioned except marijuana contain the poison *atropine* as their primary active agent.

Such plants were part of many religious and quasi-magical rituals, but by the Egyptian period were being used in healing as practiced by physicians, as well as in the magic practiced by priests. The notably less spiritually inclined ancient Romans prepared a pain-killing liquid from *Mandragora* for surgical purposes.[22] The early scientists of the Arabic world, including Avicenna (980–1037), Al Razi (1145–1209), and Al Baghdady (1121–1213) are to be credited with serious advances in the treatment of pain during the early Middle Ages. In Western Europe at the time, pain and illness "were interpreted to be God's punishment for crime and sin" and were thought to be best treated by prayer and redemption.[23] The Arabs kept the practice of drinking *Mandagora* and other drugs alive and also experimented with hashish, hemlock, and henbane. They discovered that alcohol is the active ingredient in the fermented spirits of grapes and other fruits and vegetables, and they learned how to synthesize sulphuric acid in order to distil alcohol.[24]

Western Europe may have been far behind the Muslim scholars at this stage, but however much medieval theologians dismissed pain as a servant of God's purpose, the uses of these magical herbs were so traditional, and practical that ordinary people, "mostly women," still knew "formulas for soporifics and analgesics" and presumably prescribed them in similar forms for similar cases, if less scientifically. Thus, the religious ban on anesthetics and analgesics in the West was never complete, and by the 13th century, medical texts give evidence of something called "a soporific sponge," which was used prior to surgery.[25] Some version of the "soporific sponge" has been in use in medical cases for nearly a thousand years of recorded history. Given the proven analgesic and anesthetic effects of its quite powerful herbal ingredients, it is unlikely that it was completely useless.

Still, the early physician's ability to alleviate physical pain changed little over close to a thousand years, and the situation persisted well after the discovery of what would become the first modern anesthetic. Ether was discovered in the high Middle Ages, in 1275, by the Spanish chemist Raymundua Lullius; he called it "sweet vitriol."[26] In 1540, "sweet vitriol" was synthesized by the German scientist Valerius Cordus, and at about the same time, the Swiss alchemist Paracelsus discovered the gas's weirdly enjoyable hypnotic effects, probably by experiencing them himself. In 1730, a German scientist named W.G. Frobenius changed its name to "ether."

This was the dawn of the "Enlightenment," the great boost in scientific enquiry that came with a philosophic decision in Western culture to place human, rather than divine, concerns at the centre of creation and learned interest. Discoveries came about rapidly in the wake of these new attitudes. By the end of the century, the British physicians Richard Pearson and Thomas Beddoes were using ether to treat a variety of diseases, including "catarrhal fever" (what might be called severe sinusitis today) and scurvy. By 1805, American doctors were using ether to treat pulmonary infections, but no one had thought of using it to put patients to sleep. The ancient soporific sponge of doubtful efficacy was no longer in use, and in any case, there were few surgical interventions at most 19th century hospitals.

Between 1821 and 1846, the Massachusetts General, in Boston, registered fewer than one surgical case a month, and these were performed only as last resorts. The danger of death purely from shock was so high that what we now call "elective" surgery was largely unknown. The medical history section of the Harvard University website notes that some doctors actually used a hard left to the jaw to render patients unconscious. But in general, "opium and alcohol were the only agents ... regarded as of practical value in diminishing the pain of operations." That pain was beyond what most of us can imagine today. One elderly Boston physician, reminiscing about pre-anesthesia surgery, wrote in

1897 of the "yells and screams, most horrible in my memory now, after an interval of so many years."[27] Of the two chemical agents available, alcohol had to be administered in such large doses as to cause vomiting and even death, while opium's side-effects were nearly as bad and the drug was unable to "completely blunt the feel of a surgeon's knife."

In accordance with the history of such substances, humans first used ether for less than practical purposes. In the first part of the 19th century, medical students seem to have regularly gotten hold of the compound for what were termed "ether frolics." In other words, like their Paleolithic forebears, they used it to get high. But in 1842, a formerly frolicsome student, Dr Crawford Williamson Long, remembered its effects and used the gas to remove a tumor from the neck of a Mr James Venable. Because he didn't write up his results until 1848, he was upstaged by a Connecticut dentist, Dr William T.G. Morton, who had once worked under the tutelage of Dr Horace Wells, an early promoter of another pain reliever: nitrous oxide. In January of 1845, Wells had achieved a humiliating notoriety when he was granted the right to a public demonstration of the action of nitrous oxide at the Massachusetts General Hospital. The demonstration failed, probably due to an insufficient dose, and the room filled with catcalls of "Humbug!" from a public that still regarded any claim to harmless and reversible unconsciousness as the very stuff of carnivals and mountebanks.

Through Wells' colleague, a Dr Charles T. Jackson who was a professor at the Medical College of Massachusetts (Harvard) where William Morton was in pre-med, Morton decided to do some more research on "ether frolics." He experimented on himself and on small animals, and on 30 September 1846, removed a tooth from a local merchant, Eben H. Frost, who was anesthetized by ether. Word spread, and less than a month later, on 16 October 1846, young Dr Morton anesthetized a patient for a senior surgeon at the Massachusetts General Hospital. The surgeon successfully removed a "congenital vascular malformation" from a patient's neck, and Morton announced to the excited spectators, no doubt in reference to Wells' experience in the same room only four years before, "Gentlemen, this is no Humbug!"

It was a great day for anesthesia, surgery, and especially for patients. The *People's Journal* in London wrote in early 1847, "Oh, what delight for every feeling heart to find the new year ushered in with the announcement of this noble discovery of the power to still the sense of pain, and veil the eye and memory from all the horrors of an operation. We have conquered pain!"[28] In England as well as in America, it was hailed as "the greatest gift ever made to suffering humanity!" The Ether Monument, the oldest statue in Boston's historic Public Garden, remains a touching tribute to the event.

All over the world, surgeons, realizing their work was about to become transformed, literally jumped at the chance to use the new gas. In late December of 1846, only two months after the first event in Boston, Professor Robert Liston of the University College Hospital in London, England, used ether in an operation to take off a leg at the thigh. Liston's patient remained partly conscious but showed no distress and later remembered no pain. Within days, "operating sessions intended for students and visiting practitioners but open to hospital patrons and patients' friends were suddenly as popular as music-hall turns." In mid-January, a crowd caused a stampede in the halls of Guy Hospital, climbing up to look down through the skylight, crowding about the gurney, and terrifying the patient, a 14 year-old boy.[29] By April of the following year, use of the new wonder-drug had spread from Great Britain to France, Switzerland, Germany, and Spain, and as far as Russia, Portugal, Czechoslovakia, and all the Scandinavian countries. Its practitioners, led by the brilliant John Snow in London, were already taking baby steps towards specialization; they were not yet known as "anesthetists," but as "etherists."[30]

One would think that honours and gratitude, as well as position and wealth, would have accrued to this "greatest gift." But Morton, Jackson, Wells, and Long, the central figures of the dramatic discovery of modern anesthesia, by and large reaped only poverty, public humiliation, addiction, illness, and hardship from their association with ether – so much so that it wouldn't be hard to believe that the human demand for a magically painless and reversible oblivion holds the traditional price of miraculous cures: a curse.

The first to go was Horace Wells, Morton's former tutor and partner, who had continued to fight for the efficacy of his discovery, nitrous oxide. He had already given up his practice in the 1840s, apparently after a fatality, when in the winter of 1847 he began experiments with yet another drug, chloroform. He became addicted and only a few months later, in January of 1848, was arrested for throwing acid on the clothing of a prostitute. The official website of the anesthetic nursing profession notes, "Two days later, at Tombs Prison, he committed suicide by slashing his thigh with a razor." He was 33 years old.[31]

Simple greed brought on most of William Morton's problems. Right after his groundbreaking surgery in 1846, he made the disingenuous claim that he had discovered a new substance, "Letheon." "He spent all his time and money promoting the use of Letheon and not practicing dentistry. Initially, he refused to reveal the nature of the solution." This drew a very negative response from the medical community and was a serious mistake because ether has a very distinct aroma that was soon recognized. In 1847, Morton began calling it "ether" again. However, encouraged by both the son of a patent commissioner and Charles T. Jackson, the person who had initially sponsored his and Wells' work at Harvard, Morton tried to get exclusive use of it by patenting the material. Despite the tantalizing experience of nearly getting $100,000 in 1852 and again in 1854 from the U.S. Congress in recognition of his discovery, Morton never received any money. He died of a stroke at the early age of 49 and his wife and five children were left penniless.

Charles Jackson, Morton's co-patenter, was no stranger to bitter litigation over credit and money. He was one of many who had claimed some of Thomas Edison's inventions as his own. As far as ether was concerned, at first he received some recognition, in the form of a shared prize of 5000 francs from the French Academy of Medicine. Morton had refused his share of this prize as he was bitterly feuding with Jackson and Long and claiming the discovery was his alone. Some time after Morton's death, Jackson suffered a stroke that resulted in such severe paralysis and speech impairment that his caretakers thought he had gone mad. He spent his last days in an insane asylum, surviving until the age of 75. As for the probable first person to have used ether as anesthesia, Dr Crawford Williamson Long, he also feuded over money and discovery credit. However, he lived a normal if somewhat impoverished life, continued to practice, and died at the age of 62 while trying to administer ether to a woman in labor.[32]

DANCING WITH DEATH

Marshal Joffre, commander of the French Armies in the First World War, said that it took 10,000 to 15,000 lives to train a major-general. It doesn't take as many as that to train an anaesthetist, but it does take a certain number.

W. Stanley Sykes, *Essays on the First Hundred Years of Anesthesia*[33]

Chloroform is the modern age's second most famous anesthetic, and its history isn't much more cheerful. This chemical was first produced slightly earlier than ether, in 1831, but its uses weren't solidified until about the same time. Two chemists, the German Justus von Liebig and the French Eugene Soubeiran, combined chlorine bleach powder (calcium hypochlorite) with acetone (propanone or ethanol) to create the new compound. We now know that these substances are highly carcinogenic over the long term. There were also shorter-term problems, such as serious liver, kidney, and heart effects, that were not discovered for some time. Neither scientist seems to have thought of a practical use for his discovery, so it wasn't used to any effect for about 15 years. In 1847, the Edinburgh obstetrician James Young Simpson thought of using it as a general anesthesia during childbirth after having tried it out on himself only a few weeks previously. After this, its use in surgical situations of all kinds expanded rapidly, especially in Europe; Queen Victoria, mother of so many babies, blessed its advent, as did many other women undergoing childbirth.

As is true with other painkilling drugs, inhaling chloroform can cause dizziness, intoxication, and addiction, but its most serious side-effect is sudden death from cardiac fibrillation. Because this did not affect more than about one in 2,000 to 6,000 people, it wasn't immediately noticed. Still, as early as a year after its first use, the first fatality was reported. More followed. There was a good deal of controversy and many studies in the years to follow but until 1911, no solid conclusions were reached. And even though the heart arrhythmia effects were proven at that time, the anesthetic continued to grow so much in popularity that it was used in a staggering 80 to 95 percent of all anesthetic cases performed in the UK and the German-speaking countries. It was less popular in the U.S. and Canada, but continued to be employed right up until the middle 1970s, by which time the proof of its dangers had become overwhelming. Ether only kills one person per 14,000 to 28,000, making chloroform four to ten times more dangerous.

Curare, which was to make surgery far safer than chloroform or ether, was a speculative drug in terms of any sort of use. In fact, its eventual application to anesthesia was not foreseen by the people most interested in it – even well after its final adaptation to anesthetic use by Dr Harold Griffith in 1942. Consequently, only chloroform and ether, both of which were sometimes administered after a dose of alcohol, were used in surgery.

Doctors and druggists in the 19th century considered the number of deaths due to chloroform administration compared to the number of times it was administered "an acceptable risk." Very recent deaths due to the administration of drugs like NSAIDs or the Prosac family illustrate the fact that this criteria remains the basis of licensing most pharmaceutical drugs. Even a hundred years ago, however, the public was beginning to have views that were different from the drug developers. When quoting a famous old physiologist's disdainful remarks that "many people will now suffer the short but extremely severe pain caused by the extraction of a tooth rather than run the trivial risk of using an anaesthetic," Sykes ripostes with, "the public had, at any rate, sufficient sense to realize that, although the percentage of deaths might be statistically and numerically small, each fatality was 100 percent dead, a fact which appears to have escaped the attention of the physiologist."[34]

Then, as now, purveyors and enthusiastic promoters of these powerful drugs saw both utility and wealth and fought any kind of restrictions or regulations on their products.[35] The few doctors who realized the complexity of anesthesiology and were trying to make it into a specialty were left to fume. As late as 1901, the British Society of Anaesthetics complained to the General Medical Council that there was still no compulsory training in anesthesia in any hospital in the whole of Great Britain and Ireland, no examinations on the subject, and that "in view of the fact that every doctor is liable to be called upon to give one," compulsory instruction should be insisted upon.[36]

When taxed with the dangers of chloroform, the medical profession did not turn to primary research and try to understand how the human body responded to the various new drugs. Instead, it took the rather more common research direction of trying to find its way around the problem of too many deaths from one method by introducing new chemicals or new ways to deliver the old ones. Sykes mentions that throughout the rest of the 19th century, the promoters of various new anesthetics and modalities tended to be more enthusiastic than critical of any new development in the field. Edward Lawrie, a great protagonist of chloroform, claimed that because the heart was rightly "refusing to convey any more chloroform to the brain ... If the patient had only been left alone ... the stoppage of the heart would have saved his life." Overdoses occurred due to the simple ingestion of too much of the chemical. Patients vary; they come in different sizes, metabolic rates, states of health, and vulnerability to allergens. So researchers, while investigating how to avoid overdoses by means of special, calibrated machines and the addition of oxygen, "omitted from their calculations [such important complications as] primary cardiac failure and delayed chloroform poisoning."[37]

FROM GUESSWORK TO SCIENCE

The first problem which interested me was the provision of a better
airway. Anaesthesia in those days was all too frequently associated with
bubbling, gurgling, retching, regurgitation, tongue-biting, wild
thrashing about, and sometimes deadly asphyxia.
                    Harold Griffith "An Anaesthetist's Valediction"[38]

The early use of anesthesia seems to have been carried out by eccentric
people who could approach the near-death of their patients fearlessly,
with daring or even levity. However, for truly safe, scientific, and successful anesthesiology to develop, another kind of experimenter was
required – someone whose familiarity with the dying had helped them
realize that the tightrope line between life and death is neither stable
nor clear, but instead remarkably thin and elastic.

Avoidable mistakes occurred primarily because no one was studying
the drugs in a scientific manner. Moreover, anesthesia was not seen as
an important medical specialty and was regarded as a chemical application to be relegated to inexperienced interns or students. Surgeons
habitually called upon any GP who was handy or used nurses and even
porters to administer the gas. The idea that patients were dying from
inexpert application and misunderstanding of these chemicals, rather
than from some innate antipathy towards the chemical itself, was a very
long time coming. Abetting this situation was the very language that
surrounded deaths due to misuse of anesthetics, which, until at least
the 1950s, put the blame squarely on the patient. "He couldn't stand
the anesthetic," "the anesthetic didn't agree with her," "we lost them on
the operating table," and other such euphemisms deluded the doctors
and surgeons about the real causes of surgical deaths as much as they
did the late patients' relatives.

The reasons for the long delay in real scientific use of these powerful
drugs were almost entirely philosophical. Even as late as 1868, well
after ether had come into general use, the respected researcher Ramon
de la Sagra was experimenting with the effects of both ether and chloroform on human consciousness – not in order to alleviate pain or to
facilitate more complicated surgery but to determine whether the
human soul had a physicality that could be measured by changes as it
left or entered a body under sedation.[39] This attitude typifies the priorities of many researchers well into the 19th century and explains the
long delay in surgical and medical advances.

Harold Griffith had become interested in anesthesia on the battle-field, well before he graduated from McGill in 1922. His fledgling specialty was still in a primitive state at that time, however, even in the most modern hospital operating rooms. Ether, chloroform, and nitrous oxide were the only chemicals available for normal use, and the only hospital equipment was a simple gauze mask with a pinhole pricked through it on which the physician dropped the chosen substance. It was almost always ethyl chloride, and it was used both for major surgery and as a local.

Griffith's own 1922 prize-winning McGill paper on the subject, written when he was still a student, is pretty alarming. He counseled that patients would more than likely spit, vomit, or begin to turn blue, but that the anesthesiologists must not panic; one had to continue giving ether even when it looked as if the patient had stopped breathing and was suffocating. Griffith reassures them, as an old hand who had anesthetized 400 patients well before he actually became a doctor, that "the jaw would relax" once the patient had passed out from lack of air, but if you didn't want to wait that long, "it is well to have always a mouth-gag handy and a wooden wedge to help pry open the teeth." Once open, "the tongue should be grasped with forceps and pulled forward. If this does not suffice to restore the breathing at once, gentle pressure on the abdomen may help, or... a few movements of artificial respiration." He suggested preceding the ether with morphine and atropine, and a "slow, steady induction with concentrated vapour" as soon as the patient is asleep.[40]

Harold's breezy confidence and apparent lack of concern over the state of the patients' mouths after such treatment belies the fact that deaths from overdoses of anesthetic or simple lack of oxygen were not at all infrequent. Even in official papers, they were attributed to "an act of God," or, as Dr Eli Katz put it, to "a wonderful, meaningless jargon term, *status lymphaticus.*" Of course, that was the 1920s, but even by the 40s, twenty years later, anesthesiology was still slow to catch on as a specialization. In all of Canada, only half a dozen doctors specialized in it before 1940, and of the 7,000 hospitals in North America, there were only 1,900 anesthetists registered with the International Anesthesia Research Society by 1942. Nurses often administered anesthetic in the United States and still do, particularly in the armed forces. Doctors were required in Canada, but they were general practitioners, often with less expertise than the nurses. Enid (Johnson) Macleod, who was Griffith's resident in Montreal, practiced in Sydney, N.S., between

1942–48, and said that even then, she was only called in if the GP about to do the operation thought it might be particularly tricky. One likely reason is that patients were upset at a separate bill for anesthetic and didn't want extra specialist costs.

Over time, anesthesiology became a specialization the same way surgery had. Doctors who started as GPs and who were particularly interested in it gradually got together and founded their specialty. But they encountered strong opposition from many surgeons, researchers, and hospital administrators who, then as now, did not feel that a few deaths here and there were really such a serious problem. Wesley Sykes points to the career of F.W. Hewitt, a British anesthetist who was the first to have some success in the campaign to regularize the profession. In 1907, in Great Britain, only eight out of twenty-seven medical examining bodies insisted on any evidence of instruction in anesthetics. In 1911, a mere four years after Hewitt's onslaught, all bodies demanded such expertise. The change may have come about through Hewitt's dry writing style as much as his professional influence. Back in 1903, he had written that, "while it is customary to place at the disposal of hospital patients, so long as they are conscious, the services of the most eminent physicians and surgeons of the day, it is also customary, directly they become unconscious, to hand them over to the care of comparatively uneducated and inexperienced junior officers who are left to do the best they can for their patients during what may be to the latter the most critical time of their lives."[41]

Worldwide, so many people fought to have anesthesiology elevated to specialist status that it's not possible to credit them all here. What's remarkable is how long they had to fight. Even by the 1930s, as Harold Griffith put it, it was starting to become clear that in addition to his technical skill, "the anesthetist ... must have the wisdom of a physician and an appreciation of the problems of surgeons and obstetricians. He must be familiar with the extraordinary conditions involved in all the surgical specialties. He must be a clinical pharmacologist, because he deals with all kinds of drugs; a biochemist and physiologist of sorts because he is responsible for the maintenance of vital function under widely varying conditions; and he must be a practical psychologist because he deals with patients at times of peculiar strain and stress."[42] Griffith named dozens of early anesthetists who spent their entire careers simply trying to get the profession recognized as such. In Canada alone, Samuel Johnston, Charles Robeson, William Easson Brown, Wesley Bourne, and Charles Laroque worked towards this end.

A book of this nature, trying to tell the story of medicine through one hospital, has had no choice but to underplay the remarkable contributions made to medicine, hospital care, and anesthesiology by the many hundreds of people who are as deserving of attention and praise as is the Griffith family. But even if there were space and time for all the accomplishments of the great John Snow or the much later Frank McMechan, Digby Leigh, Enid Johnson, Georges Cousineau, and so many more, a key question would remain. Why were there decades of both public and professional resistance, both here and abroad, to the idea of professional anesthesiology? A remark made by the surgeon Sir Alfred Fripp in 1908, in answer to proposals seeking to improve anesthesiology in Great Britain, may partially explain the situation. If hospitals decided to add the expense of a specially trained anesthesiologist to the cost of each operation, Fripp pointed out, that action "opened up the possibility of having to face a very large social question, of whether there was not already more than enough done for that very large class that could afford something, but could not afford to pay the full fee for their medical and surgical attendance, and who were very prone to get their services for nothing at all."[43]

In other words, in the two-tier medical system of the day, deciding to offer that level of professional care was seen to be prohibitively expensive. As it stood, private patients had the choice of getting anesthesia specialists for their cash operations. But publicly admitting that access to proper anesthesiology was critical to a patient's survival would have forced hospitals to provide it to the public at large, in the same way that they had provided antisepsis and good surgery. It seems that hospital administers believed that the relatively small number of lives that would be saved, especially since they would be concentrated among the non-paying, public patients, just weren't worth that kind of expenditure. Such arguments limiting the use of various medical techniques are still widespread. For example, professionally trained paramedics accompany ambulances on their rounds in most of North America today. Yet in the winter of 2005, Quebec's provincial Health minister had recourse to the same argument – that is, that such expertise is simply unnecessary. Although the ambulance guild insists that many more lives are saved when trained specialists are available, the minister was probably considering the economics of the proposal.

FOUNDING THE NEW PROFESSION

We watch closely those who sleep
                    motto of the Canadian Society of Anesthetists

Harold Griffith's professor, mentor, and eventual best friend following World War I – the person who sheltered and fanned his growing interest in the undervalued realm of anesthesiology – was Wesley Bourne, the first accredited anesthesiology specialist at McGill. Bourne was a surgeon who had to give a lot of anesthetics. Unlike most of his fellow surgeons, however, he became fascinated by the action of the drug on the human body. His son, the recently deceased Dr Robert Bourne, a gastroenterologist, spent his entire medical career at the Queen Elizabeth. Bourne said that when he was a boy, seventy years ago, Wesley was researching the action of these drugs himself because there was no body of knowledge about them. "He would work all day at the hospital or the University, then go up to his lab at McGill and work all night with his experimental animals – rats and dogs – measuring their reactions to the various anesthetics. He had a cot set up there to sleep, and I'd go see him there. I was fascinated too. It was in the Pharmacology Department of McGill. There was no such thing as an Anesthesiology Department."

Back in the 1920s, as Bob put it, "Dad was the senior man in anesthetics at McGill. Harold went to him for advice and they became very close friends." The two men were founding members of the various incarnations of societies intended to unite and gain recognition of the profession, from the Anesthetist's Travel Club on. Their life's work on this aspect of anesthesiology came to a head in 1952, when together they set up the World Federation of Societies of Anesthesiologists, which eventually became today's World Congress of Anesthesiologists. Its yearly meetings in Rome, London, or Paris never omit honouring the names of Bourne and Griffith, and the Wesley Bourne Chair of Anesthesiology at McGill, founded in 1945, like the Harold Griffith Chair in Anesthesia Research, are still two of the highest honours available in the profession in Canada.

Things went very slowly in the early part of Bourne and Griffith's careers, however, particularly during the period between the World Wars. Knowledge of the physiological action of the drugs was growing, as was the number of chemical options and the interest in the profession; however, formal recognition of the specialty still moved at a snail's-pace. Even the famous medical innovator, Wilder Penfield, was originally opposed creating a specialty in anesthetics. In the late 1930s, when Wilder had first come up to Canada from the U.S., where the almost universal practice was to use nurse-anesthetists, he gave a speech to young graduating nurses at the Royal Victoria hospital decrying Montreal's insistence on using doctors to administer anesthetics. Local anesthesiologists were outraged. Bob Bourne knew the story well and said, "Wilder had brought his own nurse-anesthetist up with him and was probably irritated that the rules here required him to use our MDs. So at the speech, he couldn't resist, I guess, announcing to the young women that he thought it was disgraceful that nurses weren't being entrusted with this work. My dad heard that speech and of course didn't agree at all. Then he was told to supply the great Dr Penfield, once he'd moved here to practice, with MD anesthesiologists." Bob Bourne's eyes couldn't help sparkling as he finished his story. "Dad got the very best people he had and sent them to work with the great man. Finally, one day, they met in the elevator at McGill. So Dad said, 'What do you think of our anesthetists?' He told me that Penfield replied, 'Wesley, I never knew what anesthesia was before.' And after that, Penfield certainly supported the profession."

It wasn't until another war, however, that the full transition was made. By the time Europe was bursting into flames in 1939, Wesley Bourne, Harold Griffith, and Digby Leigh of the Children's Hospital of Montreal were known as the "Great Triumvirate" of anesthesiologists in Montreal. They finally got their own department recognized at McGill thanks to the push that a world conflict always gives to new technologies. Bob Bourne said, "These three were asked to set up a method to train the armed forces medical personnel in anesthetics when World War II began." It had come to the attention of the authorities that more of their soldiers might survive that way. "So, out of their four-month course for medical officers, which was a fast, intensive training in anesthetics, grew the whole McGill department of anesthesiology. Throughout the war, Dad kept all the information pertaining to that course in his briefcase; he used to say, 'Here's my anesthesiology department, right here!' He'd been pushing to get a McGill department and proper specialty status for years, all his life, and after the war, that information came out of his briefcase and became a post-graduate course. Of course, it became much more stringent – two years of practical instruction followed by one year of internship to claim the specialty. Wesley was McGill's first professor in the field of anesthesiology; Harold was the second."

Although Bob Bourne asserts that "Harold became Wesley's best friend," like many others, Wesley Bourne refused for a significant number of years to even try to use Harold's great discovery, curare, because he thought it was too dangerous. Although this must have been a serious blow to Griffith, it wasn't enough to affect their friendship. "See this picture?" Bob said, indicating a fine studio portrait of Wesley, with his compact body and chiseled features still radiating handsome vitality at sixty-four. "Harold always had that picture with him; I mean, even when he went into the nursing home at the end of his life and was allowed to keep only one or two pictures and mementos. His wife Linda told me he kept this picture near his bed." It's inscribed, "To Harold Griffith, with affectionate regards, Wesley Bourne, 15 June 1949," dated to a year shortly after their lifelong dream for the profession had become a reality.

SLOW, STEADY PROGRESS

Operations on the chest [had been] virtually confined to ... procedures such as the removal of part of a rib to drain the pus from an empyema, or ... the deliberate removal of ribs to collapse tuberculous cavities in the lung ... [Dr] Bourne preferred to use high spinal anesthesia ... but the risk was high, as a miscalculation could result in paralysis of the diaphragm on which ... spontaneous respiration depended.

Richard Bodman and Deirdre Gilles[44]

Discoveries on the chemical and technological front happened so quickly after the 1920s that anesthesiologists worked feverishly to get their profession recognized. Daredevils were constantly introducing new drugs and techniques; it was up to the serious professionals to decide how, when, and if to use them. For example, in 1923, the newest anesthetic chemical to gain attention was ethylene. It was "clinically very similar in its effects to nitrous oxide: rather more potent but not nearly as strong as ether or chloroform." Harold Griffith adopted it with enthusiasm and published four papers on its use between 1928 and 1931. Harold combined a definite touch of the daredevil with a somewhat larger dose of the cautious, professional anesthesiologist. When he began experimenting with ethylene, he combined its use with endotracheal intubation, a new and difficult technique, and used it only for operations on the head and neck with the final refinement of adding ether for abdominal surgery to relax the muscles. This was a level of complex expertise virtually unheard of in most hospitals of the day.

Medical researchers were still searching for new chemicals and techniques to put people to sleep because of "the difficulty of maintaining unobstructed respiration while operating on the head, the face, or the throat." This considerable problem "had exercised the minds of surgeons ever since the introduction of anaesthesia in 1846."[45] A deeply unconscious patient's throat tends to collapse, which obstructs breathing, and she can suffocate. Even if that can somehow be prevented, the anesthetic gases have to be delivered into the lungs to keep the patient asleep while the surgeon operates with the mouth open to permit the gases to enter. Throughout the late 19th and early 20th centuries, many ingenious devices were invented to enable surgeons to introduce a tube through the mouth and larynx into the wind-pipe or trachea, hence the term "endotracheal or intratracheal" tube. The gases fed into this tube go directly from the trachea into the lungs where the drug can be absorbed by the bloodstream.

Back in 1909, Meltzer and Auer, two U.S. physiologists, had pioneered a technique they dubbed "intratracheal insufflation." They blew ether and air directly into the trachea of anesthetized dogs from a catheter passing through the mouth and larynx. They discovered that "if sufficient ether was administered the animal could be kept alive without the necessity for respiratory movement." A New York surgeon, Charles Elsberg, repeated these experiments on people and described it in the first American textbook on anesthesia. More pioneers followed, including Francis Nagle, chief anaesthetist at the Royal Vic, who claimed 300 intratracheal ether insufflations in 1913 alone. Charles Robson and Harry Shields, working in Canadian military hospitals in WWI, became adept at the new technique. By the early 1920s, it was a fairly common practice in Canadian hospitals; Harold Griffith greeted it with enthusiasm after his experiences with wet handkerchiefs and dying soldiers.[46]

Of course, the First World War greatly accelerated the pace of medical discovery. A "facial unit," the precursor of the specialty of faciomaxillary surgery, was established at Queen Mary's Hospital in Sidcup, near London, at the end of the war. Ivan Magill and Stanley Rowbotham, two medical officers with no special experience in anesthesia were recruited to run it. They used Elsberg's method of passing a urinary catheter down the throat to do ether insufflation. There was a problem, however. The catheter was so narrow, "the patient could breathe out around the tube, blowing the ether into the surgeon's face. This was neither efficient nor popular."

Dierdre Gillies, Harold Griffith's colleague and the author of this comment, was putting it mildly. Ether intoxication, a rather nasty experience that can include vivid hallucinations, was a serious problem because patients were exhaling these stupefying gases into the faces of the people who were supposed to be alertly performing operations on them. So Magill and Rowbotham tried passing two catheters, one in each nostril. The patient took in the ether through one and exhausted it through the other. This freed the throat so it could be packed with gauze to allow the surgeon to see what he was doing "without the exhaled ether bubbling up through blood and saliva into his face." This method was then further refined by replacing plain air with nitrous oxide gas stored in pressurized cylinders. In 1921 alone, Rowbotham and Magill did 3,000 intubation anaesthetics on the war veterans with catastrophic head and facial injuries that only a few years before had been largely inoperable.

As anyone who has seen an episode of ER knows, it remains true to this day that, "It is not easy to pass a catheter into the larynx of an anaesthetized patient," as Griffith put it. He was summarizing the sentiments of his fellow doctors, most of whom never even wanted to try the procedure. In 1928, a decade after the war was over, Griffith read a paper on "intertracheal anaesthesia" to a gathering in Boston. He later recorded that, "of the hundred or more anaesthetists who were in the audience, probably not more than ten had ever passed an endotracheal tube, so they weren't much interested in what I thought were the fine points of my presentation."[47] These new procedures were much safer for the patients, but they were difficult for the doctors. The fact that Griffith enthusiastically mastered each and every one when it was still just being introduced says something for his interest in developing anesthesia as a specialty.

MANAGING AIRWAYS

Anesthesiology is the difference between a clinic and a hospital. In terms of human health, there's a huge gap between being able to manage airway problems, and not being able to.

Dr John Hughes

"A clinic," Dr John Hughes goes on to explain, "is really just a glorified doctor's office. Advanced cardiac life-support, the ability to go in and stop bleeding from aneurisms or accidents, removing foreign objects or repairing seriously damaged tissues, all those things and more need *real* hospitals. And one fool-proof definition of a hospital is: it's a place where professional anesthesiologists can manage the patient's airway. These are the first things you learn in med school, and this is the basis of the triage you do in an ER. It's our ABC: Airway, Breathing, Circulation. Is it working or not? You can even say that anesthesiology is a paradigm for medicine itself. Because from that first day as a med student, the first lecture, the first minute on the job, you have to understand that five minutes without air, and we humans are done for. No drug, technique, or fancy machine is going to do a damn thing for us if we can't breathe. That's why we rush people to real hospitals, and not to clinics, in an ambulance. Above all other things, we have to make sure they can breathe!"

Harold Griffith was so clear on this concept that he was one of the first to take on the terrifying responsibility of doing the patients' breathing for them. He was also one of only a few doctors in Britain, Canada, and the U.S. who was experimenting with new gases and new ways to administer them. Sometimes the gas would paralyze or inhibit natural breathing. In that case, an attending physician, generally not yet a skilled anesthesiologist, took hold of a simple rubber balloon attached to an oxygen tank and the intubation tube and by flexing and unflexing kept the lungs pumping and expelling throughout an operation. That procedure is called "insufflation." But in order to do this, you must intubate the patient. A catheter going in through the nose or mouth must also introduce both the anesthetic gas and also the life-giving oxygen, as each is needed.

Despite its advantages, many doctors continued to resist intubation for decades. Innovators like Griffith, however, studied the medical journals, which featured illustrations of many new instruments, such as laryngoscopes, that could help the physician visualize the larynx. These doctors also learned about every advance, including "blind nasal intubulation," which was pioneered by Ivan Magill. The new "Magill endotracheal tube" was a simple piece of rubber hose that Dierdre Gilles says Magill used to keep in a biscuit tin. It was publicized at a joint meeting of the BMA (British) and CMA in Winnipeg in 1928 and was adopted by Ralph Waters at Wisconsin and John Lundy at the Mayo.[48]

Fortunately, even back in 1928 when Griffith's paper on inter-tracheal anesthesia failed to make much of a hit, there were a few enthusiasts in the audience. Ralph Waters, an anesthesiologist just starting his work at the University of Wisconsin, came up to congratu-late young Harold and later traveled to Montreal just to see the tech-nique, inviting Harold to join him and Lundy in their new, rather jolly group, which became known as the "Anaesthetists' Travel Club." This gradually turned into the distinguished Academy of Anesthesiology. The members of this original group of quirky inventor/doctors all became fast friends. Griffith had his own spin on Magill's method, which turned out to be even more widely accepted. Using a Chevalier Jackson speculum, he introduced a silk or lisle catheter of "such a size that it will nearly fill the trachea ... up to F32, which is the largest size I have been able to obtain." Later he got F36s. He had the patients re-breathe into the small rubber bag to which the catheter was attached. "I usually keep my hand on this bag, into which the gases are now directed from the machine, and thus even when the patient's head is completely covered, I can follow the depth and rate of respiration and can control the intra-thoracic pressure." [49]

In other words, the patients' lives were literally held in Griffith's hands, and he had to focus every atom of his attention on every tiny tremor or change in any physical aspect as he adjusted their breathing for them. Today, we expect anesthesiologists to be carefully monitoring heart rate, breathing, pupil reaction, and blood pressure levels, all of which are minutely measured on the many machines that surround a modern operating table – machines that were developed following the animal research of people like Wesley Bourne. Before that, surgeons concentrated only on whether the patient was sufficiently unconscious and still alive. In these early days, Harold and the other new anesthesi-ologists were the only ones interested in varied and detailed responses of the human body to the surgical assault. They had to have minds that would naturally delve into a really holistic view of the patient and all his or her reactions so that the profession could begin to reliably recog-nize the signals signifying a dangerous tilting of the delicate balance between life and death.

They also had to invent their own equipment and technologies. For example, the urinary catheters that made such a difference in surgical safety were not readily available. Harold spent many of his off hours searching for them before he found the best kind, which was made of silk or lisle and manufactured by the Porges Company in Paris. For years, Harold Griffith told the story of how his supplier had confided to him that the shop floor girls at the French factory kept asking, "What kind of men are these Canadians who need such huge catheters?" He experimented with many different kinds, with what disappointing or even gruesome results we can only imagine, including "double tubes, Hargrave's woven wire tubes, and Flagg's flexible brass tube." But the simple gray lisle catheter worked best. Amazingly, the design remains the very same to this day except for an inflatable cuff that was added to make the system airtight. A colleague named Arthur Guedel, Griffith recounted, praised this refinement, but they had to manufacture them by hand, at home. Eventually, Griffith was able to buy them through the Foregger Company, but even then, they were actually being made as a cottage industry by the daughter of their colleague, Ralph Waters! This picture of a tiny group of interested specialists enlisting each others' friends, connections, and even children to help develop the profession, right down to the homemade manufacture of specialized surgical equipment, is typical of what was going on in many branches of medicine in the 1920s to the 40s.[50]

During this period, the chemical and equipment company researchers were also likely to be medical doctors and together, they and the practicing doctors would roll up their sleeves and simply invent whatever chemical or mechanical device they needed. Such work created a camaraderie, a vision of shared purpose – the improvement of medicine and care of the patient – that led doctors to regard research chemists and inventors, as well as the drug companies and their representatives, as close allies and trusted colleagues. A typical example was Dr Karl Connell, a surgeon at the Roosevelt Hospital in New York between 1900 and 1930. Like Griffith, he was frustrated by the primitive nature of anesthesia administration. In the early years of the century, he invented his own machine to administer Horace Wells' favourite anesthesia, nitrous oxide. During the First World War, he was called upon by the Chemical Warfare Service to devise something to help protect allied soldiers from poison gas attacks. His subsequent Distinguished Service Medal cited the fact that, "Practically alone and unaided and at great personal risk of his life, *he exposed himself unhesitatingly to the highest concentration of deadly gases while working with experimental models of masks.* Major Connell invented, tested out and perfected a new type of gas mask superior to any then in existence."[51]

This medical and inventive paragon retired from his surgical position in 1930, only to turn his rustic, isolated fishing cabin in the

Catskills into a production factory "for the world's best anesthetic administrating machines."[52] Connell had to work very closely with the chemical companies that produced anesthetic drugs as well as with large laboratory suppliers like Zeiss. Soon, in most doctors' minds, the remarkable advances that this multi-faceted partnership brought to all concerned meant that any clear distinction between the ultimate aims of the inventors, the companies, and modern medicine itself became blurred. Such comradeship produced many wonderful innovations, but it also led to the gradual corruption of drug standards and testing methods by the drug companies – a side effect that has only become clear 60 or 70 years later.

Throughout the 1930s, however, in the hey-day of true inventive collaboration, all three segments of the new scientific medical community were heady with enthusiasm for new materials and new delivery systems, sailing together into the unknown with as much daring as the era's dashing airplane pilots. There survives a lively correspondence between Connell and Harold Griffith, which illustrates how the former tried to devise new materials to meet the requests of the latter. On 8 July 1935, Connell writes that Griffith's order "has been held up to give you a new dead weight blow-off in place of the spring valve...Knowing your scientific interest, research mind, and sound analysis, I await with interest the results of your use of the [newly designed] rubber parts."[53]

NEW AGENTS TO MOCK DEATH

The agent which I still use most frequently, cyclopropane, can be given so badly that both the immediate and future recovery of the patient are in jeopardy. And this is true of almost all the many agents which we now have available.

Harold Griffith, describing his clinical record
of 350 cyclopropane administrations[54]

In 1931, after over 1,500 administrations of a drug called cyclopropane, using the lisle catheters and a hand breathing apparatus, Griffith again summarized his experience in an article. He emphasized that not only was this new drug extremely necessary for head cases, it was also useful for abdominal surgery, which was a huge problem for surgeons because the unconscious abdominal muscles clench and are difficult to cut. For these and other reasons, he wondered why endotracheal anesthesia was still looked upon almost as a curiosity in many American clinics. Griffith described great success in resuscitating newborns, which must have been very useful in this period because mothers were still being given heavy does of chloroform or ether before birth.[55]

Griffith continued to write about the astonishing amount of opposition to intubation methods, especially from specialists who "thought it was going to do damage to the larynx and trachea." The surgeons at Boston's Massachusetts General, for example, still famous for their introduction of ether to the world in 1846, were so married to that drug that "they would use nothing else and were violently opposed to endotracheal anesthesia, and generally preferred to use nurses as anesthetists." Despite the slowness of many to adopt it, however, "the endotracheal tube eventually revolutionized the whole course of anesthesia," as Harold's colleague Diedre Gillies puts it.[56]

Griffith wasn't interested in methodology alone. He also pioneered new gases and chemicals, the most successful of which was cyclopropane. Although far superiour to ether and choroform, cyclopropane had many downsides, including serious expense, flammability, and difficulties in administration. But Griffith loved cyclopropane and used it "for the rest of his working life."[57] By 1940, for example, he was using it in 90 percent of his cases.[58] Each doctor had his own methods of administering it because it was so dangerous. Bodman and Gillies say that while "very potent and safe in experienced hands, in the higher dose range cyclopropane caused respiratory depression," meaning that patients could stop breathing. But since Griffith "always used it for major surgery with an endotracheal tube," he kept the patient going with hand pressure on the breathing bag. The two leading proponents of cyclopropane in the U.S. were Ralph Waters and Arthur Guedel. These pioneers used very different procedures, both of them pretty terrifying. Waters used little premedication and depended on an "artist's skill" to judge just enough depth of anesthesia that would enable him to avoid intubation. This method left some doubt as to whether the diaphragm was relaxed enough to permit safe surgery. Guedel went the opposite direction. He used heavy premedication with Pentothal and forced a huge, 75 percent, concentration of cyclopropane "through a protesting glottis." This method depended on a "leakproof system." If anything went wrong while changing the bags, a patient could go into dangerous apnoea.

The danger of death caused by respiratory depression or cessation could be remedied by any of these methods, but insufflation had an extra advantage that Griffith was one of the first to recognize. "One of the greatest advances [in the profession of anesthesiology]" he later wrote, "has been the recognition of the importance of ventilation, which was not recognized at all in my earliest years; patients were left to wallow in their own carbon dioxide." The statistical results of thousands of surgical cases wallowing in CO_2 – death and brain and nervous system damage of various degrees, including a form of mental retardation – can only be imagined. Nobody was keeping records at the time.[59] Perhaps this is one explanation for another common statement of the era: "He/she was never the same after that operation." Debates over how to manage these problems continued to rage in the specialty for at least twenty years.

The problem of flammability was not yet solved. These new gases were so explosive that they could be set off by simple static electricity. Harold Griffith described an occasion at the Homeopathic/Queen Elizabeth when an orderly removed a cloth covering from an anesthetic machine on a cold, dry morning. A static spark caused a loud explosion, fortunately with no injuries. After that close call, Griffith had a humidifier installed in the operating room and never again used a cloth cover on the machines. He also used an inter-coupling device to prevent sparks between the table, the patient, the machine, and the floor. Even in the 1970s, however, his colleague and protégé Dierdre Gillies continued to complain that, "In spite of reports (from the AMA and the Bureau of Mines), many anesthetists remain woefully ignorant of the hazards associated with explosive anesthetic agents." So the explosions associated with the early days of the specialty occurred on occasion.

CURARE'S DARK HISTORY

Curare...one of the most sinister poisons known to man, the 'flying death' of the Amazonian jungles. Made by witch doctors...smeared on arrows or blow darts, it strikes down animal, bird – or man – in a peculiarly horrible death.

Weekend Magazine[60]

Of all the drugs that mimic death, only the most recent was actually developed under relatively stringent scientific conditions. However, its history is no more free of the mysterious and dangerous than that of its predecessors. Curare, by far the most important component of modern surgery today, was not discovered in a laboratory. Instead, it was discovered, purified, and applied to highly pragmatic uses by a people who lived in tropical forests far from modern surgical hospitals. Without these peoples' knowledge, which was acquired over many generations through dangerous experimentation, as well as their voluntary help, modern surgery could have remained in the dark ages to this day. Curare's simple gift is to make operations done on the respiratory system, head, and torso not only possible but, for the first time in human history, relatively safe. All the diseases and injuries of these key parts of the human anatomy finally became accessible to the surgeon's hands because of this one drug.

The first name generally associated with this remarkable nerve poison is the Spanish explorer Franzisco Lopez de Gomara. His report on both its ingredients and effects, written in 1553, was typical of the stories of the wonders to be found in the New World. Not only did he describe a true witch's potion as a closely guarded secret brew of serpents' fangs, ants, spiders, and poisonous plants, he also claimed that only old women were allowed to make the sinister liquid because anyone who did so rapidly died from the vapours given off during its boiling. How quickly these expendable members of society succumbed, Gomara claimed, was a measure of that batch's effectiveness. Subsequent reports by the Spanish physician Nicolas Monardes in 1574 and Sir Walter Raleigh, twenty years later, only added to the ghoulish drama surrounding curare, or *wourali*, as it was then known. A string of Jesuit priests kept these stories alive in the 17th century. One, Fr. Joseph Gumilla, wrote a widely circulated book in 1741 that the early 19th-century explorer Alexander von Humboldt referred to, with disgust, as "collected folklore."

Real scientific interest took off in 1743 with a report from the French naturalist Charles Marie de La Condamine. He asserted that the mysterious brew was entirely vegetal, made from thirty different herbs and roots, especially "certain vines." He was the first to test the speed with which the toxin took effect, which he repeated with a carefully preserved sample in Europe before fascinated scholars. When the American Edward Bancroft and the Italian Felice Fontana went among the Acawai Indians of Guiana, Bancroft gave fairly exact descriptions of methods of preparation, solubility, and possible antidotes, which were "very much more accurate than previous accounts."[61]

But it was the famous naturalist, explorer, and scientist Alexander von Humboldt who brought the study of the poison into the modern age. He witnessed its manufacture during a rather riotous harvest festival while exploring near Esmeralda on the upper Orinoco in May of 1800. His observations only became public twenty years later, in 1819, with the publication of his expedition notes. Charles Waterton, an eccentric British squire, did not know about von Humboldt's experiences when he went on a journey to Central America in 1812. Waterton was in search of bird life but became fascinated by the highly effective and mysterious arrow poison. He wasn't a real scientist and, unlike von Humboldt, appears to have made no attempt to gain permission from the local tribal chemist in order to learn how the substance was made. Between bouts of fever, as soon as he could collect enough, he injected several animals, including an ox, which died within two minutes.

Waterton also described wourali as a concoction of snake fangs, plants, and poisonous insects, requiring many months to prepare. He had seen it paralyze and kill very large animals with a single arrow, yet the animal's flesh could be eaten at once – so it didn't seem to be a poison in the normal sense of the term. Once back in England, Squire Waterton used this substance in experiments on just about any unfortunate creature he could find, all of which died at rates whose variations he noted carefully in notebooks. The most famous subject was a she-ass who "died in apparently ten minutes. An incision was then made in its windpipe, and through it the lungs were regularly inflated for two hours with a pair of bellows. Suspended animation returned," although the animal sank again into apparent death when the artificial respiration ceased. Waterton and his assistants kept the arduous inflation practice up for another two hours – at which point the ass recovered completely! As a reward, she was named Wouralia, and ended her days as a pet on the Squire's grounds.[62]

This seems a very perspicacious experiment for a dilettante that foreshadowed intubation and artificial respiration, practices of modern anesthesiology that were not to be developed for more than a hundred years. It didn't create much of a stir in respected scientific circles at the time or even much later, however, probably because Charles Waterton was such an archetypical eccentric. He looked so disreputable that he was frequently mistaken for a servant on his own estate, and in later life was often to be found perched like an aged vulture on the top of his tallest trees. "On one occasion [he] made himself a pair of wings and was only dissuaded with difficulty from launching himself from the roof of a building to try them out."[63]

Although the Waterton tradition added to the carnival atmosphere surrounding anesthesia, a more scientific approach was simultaneously dawning. Alexander von Humboldt never forgot his experiences during his own scientific explorations of the same area in 1807. In 1837, he helped support two young scientists, brothers named Richard and Robert Hermann Schomburgk, in their bid to return to Guiana.

Von Humboldt had written, 30 years before, that only one plant, not 30 as La Condamine claimed, was needed to make curare. He recounted how he had respectfully watched as the man he termed "the local chemist" brewed curare in a palm-leaf hut which was "set up like a chemical laboratory [where] the greatest order and cleanliness prevailed ... Large earthenware pots [were used] for cooking the plant juices, shallow vessels with a large surface area to help evaporation, and cone-shaped, rolled-up banana leaves for straining the fluids which contained more or less fibrous substances."

He learned from this "poison master," whose every word and gesture he recorded, that, "the...poison was contained in the bark and part of the sapwood...The poison master laid great stress on [the] funnel more than on any of the other equipment in the laboratory." Von Humboldt went on to describe every aspect of the manufacture, from the "cold infusion of the crushed mavacure bark to the evaporation of the poisonous liquid and the addition of the thickening agent.[64]

Like so many other scientists before and after him, Von Humboldt tasted the concoction, which he found "very pleasantly bitter." He did this with confidence, following the directions of his teacher. He wrote, "There is no danger ... so long as one is sure that one's lips and gums are not bleeding ... curare only has a lethal effect when it comes into direct contact with the blood. Therefore, whatever the Orinoco missionaries may have said, the vapours from the cauldron are also harmless ... and La Condamine is wrong when he asserts that Indian women condemned to death were executed by the vapours of ticunas poison."[65]

Von Humboldt encouraged several other young scientist/explorers, including Jean-Baptiste Boussingault and Francois Desire Roulin, to go and learn from the Indians. They did, and the latter managed to isolate an alkaline curare base in Bogota in 1827. Von Humboldt's original protégés, the Schomburgks, conducted an exhausting expedition lasting several years. Richard observed another manufacture of the poison and managed to figure out the actual recipe for *wourali*, which in this case added two other *Strychnos* species to the main ingredient von Humboldt had written about 35 years before. Richard, like Alexander, also tried it on himself to cure a fever because he had no quinine. He "stopped when he realized the danger of an excoriation of the tongue or throat."[66]

In France, physiologists and pharmacologists performed more serious experiments in an effort to understand how the poison affected motor activity and whether it destroyed the ability of muscles to contract. Because it only seemed to affect the peripheral ends of the motor nerves and did not destroy the muscles, one recommended the use of curare in the treatment of tetanus. The scientific amateurs that abounded at this time avidly read these accounts, whether in crude versions in the popular press or the heavy, specialist tomes and periodicals published by the Schomburgks and von Humboldt. A veterinarian neighbour of Squire Waterton's obtained some *wourali* from him and tried it on a horse suffering from tetanus. The horse appeared to recover but died the next day from overeating. Humans suffering from the same disease were given the drug by Waterton and other amateurs throughout this period and well into the 1850s, to no avail. After that, interest waned for such a long time – 80 years – that it was as if *wourali* had never been discovered at all. Only a few chemists, including Rudolf Boehm in Leipzig in 1895, continued to try to isolate and clarify the curare alkaloids – for what use he didn't yet know. In the early 1930s, Heinrich Wieland in Munich and Harold King in Britain, among others, managed to obtain crystallized curare alkaloids. Harold Griffith and his Homeopathic Hospital colleague Enid Johnson were the doctors who, just a few years later, would make the South American arrow poison respectable. Obviously, the odds against it becoming so were formidable.[67]

MORE HORRIBLE HISTORY

We have established the value of a new therapy that is going to rescue shock therapy from being abandoned.

Psychiatrist Dr Abram Elting Bennett[68]

Even into the late 1930s, curare still remained shrouded in superstitious popular legend and consigned to scientific oblivion. That's when Harold Griffith, along with a few other curious anesthesiologists, began trying to figure out how it really worked. The reason for their revived curiosity was the poison's odd ability to paralyze without killing or in any way damaging tissue. In fact, the victims, although unable to move and eventually even to breathe, remained fully conscious and aware of pain, as Scott Smith's experiments later proved.[69] And like Waterton's she-ass, they could in theory be kept alive and eventually re-animated by the insufflation that researchers like Griffith were pioneering as a standard anesthetic technique.

Why was that paralysis so important? Simply because it's dangerous to cut into the chest, throat, and abdomen when they are tensed but relatively safe when they are relaxed. This is why, as the famous 19th-century British surgeon Sir John Erichson wisely intoned, "The abdomen, the chest and the brain will be forever shut from the intrusion of the wise and humane surgeon."[70] The problem was that in order to get the depth of unconsciousness required to make the muscles relax adequately, so much anesthetic had to be given that the patient was in serious danger of hypoxia, or suffocation.

In what seems today to be a rather dark episode, curare was rescued from oblivion because of its ability to render the muscles of people receiving electro-shock therapy flaccid and paralyzed. The psychiatric profession had begun using electric shock therapy early in the century for ills ranging from serious psychoses to simple senility and even mild "midlife depression." It was even used on "spastic" children with illnesses such as muscular dystrophy.

The powerful electric shock therapy administered at the time frequently induced convulsive seizures so violent that patients' bones were broken, fractured, and dislocated at rates as high as 43 to 51 percent. Some psychiatrists, like Dr Bennet, quoted above, used spinal anesthesia prior to shock treatments "in desperation," but finally, the incidence of injury and death from such methods was simply too high, even for people judged incurably insane. Dr Bennett turned his hopes to curare so that electro-shock therapy could "survive."

In 1938, Bennett obtained a quantity of crude, homemade curare straight from an Ecuadorian explorer and began using it experimentally on mice. He quickly followed up by using it on "spastic athetoid children." "Within a few months," Bennett wrote, "refinements of standardization techniques were made by Holladay of Squibb by his ingenious rabbit head-drop test. This proved to be a highly accurate dosage, directly transferable to man." The new preparation was called "Intocostrin." The strong partnership between corporate and hospital or academic researchers shows itself clearly when Bennett reported the

gruesome observation that, "following an observation in Nebraska
State Mental Hospital that pelvic examinations upon disturbed female
psychotic patients could be very easily made because of the complete
muscular relaxation after an injection of curare, it was thought that
curare would be useful in producing muscular relaxation under general anesthesia. This matter was discussed with Dr Lewis H. Wright of
E.R. Squibb & Sons. Upon his suggestion, Dr Harold Griffith, of Montreal, together with Dr Enid Johnson, first used curare in anesthesia in
January, 1942."[71]

Griffith himself, writing much later, admits, "When the idea of [the
use of curare] was first suggested in 1940, I passed off the idea as fantastic and laughed ... but ... in October 1941, when [Dr Wright] of
Squibb told me Dr Bennett had administered the drug to hundreds of
psychotic patients without harmful effects, I decided an anesthetist
could control respiration and give it a try."[72] Using curare as a muscle-
relaxant and a relatively light dose of an anesthetic like cyclopropane,
Griffith was able to achieve the effects of extremely deep anesthesia
without its usual dangers. His first patient was a "muscular young man"
admitted to the Homeopathic Hospital of Montreal for an appendectomy. The operation was a complete success and led to a revolution in
the entire discipline. It gave surgeons all the advantages of deep anesthesia without its dangers. As Eli Katz, who ran the ENT department
between the 1950s and 70s said many years later, "Curare made a lady
out of anesthesiology."

In the early 1950s, when Katz began working at the Queen Elizabeth,
he remembered that, "even in my first year of internship as a GP, I was
expected to give anesthetic. No one worried about lawsuits in those
days. People just died during the operation; no one even kept track of
how or why. And these were explosive gases, too, so of course they blew
up regularly, but no one kept track, so I can't give figures." Starting virtually from scratch, Katz established the hospital's Ear, Nose, and
Throat Department. "Dr Harold helped buy the instruments. I had
accumulated some before the war. In those days, tonsillectomy was the
fad [even though] we were pathetic at anesthesia. We had to suction
out the blood and ether, bend over the exhaled ether, try to stop all the
bleeding in the throat so we could use the mask – it was a mess. That's
when curare came out. It relaxed the muscles ... We started out using
ether or chloroform, and bleeding was the big problem. This was at the
beginning of the period when Harold Griffith and Enid Johnson began
using curare, injecting it to relax the larynx so they could intubate.

That's what I mean by saying curare made a lady out of anesthetic ... It revolutionized surgery, especially in the throat." Katz admitted that before curare, "we had a much higher death rate ... And with the other drugs, there was also a much longer recovery period. There was a big difference once we started using oxygen. The patient would be conscious sooner. Of course, we had to be very careful, make sure they were breathing."

So the benefits were real and immediate, especially in thoracic and throat surgery. The reason Griffith gets credit for pioneering the use of curare is not because he discovered that curare could be used in the Intocostrin form – Squibb and A. E. Bennett pioneered that. Harold was unique for another reason. When it came to the complications of extended surgical use in the early 1940s, no one knew how much of the drug would be safe. Other anesthesiologists were deeply interested in curare and were trying it out for regular surgical purposes on experimental animals. Throughout the early 1940s, researchers such as Dr Stuart Cullen of the University of Iowa used hundreds of dogs and other animals in Intocostrin experiments. They all died. Reluctantly, these hopeful innovators were forced by their results to judge curare far too dangerous for surgical use. In fact, it earned such a bad reputation that even some of Griffith's closest colleagues, such as Wesley Bourne, wouldn't touch it for many years.

Dr Franco Carli, the holder of the Harold Griffith Chair of Anesthesiology in the McGill teaching hospitals today, says that, "Only a homeopathist, like Harold, could have figured out how to use curare." Carli points out that the *quantity* of the drug that is still used today to provide the desired muscle relaxation, "is infinitesimal. Simply ridiculously small! No classically trained doctor would consider that such trace amounts of a chemical could in any way be usefully therapeutic. But of course, homeopathy is based on the theory that absolutely tiny, trace amounts of a substance can have important effects on the human body." In short, in his experiments, Harold took virtually molecular amounts of the chemical in solution very gradually *upwards*. Meanwhile, his colleagues were administering what allopathic medicine would consider "normal" dilutions of the chemical, which invariably were too strong even for small animals. Homeopathy was very much sidelined in medical circles in the 1940s, and Harold never formally stated that he was using homeopathic theory when developing curare; maybe he did so without thinking about it. But his statement towards the end of his life about his early training, when he said, "I remain convinced that there is much truth in homeopathy," makes it clear that he retained an inner respect for that system. Dr Carli puts it more succinctly. "We owe this breakthrough to the way Griffith had been trained – to always use *less* of a chemical instead of more."

For this contribution, Harold received many local and global accolades and honours. For example, since his retirement, every meeting of the World Congress of Anesthesiologists has hosted a "Harold Griffith Symposium." He also left a living legacy: Deirdre Gillies, the brilliant young anesthesiologist he trained and who kept his memory alive long after he retired from the Queen Elizabeth. She was a classically trained British anesthesiologist, and John Hughes remembers that, "she inspired in everybody the feeling that if you were the patient, she'd be the one you'd want at the head of the table doing your operation. No matter how grim the situation, you knew that fear would impede neither her judgment nor her execution." Gillies stepped seamlessly into Harold and Jim's shoes when they retired in the late 1960s as chair of the chiefs of staff. "She was like a parallel government to the board," smiles Hughes. "And it was her whole life. She never married; the Griffiths were her family. It was still common for doctors and nurses in that generation to be totally devoted to their work."

As for her mentor, Harold Griffith, he went to his grave modestly deprecating his part in the discovery that had revolutionized surgery and made his name in the world. He certainly didn't try to patent the technique or claim exclusive discovery. And interestingly enough, unlike his predecessors in ether and chloroform, Griffith sidestepped the anesthesia curse. Today he is remembered as a giant in his field, arguably the most important and honoured anesthesiologist who ever practiced, even if he didn't make much money from his efforts. Unlike Morton and Jackson, he doesn't seem to have been interested in that aspect of research. Along with is father, A.R., Harold wasn't inspired by the more modern quest for personal fame and big financial rewards and, thanks to all the writings they left behind, we know where they got the curiosity and confidence to found and revolutionize a specialty. The diaries, papers, and lectures of both father and son, now preserved at McGill University, record Harold as an adolescent combining work and play to figure out how to run a debating society or float a raft well before he had to figure out what kind of catheters would work for intubation. Harold left a clear picture of himself as a small boy following A.R. around the Montreal Homeopathic. He watched sick people getting well after having been administered infinitesimal doses of herbs and chemicals, which, like most homeopathic medicines, would have killed them in larger doses. The impression left on him when he saw his patients fighting off the influenza pandemic after infinitesimal doses of homeopathic medicines is also clearly recorded. The testimony given by his daughters and grandsons describes a person with unusually pragmatic instincts whose achievements flowed out of a lifelong desire to be of service.

As noted at the beginning of this chapter, this particular combination of internal values and the ability to act on them in the external world remained the same whether Griffith was administering his hospital, dealing with a patient, or playing with his family. That's probably why their high standards seem to have imprinted themselves permanently on the institution he and his father headed for so long. It's also nice to imagine that those staunchly altruistic values saved him from the curse that, up to then, seems to have haunted his very tricky specialty.

4

Medical Bills

HOSPITAL HALCYON: THE ROARING TWENTIES

1926: I might state that a number of subscribers have very generously
anticipated the payments of installments, which under the terms of the
campaign were spread over four years, and I would like to take this
opportunity of expressing our thanks to them.

S. B. Hammond, Treasurer's Report, The Homeopathic Hospital
of Montreal, 1926[1]

A hospital researcher and doctor such as Harold Griffith could bring
about revolutionary advances only if the hospital where he worked
received unstinting social support and generous and dependable funding. Traditionally, the Homeopathic had depended for that support on
an interestingly diverse number of sources, including generalized charity, often of a religious nature; user fees from those who could afford it;
and unpredictable influxes of occasional large gifts from wealthy and
influential members of society. These contributions were supplemented by small, steady, and therefore increasingly vital annual governmental stipends, both municipal and provincial. Such support
naturally fluctuated from year to year and made annual planning, to
say nothing of long-term decisions to increase staff or expand the facilities, nerve-wracking.

This diversified funding system worked well as long as economic conditions were favourable. Throughout the 1920s, local and community
hospitals were becoming organized, professionally rigorous, well-
equipped institutions, although they didn't yet have the reputation for

excellence that would come with surgical advances and antibiotics. But in order to support the technological revolution that promised real power over many diseases, hospitals had to attract more paying customers. Without appreciable government stipends, they needed well-to-do medical consumers to subsidize their technological ambitions as well as their traditional responsibility – non-paying consumers. Better food, bed rest, and cleaner, quieter surroundings were what they had always been able to offer the poor and semi-poor. To attract the upper middle classes, they had to provide amenities that could equal or surpass the comforts of being nursed at home by family or servants. In the United States, a greater number of hospitals intended uniquely for the poor had been kept separate from facilities for the paying patient. Some American and nearly all Canadian hospitals welcomed both kinds of clients; while housed in separate wards or clinics, they were under the same roof. It was the latter type of hospital that began to invest in nicer furnishings for the private wards and, increasingly throughout the 1920s, in special buildings, wings, or pavilions for the exclusive use of the wealthy. This was a true two-tier system (to use the current term), much like the one found in the U.S. or Mexico today.

Typically, the buildings or wings intended for paying customers were architecturally separate from the rest of the hospital. For example, the Ross Pavilion of the Royal Victoria Hospital in Montreal was built in 1920 on a hillside with a magnificent view. It was connected to the main facility below by a very expensive tunnel that ran through a landscaped woods with formal gardens, a teahouse, and a special parking court. While normal patient wards still had up to forty beds that were dependent on bedpans and communal baths down the hall, the Ross Pavilion offered the paying patient either two-room suites with baths and a private balcony or large private rooms with adjoining baths. Despite luxuries of this type, many rich people still patronized the hospital in their own neighbourhood or went to the one their physician recommended. So the humble Homeopathic, like many other small, community hospitals, also invested in larger rooms with more air, light, and better furniture in hopes of being able to attract and keep the custom of local paying patients.

Throughout this period and because of these two-tier accommodations, hospitals were able to steadily increase private fees. As well, the public's confidence in hospital services was expanding almost monthly. As governments began to recognize the considerable fiscal advantages of having public health institutions help them avoid the expense and

chaos of seasonal epidemics, their grants to the public wards and indigent patients slowly crept upwards. At this time, contributing to the
local hospital was looked upon as society's most effective and praise-
worthy form of public charity – typified in the media by the x-ray
machine Kris Kringle supplies at the end of *Miracle on 34th Street*.

Benefactors like Kris abounded and many of them endowed wings
and departments or left entire fortunes to the hospitals that had provided care for their loved ones. As noted ahead, medical care outside
hospitals was booming as well. In the 1920s, even small-town practitioners' incomes reached an all-time high when compared to those of
other professionals. Consequently, all across North America, the
majority of doctors opposed serious increases in government funding
or control over their profession. Hospital boards and administrators
were also fairly satisfied with their finances. However, serious problems
were brewing with consumers.

The highly mixed economic foundation on which this expanding
hospital system was based was developed almost entirely on the capital-
ist model for private businesses. Hospital boards simply glued their traditional social contract to provide non-profit, donated, or partially
donated care to the poor to an economic model that was designed to
generate profits for industrial enterprises. The expectation, as David
and Rosemary Gagan put it, was that "continued public generosity,
medical efficiency, a starkly economical free service – neither more,
nor less, than the poor deserved – and the expansion of professional
philanthropy ... would carry the hospital's historical burden of charitable care and treatment without detriment to its new [and increasingly
expensive] scientific mandate."[2]

However, events during the 1930s changed this expectation. Economic pressures as well as unexpected levels of immigration, unpredictable demographic shifts and social transformations, and changing
patterns and types of diseases, "repeatedly inflated the quantity, the
scope and the costs of the public hospitals' charitable obligations." The
Gagans note that despite the apparently rosy economic indications of
professional salaries and institutional expansions in the 1920s, it was
precisely at this period that the unexpected strains on that basically
unsuitable business model began to catastrophically "sap ... the public
and private resources available to sustain hospitals' legal responsibilities for medical charity." What looked like a diversified, flexible system
turned out to be too rigid to accommodate the rapidly increasing
influx of middle-class users. The only economic choice available to

hospital boards was raising their fees to private patients, so fees sky-
rocketed. They were desperately needed as the new scientific treatments became more expen- sive, but they were also intentionally
inflated and manipulated by the boards, which used this money to
cover their mushrooming charitable costs.

"Throughout the 1920s," as the Gagans note, "hospitals inflated the
fees of paying patients and implemented a catalogue of diagnostic sur-
charges that further elevated the cost of hospitalization."[3] If an institution's financial stability depends upon identifying and housing as many
sick people as possible, it's easy to predict it might find itself in a conflict of interest. Surgery was the "jewel in the crown" of the modern
hospital and its major money-maker, so determining how many people
actually needed it, as well as diagnosing an illness that required hospitalization in the first place, tended to increase in direct relation to the
institution's financial needs. Today, this tendency is termed PID, or
"Physician Induced Demand." PID statistics are currently used to determine the availability of medical services granted by U.S. Health Maintenance Organizations (HMOs). So nervous are the managements of
for-profit HMOs about the possibility that a surgeon might over-pre-
scribe surgery, for example, that they often step in to try to curtail or
delay needed interventions. Basically, the current tendency to under-
treat, especially in a for-profit system, and the historical problem of
over-treating shows that any hospital financing body, past or present,
whether it raises finances via its own board, a private HMO, or a provincial government, is in the same situation of conflict of interest in terms
of granting services. It may tend to either under-use surgery and hospital treatments or over-use them, depending on whether that use
enriches or impoverishes the funding institution.

In the 1920s, when this problem was first surfacing, doctors, nurses,
and administrators were surveyed to determine who was responsible
for the growing trend towards "excessive hospitalization that contributed to overcrowded wards, higher operating costs and increased
patient financial liability."[4] This was the beginning of what we now term
"Evidence-Based Medicine," that is, statistical analysis of both treatments and management practices, conducted to eliminate subjective
assessments and to objectively determine effective and efficient practices. Survey respondents in the early 1930s blamed doctors for hospi-
talizing people for their own convenience and over-medicalizing such
things as childbirth. They equally blamed patients for staying too long
because they were more comfortable in the hospital than they might be

elsewhere, although this last is probably less of a problem in the Canadian system today. To a lesser extent, they also blamed the administrators who needed the funding a large number of admissions provided and who hesitated to risk the legal repercussions of second-guessing the doctors. This roster of hospital workers polled more than 70 years ago agreed entirely on one thing: "for a variety of reasons, on any given day, the well-being of one-fifth of Canada's hospitalized patients would have been better served in some other environment."[5]

Among other similar studies across the country, a 1936 analysis of patients in Ontario hospitals "identified unnecessarily lengthy pre-operative hospitalization when no useful diagnostic work was done, disagreements among surgeons over appropriate therapy and unjustifiably prolonged convalescence from herniotomies and appendectomies in particular, [all] as evidence of medical inefficiency." This inefficiency was blamed for the hospitals' inflated costs. And although indigent patients were the "principal ... recipients of inappropriate, ineffective, untimely or unwarranted surgery" paying patients were not immune.[6] The ultimate cost fell upon the middle group, the "patients of moderate means," who were hospitals' main support and who, gradually throughout the 1920s, were not just falling through but totally disappearing from the cracks in a system that had been set up for the very rich and the extremely poor.

Describing the formalities of hospital admission for the typically frightened, sick, or injured human being who was about to become a patient, the Gagans state that at this time in Canada, as in the United States today, "The most important formality was the issue of payment." In fact, "What individual patients or their guardians were willing to pay for hospitalization determined the level of accommodation and the services to which the patient was entitled, in hospitals where even the public wards held two distinct classes of patients."[7]

Nurses still alive today remember how in the private wards at the Homeopathic, wine glasses and special linens had to be properly apportioned, with small glasses for sherry, large for red, and so forth. Indeed, as an article entitled, "Private Room Service in Keeping with Present Day Needs," which was published in the 1935 edition of *Canadian Hospital* put it, "any reasonable request [should] be fulfilled" for the paying medical consumer. For the non-paying consumers, however, hospitalization "was synonymous with varying degrees of institutional intractability, discrimination, judgmentalism, dehumanization, and *noblesse oblige.*" The Gagans note that as early as the 1920s, "the potential of the strategy of making the rich more or less voluntarily pay for the poor had already been exhausted, at least in terms of consumer tolerance." And then the Great Depression "finally exposed – to the point of impending total collapse – the historical tenuousness of hospitals' financial structures, social assumptions and public policies." The profit-centred industrial model proved to be "inconsistent with the economic circumstances of half the population, who simply could not afford health care."[8]

THE VERY DIRTY THIRTIES

1932: While the Hospital is in need of considerable new equipment, it was considered advisable to keep these expenditures reduced to the smallest possible amount, and you will notice that the Fixed Assets were increased by only $363.87.

S. B. Hammond, Treasurer's Report, The Homeopathic Hospital of Montreal, 1932[9]

According to most analysts, including C. David Naylor, another of Canada's premiere medical historians, the palmy days of 1920s medical funding would have eventually collapsed even without the added impetus of the Depression. He agrees that, "Doctors, like Canadians in all sectors of the economy, did well in the 1920s. Whereas gross medical incomes were reputed to have climbed above an average of $2,000 per year for the first time in Ontario during the early 1900s, a survey of 500 Ontario physicians' gross receipts for the last five years of the 1920s revealed an average annual inflow of $6,262. Manitoba rural practitioners were reported as grossing an average of $5,010; while in Winnipeg, generalists averaged $6,523 and specialists earned $11,368."[10] This last figure is staggering in terms of buying power at the time and reflects the commonplace experience of most Canadians and Americans: that the largest and fanciest house in small and medium-sized towns throughout the first half of the 20th century was normally owned by "the Doctor." Even though doctors practicing in hospitals did not generally do quite as well – Harold Griffith's salary didn't hit five figures until the 1960s and never went above $30,000, even in the 1970s – their professional situation seemed to improve year by year. Small wonder they opposed any changes along the lines of Germany, which had massive government funding in place by 1911, or Britain, which was moving in the same direction.

Even in their first halcyon period, however, doctors who were truly interested in the technological revolution and in generalized, egalitarian health care recognized problems. They knew that their charitable funding was unpredictable and might not enable them to equip hospitals, deal with public health emergencies, or fund innovations in a stable fashion. Naylor quotes an article by Dr J.H. MacDermot in the *Canadian Medical Association Journal,* (CMAJ), in 1929, as fairly representative of attitudes across Canada. By this time, they were sufficiently confident in their hold on the public's trust and esteem to entertain the idea of collaborative funding – provided they remained in the driver's seat. Dr MacDermot described the medical profession's attitude as "expectant." "We are not supporting ... any scheme; nor are we opposed to health insurance. We should be willing ... to support and help to implement any wisely designed measure calculated to improve social conditions, to lessen sickness and to prevent disease. We should be ready ... to advise the Legislature as to what is sane and wise, and what would be short-sighted and dangerous legislation."[11] This attitude was already very different from that found in the U.S., where doctors and their associations were vehemently opposed to any direct government funding of health care.

The Canadian attitude of waiting for the government to present them with a sweet deal in which the profession retained control, Naylor goes on to say, "was about to be transformed" by the stock market crash on Wall Street in 1929 that lead to a worldwide depression. In Canada, only three short years later, a quarter of the workforce was unemployed. Not just patients but formerly prosperous physicians were facing desperate situations. As Dr Lewis Andreas, recounting his professional experiences during the Depression in Studs Terkel's famous book, *Hard Times,* put it, "One found oneself with a lot of training, knowledge, skills, ready to spring forth on the world – and no customers. People weren't going to doctors because they just couldn't afford it."[12] A survey of practitioners in Hamilton, Ontario backs up the American's assertion. Between 1929 and 1932, "the total volume of [medical] services delivered fell an average of 36.5 percent. In 1929, 77.5 percent of work done was remunerative; but in 1932, half of the patients were non-paying." In fact, "Almost one-half of the doctors in the Hamilton survey sample claimed to be unable to provide the necessities of life for their households." In rural Saskatchewan, doctors found themselves joining queues for relief rations from Ottawa. "There was also a definite awareness that many patients, whether paying or non-paying, were putting off visits to the doctor, even though their illnesses were serious."[13]

Under the then-current business/charity system, the state or province, or, in the case of most American and some Canadian hospitals, the municipality, was supposed to provide free rooms and medicines for "the indigent," and physicians were supposed to offer their diagnosis and treatment for free. Then, as now, in a two-tier situation, the people who were not provided for at all were not the truly destitute, but the working poor, the lower middle-class, and the recently unemployed. In Chicago, for example, the situation for Dr Andreas became so serious that in 1932, he became involved in revolutionary efforts to vary the sources of medical funding. He was a founding member of Chicago's first medical center to offer a group practice and low fees and his experiences in Chicago were repeated across the continent. As he pointed out, "The poor got some care; they could go to free dispensaries. The rich got good care because they could afford it. There was this big middle class that was not getting any care." People who were too proud to accept treatment in a charity ward but too poor to afford care had two stark choices. They could let their conditions deteriorate, or they could continue seeing their doctor in hopes that "an economic recovery would restore their ability to pay."[14]

Semi-professionals, teachers, health care workers, and factory and shop workers were hit hardest. Andreas recounted, "They put off care until things got real bad. They probably lost their lives." With municipalities also caught in the debt spiral of the period, the only hope for funding was other levels of government. As Naylor puts it, "Doctors faced a growing number of bad debts and falling incomes. If properly arranged, state health insurance could provide the practitioner with guaranteed payment from his augmented proportion of non-paying patients; badly handled, it could leave the doctor enmeshed in the state regulatory apparatus, and no further ahead."[15]

Community hospitals faced the same dilemma and went into pure survival mode. The luxurious private pavilions were one of the first casualties of the general financial collapse. Not one was built after about 1931, and society had changed so fundamentally by the end of the Depression that none have been built in Canada since. There followed a "wholesale retreat of paying patients from the hospital" throughout the 1930s, and even small institutions that had hitched their wagons to the star of two-tier care spent the entire Depression trembling on the edge of bankruptcy and closure. By the late thirties, of those paying patients staying an average of two and a half weeks, at a cost of $120 a week, only 30 percent reported having little difficulty in paying their hospital bills and as many as 15 percent were experiencing extreme financial duress – on the level of losing houses or apartments, life savings, educational opportunities, and so on. As medical technologies proliferated and treatment costs continued to soar throughout the subsequent decades, it became a very rare family that could face the news of a required operation or extended hospital stay without as much fear for their financial as for their physical survival.[16]

The tersely defensive Annual Reports of the Homeopathic don't give details about how bad things got during this time; these can only be found in departmental minutes. By the mid-1930s, for example, nurses were tearing up their old uniforms to make the bandages that their institution could no longer afford to buy. Much more seriously, and despite warm allusions in the annual reports to their nurses' heroic work, the Homeopathic Hospital Board attempted to revoke the nurses' right to free medical care and did succeed in shortening their paid sick leave.

This was not a trivial economy for the hospitals, nor was it a minor concern for the nurses. The students, especially those who were young, suffered serious health problems, including occupational ailments and a death rate significantly higher than the normal population, mostly from the infectious diseases to which they were exposed but also from septicemia from needle or scalpel wounds as well as injuries caused by lifting. Their health was a constant "source of anxiety" to their institutions. "But the concern about students' general well-being was invariably compromised by administrators' concurrent worry about its financial toll on the hospitals' inadequate funds." In a scathing 1919 report, the Vancouver General's Malcom MacEachem blamed the ill-health of his hospital's nursing students on the lack of a "well-organized medical service which adequately discovers any disease or physical unfitness, as well as treating such conditions as arise during the training."[17]

The Montreal Homeopathic was very unusual in that A.R. Griffith had always insisted that the students in the Philips' School receive free medical care in-house, paid sick leave, and protein-rich free meals. It was due entirely to A.R.'s stubborn refusal to budge on these issues that the Homeopathic Board of Directors was unable to destroy their nurses' right to free medical care during the Depression, and the nurses were well aware of the fact.[18] There are repeated mentions of the nurses' gratefulness for "loyalty" in all the subsequent Annual Reports, with Dora Miller's, written in 1936, reading, "I take this opportunity to again thank our Medical Staff for their continued interest and help with the lectures and the care and attention given the nurses when ill. The health of the student is a matter of deep concern to us; monthly weight charts are kept, x-rays are taken, physical examinations made when necessary, and the nurses are expected to report at once any indisposition. With this preventive programme we try to anticipate any trouble that might arise."[19] Although it would seem entirely appropriate for any hospital to provide these services, it was actually quite unusual. In many other institutions, "training as a nurse brought with it no guarantee of access to ... medical care." The Gagans state, "Few hospitals provided the health care required by sick nurses who, allegedly, were often left unattended in their rooms for hours without food or medicine."[20] Seldom were they seen by doctors and most diagnosis and treatment was left to the head nurse. With twelve-hour shifts requiring a great deal of hard physical labour – making beds, carrying trays, lifting and bathing patients, washing and disinfecting all surfaces, including floors – exhaustion as well as exposure to disease were factors in what the few studies of the period discovered was a worrisome level of ill-health among nurses.

EXPLOITING THE HELP

Much of the literature dealing with nurses' training in this period, and their treatment by hospital boards and doctors, is openly critical of the tendency towards exploitation and lack of respect. Educational needs, such as lecture and study time, were neglected in favour of long hours in ward work so that 'the practical always outweighed the theoretical.'
W.G. Godfrey, *The Struggle to Serve*[21]

When nursing first became a professional option in the late 19th century, it attracted hordes of young women whose career choices up until then had been exceedingly meager. But by the 1920s, word about the dangerous, heavy work nursing entailed began to affect recruiting. An even more worrisome consideration to the prospective student was the fact that once nurses graduated from the many nursing schools, they encountered serious difficulties in finding long-term employment. The lack of work available for the thousands of nursing school graduates that were being churned out every year was the result of the dirty secret mentioned in chapter 2, Growing a Culture. The secret was, as the Gagans aptly put it, that, "hospital nursing education was at best inadequate; and at worst a form of slavery."[22]

Hospitals depended on the pool of unpaid labour provided by their nurses in training. Once nurses graduated, the Boards were obliged to pay them for their formerly free work. Therefore, graduate nurses often could not find work even if their own hospitals were under-staffed. They had to turn to private practice and many became chroni-cally under-employed. Recruits began to stay away, and the resulting shortage was exacerbated by the cost-cutting programs that hospitals introduced during the Depression. The Montreal Homeopathic had been unusual in hiring its own nurses almost at once, with an average of those employed full-time jumping from one taken on every three or four years in the teens to a steady two or three being hired every year by 1929. Reports and minutes make it clear that this unusual policy was in direct response to the lack of opportunities for graduates. The two or three hired were nonetheless taken from graduating classes of five to ten students. Most graduate nurses still had to turn to private practice, although an almost equal number of young women graduating from the Homeopathic – three or four on average – married and left work altogether.[23] Still, the Homeopathic remained unusually considerate of nursing interests and as early as 1932 began limiting student enroll-ment in favour of graduates. That year, the lady superintendent wrote, "Due to the surplus of graduate nurses, it seemed advisable to admit to the school the fewest possible number of students [9 out of 40 stu-dents] and only those of the highest qualifications, relief being done by graduates."[24]

Elsewhere in Canada, graduate hiring rates were considerably lower. Nurses were most often abandoned by hospitals on graduation and had to search for whatever part-time work they could find in private prac-tice or the remaining charitable institutions for orphans or the dis-abled. As early as 1932, the work shortage had become serious enough to inspire a joint survey by the CMA and the Canadian Nurses' Associa-tion. It was conducted by George Weir, chair of the University of British Columbia's Department of Education. David and Rosemary Gagan point out that his findings were remarkably progressive. "Weir's man-date clearly linked the unemployment crisis among graduate nurses and the CMA's growing obsession with the health-care crisis facing doc-tors' middle-class paying patients, to systemic problems [within the entire] economic, educational and sociological system" surrounding both nurses and hospitals.[25]

One thing Weir discovered was that too many "slow" or inadequate students were being admitted to the schools. In particular, the grueling twelve-hour shifts on the ward and in the classroom were "too physically and mentally exacting for the average student nurse," let alone for the less intelligent or poorly educated recruits that were often hastily accepted by hospital boards strapped for free labour. In this, the Montreal Homeopathic did meet or even exceed the latest requirements for educating nurses: Weir's 1932 recommendations included one qualified instructor for every 50 to 75 students working in hospitals that had created separate departments for surgery, maternity, pediatrics, and infectious diseases. Almost a decade earlier, by 1924, the Homeopathic had one formal, full-time instructor for every fifty-one students, not counting department heads, nurse-superintendents, and doctors, each of whom gave several courses a month.[26] Rosemary and David Gagan note that this was far from typical. "Most training schools in Canada relied on graduate nurses to lecture on the many topics spread over the course of study." They report that, shockingly enough, "as late as the 1930s, there was not [one] full-time nursing instructor in the Maritime Provinces." Weir had also insisted that shifts be reduced to eight hours with "less time allocated to housework and more to medical theory" and demanded "hygienic and sanitary [housing] conditions in residences separate from the hospital and ... [not] in the same building as patients."[27]

This was not Weir's idea alone. The Royal Victoria had constructed a residence connected to the hospital by a bridge, but in a separate building, as early as 1905, following a fire in the student nurses' quarters as well as repeated problems with illness from the open infectious disease wards on the same floor. Most hospitals started building such residences in the late 1920s and 30s. Already in 1926, A. R. Griffith was pushing his investors for funds to enable the Homeopathic to open just such a separate residence/school and the Nurses' Residence Fund became a constant topic in the Annual Reports from then on. The Montreal General was building their separate school that same year, and Hopital Notre-Dame and Hopital Ste-Justine got theirs in 1931. Good housing for nurses was obviously all the rage. Bad as things were in 1931, Griffith still hired architects to plan the separate residence for his nurses.

By 1935, however, Homeopathic nurses still did not have their own
separate residence/school. Worst of all, even their second-floor quarters in the Montreal Homeopathic's new building on Marlow Street,
which had been opened with such optimism only eight years before,
were being divided into private and semi-private patient beds, in order
to bring in a little more money. The Hospital was so in arrears on its
debts that the bill for the architectural plans drawn up four years
before had not been paid and a special installment arrangement had
to be worked out with the architects in order to avoid court action.[28]
A.R.'s increasingly despairing requests for funding for such a residence, which continued from 1927 until his death in 1936, underline
the perceived necessity of a separate residence for hospitals that
wanted to be considered modern and professional. In 1938, well
before the Depression was over, the Homeopathic somehow managed
to triumphantly open their new Philips' School of Nursing in a large,
modern building that still stands next to the old hospital. So many
other ambitious projects, to say nothing of normal procedures, were
abandoned during the same period that the Homeopathic's commitment to the quality of its nursing can be inferred by this act.

The nurses involved knew who their allies were. When A.R. Griffith
and his chief of surgery, J.T. Novinger, died within several months of
each other, the lady superintendent of the Nursing School wrote,
"words are inadequate when one attempts to tell what these two kind
and staunch friends meant to us as a group and individually. Always
interested in our problems and concerned for our welfare, they never
failed to cheer and encourage us."[29] The Homeopathic had always
managed to find the money for continuing education somewhere. In
1947, for example, before the boom years of the early fifties, the
Report of the Medical Superintendent noted that various doctors had
attended medical congresses in Winnipeg, New York, Atlantic City, and
St. Louis and that nurses had been sent to the International Congress
of Nurses in Atlantic City. The hospital also entertained "many visiting
doctors and nurses from many parts of the world."[30] Even today, Montreal's largest teaching hospital, the Montreal General, would love to
have such support. According to Pat Titterton, their head nurse had to
fight in the 1990s to get the administration merely to reimburse nurses
for the time lost going to conferences and colloquia.

The Queen Elizabeth's on-going desire for continued professional
training was solidified in 1958 when a formal Education Fund was instituted by the Medical Board.[31] In 1966, just before they retired, Harold

and Jim Griffith managed to raise $165,000 to endow this fund, stipulating that it must continue to cover all employees, not just doctors. In practice, it appears to have been primarily used for the continuing education of nurses. In 1972, the fund was christened "The Griffith Foundation" by the president of the hospital, Hollis Martin. By then, it was worth between one and two million dollars. It stood at seven million when the hospital was closed. It sent nurses to important conferences and helped them achieve new levels of specialization up until the 1995 closing and since then, has funded two chairs, the Harold Griffith Chair in Anesthesia Research and, in 2004, The Queen Elizabeth Hospital of Montreal Foundation Chair in Pediatric Anesthesia, which alone cost $1.6 million.

The Griffith Fund was really an extension of A.R. Griffith's commitment to the findings of hospital reformers such as Weir, who had demanded that training schools become primarily educational facilities "rather than the agent of nurses' continuing exploitation as a source of cheap labour." As Weir put it, this step would free the profession from "membership in a cult of intellectual serfdom ... as hewers of wood and drawers of water." Weir had also suggested that hospitals begin limiting student responsibilities within the hospitals and that they prioritize the hiring of graduate nurses to fulfill those duties. Despite the fact that this analysis, as well as Weir's suggestion that universities be more involved in training nurses, was in general welcomed by both the nursing and hospital professionals throughout the 1930s, hospitals continued to be in such dire financial straits that survival was more of an issue than reform. So, despite everyone's desires, "graduate nurses still struggled to find employment, [and] the debate over the suitable balance between student and graduate nurses remained largely unresolved."[32]

THE STATE'S POOR

The free services of physicians are not asked for, or given to, or
exploited for those who can and should pay, or for whom *payment should
be made.*

New CMA ethics code, 1937[33]

Many hospitals probably wanted to be more generous to their nurses, but in the 1930s they were quite literally starving. At the Homeopathic, for example, money for the new school was somehow found, but the once all-important rich diets and kitchen supplies, for patients and staff alike, were cut back fairly ruthlessly, with the administration asking for suggestions on how to do more. Liquid diets for patients were found by a 1937 study to be below the volume of those in some other Montreal hospitals, but nothing was done about it, presumably for economic reasons. The hospital's growing debts were covered by borrowing more from the bank to service the interest.[34] In the 1920s, the Montreal Homeopathic had sought tens of thousands of dollars from its many wealthy donors for new x-ray departments and building projects. By 1937, the nurses were holding bridge nights to get one wheel chair or a single electric breast pump. Researcher Ken Hechtman, in an unpublished analysis of this period, notes that most community hospitals had to resort to measures bordering on the illegal as well as the unfair. "The short answer for how they got through the Depression is simple. They put off the creditors and squeezed the nurses."

It couldn't have gone on much longer. Naylor agrees that, "As the Depression wore on, Canada's medical profession turned to government with hope and trepidation, seeking economic salvation on the best possible terms." But despite this, doctors steadfastly refused to relinquish control of either the health profession or the hospitals to government. This situation was even more extreme in the United States and at first government intervention did prove to be a failure. In the hardest- hit provinces such as Saskatchewan and Alberta, for example, experimental salary schemes intended to help doctors only confirmed their darkest fears. The relief provided to doctors by the Calgary City Council in 1936 amounted to an average of 33 cents a call and was revised *downwards* four months later. In Saskatchewan, "drought conditions contributed to the spread of salaried-contract practice" with 75 "municipal doctors" working in the province by 1938 and receiving salaries of between $600 and $900 a year – not a living wage even then. Bankrupt municipalities couldn't manage to pay even these starvation wages, however, and "some offered payment in kind from municipal stocks of hardware and cordwood."[35]

This fiasco hardened most of the profession's attitude against government-funded medical care and salaried systems. Salaried clinics organized along socialist principles, such as Lewis Andreas' in Chicago, remained rare, although there were a few in the Canadian prairies and even beyond. In the Homeopathic's hometown of Montreal, there were powerful voices in the 1930s urging more government involvement in what was then termed "socialized medicine," including that of the famous chief of the tuberculosis unit at Sacre Coeur, Dr Norman Bethune. Before leaving for his work in Spain during their civil war, Bethune helped create a weekly clinic for the unemployed in Verdun, next door to the Homeopathic's own bailiwick. He also organized local progressives into "the Montreal Group for the Security of the People's Health," which proposed several modes of prepaid health care, "including fee-for-service and salaried clinics," with the best plan "extended to as many citizens as possible."

Bethune's American colleague Andreas characterizes this small but ardent movement. "[We felt] it was up to us to create a substitute for the society that was disappearing. Some of us figured it was collapsing. We were arrogant, perhaps, but ... [we had] splendid ideas about what we could accomplish." However, Naylor notes that despite all the highly creative tactics brewed up by socialists like Andreas and Bethune in clinics and medical schools, despite all the highly original bookkeeping, professional compromises, and charity drives in hospitals such as the Homeopathic, "the response [to any form of socialized medicine] from the profession at large was lukewarm at best." This was because the pressure on governments concerning all kinds of social programs, including social security and unemployment compensation, was becoming so intense that the charge did not have to be led by doctors alone. Society really was changing, quite rapidly.

"These simple things we stood for," Dr Andreas said years later, "group medicine and prepayment – have been achieved," even in the United States.[36] In Canada, as early as 1936, Montreal had organized one of the country's most comprehensive health relief plans; other Canadian and American cities followed. By this time, there were also signs of general economic recovery and falling unemployment rates.[37] Ironically and perhaps predictably, as soon as the economic pressures were off, doctors in most parts of Canada went back to claiming they were happy to work for free on indigents and didn't need the government interference of mass insurance programs. The majority of doctors at Montreal's Homeopathic maintained this position right up until the forced introduction of Medicare in the 1960s. Only doctors in the Prairies continued to labour under poor conditions. Because the economy there was very slow to recover, they generally remained more open to the idea of socialized medicine and subsequently, the Prairies became the birthplace of Canada's single-payer Medicare system.

All across the continent, the Depression experience profoundly changed professional attitudes towards the position of doctors and hospitals in the marketplace. "These wounds were permanent," as Lewis Andreas put it. Many doctors, including his father, lost all their property and savings and never restored their practices to their former glory. Others, like Andreas himself, were unable to find the funds to specialize as they would have wished and their careers were permanently curtailed. The hospitals, of course, lost departments, wings, and personnel. A. R. Griffith didn't even live to see the Homeopathic get its nurse's residence and must have gone to his grave wondering if his hospital would survive at all. The general response to this traumatic experience was "a new corporatism, [which] became evident in the professional ranks." Provincial medical associations, such as the Ontario Medical Association as well as the previously established Canadian Medical Association, expanded mightily and began to become skilled at highly politicized lobbying before the various parliaments. With this rapid growth came the power and money that enabled this lobby to defend their members' interests. They also began to aggressively seek social and legislative changes, including forced mass inoculations; government funding for drugs, equipment, and training programs; and care for the poor. All of these programs greatly improved the public health but they also worked powerfully in the profession's interest and contributed to its increasing influence and autonomy in the coming decades.[38] These increasingly scientific, political, and corporate-style innovations have continued to characterize the medical profession today and even the most neglected and marginalized of health professionals, nurses, have also gradually become corporatized, as well as unionized.

In short, the Great Depression was the crucible in which the medical profession's pious, altruistic past was subsumed. It re-emerged clothed in the science- and market-oriented garb that typifies the medical world today. It's actually rather shocking to see how quickly doctors and hospitals were ready to drop their exalted social values when times became lean in the 1930s. Throughout this period, the profession worked hard to shift nearly all of its former charitable responsibilities onto the shoulders of government. They did this rather neatly: they simply re-defined who should be termed "indigent" – that is, who really deserved the selfless, donated care of a professional physician – and who didn't.

Back in 1868, the Canadian Medical Association code promised that medical services would "always be cheerfully and freely accorded to indigents." This same code, as revised in 1937, seven years into the Depression, was changed to read: "While what have been called God's poor should always be cared for with charity, the growing numbers of what might be called the State's poor, or the State's wards, should be cared for on some basis that allows proper remuneration for services."[39] Only a year later, in 1938, at the Rowell-Sirois Royal Commission hearings on where health care responsibilities should lie, that is, with the profession or with the federal, provincial, or municipal governments, "the CMA brief went to some lengths in spelling out the need for federal support in paying the medical bills of a list of groups, ranging from the 'indigents and unemployed' to 'war veterans and old age pensioners.'" Naylor remarks that, "in the light of the revised CMA code of ethics, one senses that 'the State's poor' now far outnumbered 'God's poor.'"[40]

HITLER SAVES THE DAY FOR PUBLIC HEALTH

In the late thirties, I'd say our society was saved again. By Hitler. Because the stopgaps [of government programs and support] weren't working, and things were sliding back. The war, in a sense, ended the Depression. It's like an incurable disease in which there is a remission.

Dr Lewis Andreas, from *Hard Times* [41]

Anyone who has read *The Tin Flute*, Gabrielle Roy's novel of the tribulations of working- and lower middle-class Montrealers during the Depression, remembers how its young male characters, who had little work or hope for the future, kindled with joy at the thought of getting into the army at the beginning of World War II. Their happiness over the prospect of simply being fed and clothed dissolved into despair when many were rejected for service. They were unfit because their health had been destroyed by the diseases of poverty – TB, malnutrition, and brutal work injuries. The Canadian government, having first learned the woeful state of the national health during the recruitment process of the First World War, was much more rigorous in weeding out those who were too ill to perform in battle during recruitment efforts for the Second World War. Few people today realize that the social situation had become so serious in North America by the late thirties that many cities found it hard to find able-bodied soldiers. But to the advantage of the millions of men being mobilized for that war, the newfound ability to identify chronic ill health was accompanied by a more progressive government response to the demands of the medical profession for better hygiene, training programs, and access to new drugs.

Solutions to both hospital and public health care funding dilemmas that had been theories in Canada throughout the Depression gradually took concrete shape in the 1940s. Naturally, they varied from province to province. In general, however, by the time the Second World War was providing work, investment, and an end to economic hard times, physicians, hospital administrators, and the public had all accepted a much greater role for the same government that was defending them from their enemies, both in funding and in administering their medical care. Of course, the entire medical complex, from hospitals and doctors down to nurses and orderlies, still depended on paying customers and charitable contributions. By the end of the 1930s, the major public health miracles of the War years, including antibiotics and advanced anesthetics, had joined antisepsis and medical professionalism to create the truly modern, scientific hospital. Harold Griffith, along with many other young, would-be specialists, was traveling, experimenting, and founding new professional groups. Both hospitals and the medical profession had begun to wake up and expand, backed by the impetus of the booming war economy. By the time recruiting and weapons production were in full swing in the early 1940s, hospitals were about to enter what might now be called their unalloyed golden age; many of their former problems simply dissolved away.

The lack of employment for graduate nurses, for example, which had been plaguing the profession for at least two decades, was miraculously replaced by more jobs than they could handle. Qualified graduate nurses were snapped up by hospitals trying to replace the almost 4,000 taken to serve in the armed forces. This naturally boosted recruiting, income, and hospital status for the profession as a whole. "Considering hospitals' previous resistance, the substitution of graduate for student labour was accomplished remarkably quickly, although at significant expense," Rosemary and David Gagan note.[42] Some still resisted. The Calgary General, Halifax's Victoria General, and Victoria's Royal Jubilee held onto their student labour at rates as high as eight to one. But most of the other large hospitals – and good small ones, such as the Homeopathic – reversed the old pattern, with graduates quickly outnumbering student nurses almost two to one. Almost a decade after they were first suggested, many of Weir's progressive 1932 recommendations were suddenly and almost violently accomplished as a consequence of these changing economic conditions. For example, his criticism of academically and financially marginal schools led to the closure of twelve out of nineteen schools in British Columbia alone.

The profession also benefited from the same medical and surgical advances that accompanied the war as nurses, too, began to specialize. And finally, the grueling twelve-hour shifts were mitigated to eight between 1942 and 1951.[43]

After the First World War, "incredible traces of Victorian prudery," as Harold Griffith put it, had still hampered how women in professional positions functioned, even at the Homeopathic. He recounted how when he came to the Hospital as a resident in 1919, "if in the operating room it was necessary to expose the genital organs of an adult male, the procedure was posted as a 'screen operation.'"[44] A screen was set up between the scrub nurse and the surgeon; she had to hand the instruments to the doctor around the edge, thus sparing her any untoward sights. Moreover, if a student nurse, of whatever age, wished to get married, she was unceremoniously kicked out of school. This was a holdover from the Florence Nightingale days. The need to remove professional nurses from any residual mental association with the untrained wives, girlfriends, former patients, camp followers, and prostitutes who used to provide so much of the nursing required by society's sick and wounded dictated an almost inhuman level of probity in the profession. This policy was retained until Harold got full control of the hospital in 1941, by which point not just the Homeopathic, but society at large, was finally starting to fully recognize women as educated professionals.

The difficulty of the work and a vast increase in employment opportunities for women during the war years reversed the former situation of surpluses, making nurse shortages a feature of the modern era. Although the situation would pass, by 1947 small schools like the Homeopathic began to fear the possibility of closure because of lack of students. After warning that their beloved school might be closed some day, Harold Griffith more or less summed up the progressive wisdom regarding the nursing profession during the post-war period. "Occasionally we hear criticism that the hospitals for their own benefit 'exploit' student nurses. We would like to state very emphatically that our student nurses have always been considered as students undergoing training, and never as a source of cheap help for the Hospital. A survey taken by the Canadian Nurses' Association during the past year shows that our Hospital has one of the highest ratios of graduate nurses to students of any hospital in Canada ... [Yet, given the smaller supply of students,] ... it is altogether likely that in the future, much routine nursing care in hospitals will be carried out by nurses' aides instead of by student or graduate nurses. For this reason the Montreal School for Nursing Aides has been established, with our Hospital as a participating member."[45] The Queen E became the one of the first hospitals in Canada to begin graduating qualified nurses' aides to meet the new labour shortage.

As for the patients' experience of hospital care, the excesses of luxury were never to completely return, but because the hospital system was still divided by ability to pay, many of the comforts created for rich clients prior to the Depression began to be considered necessary to the psychological welfare of the middle class patients who were gaining prosperity throughout the 1940s and 50s. Thus, the elevators, communications systems, laundries, central heating, refrigeration, plumbing, and lighting systems that were once the purview of the private wards started to become generally available in the late forties. To keep up with the amenities available in so many homes and offices, they had to be constantly upgraded, too.

Moreover, as the discipline of psychology developed, such institutional luxuries as solaria, libraries, special furnishings, therapy departments, special diets, and "soothing colours" were increasingly considered essential to the healing process. All this contributed to every hospital's annual expenses. Construction costs in particular mushroomed as much as 1,000 percent in one decade; medical technology, then as now, "marched to its own drumbeat: the cost of an x-ray unit was $300 in 1900, $3,000 in 1920, $7,500 in 1930, and at least $10,000 in 1940," all in a time of low annual inflation. Because "the link between institutional wealth and institutional progress simply became inexorable," as Rosemary and David Gagan point out, "it is hardly remarkable that the aspirations of hospitals, large and small, always outdistanced their resources."[46]

This attitude became the downside of post-war good times for every hospital attempting to serve their clientele both during and after the Second World War. North American society in the 1940s through the 1960s was not only prosperous but the medical successes hailed in every form of media made it increasingly demanding. By the 1950s, every family expected their hometown hospital to provide them with miraculous healing at a reasonable cost. At the Homeopathic, as everywhere else, prosperity brought more and larger fee increases as well as what the Gagans call the never-ending and "unapologetic solicitation of the public for voluntary charitable financial support" that is part and parcel of every hospital's dealings with its constituency.

HAPPY DAYS

So altogether, this report is a happy one as regards the quality of the
work being done in all departments of the Queen Elizabeth Hospital.
We are happy too, about the generous financial support of many friends
and about the unselfish way in which workers in the campaign gave
freely of their time and effort. All these things make us grateful, and
spur us on to continued service.

Harold Griffith, 1952[47]

Only five years before writing the ebullient words quoted above, Harold Griffith had been discouraged. In the 1947 *Annual Report*, he
wrote, "Hospital work involves many busy days and long, weary nights.
Without the help, so freely given in so many ways, our task would be
impossible." The sigh is almost audible when he concludes, "We will try
to carry on the work in a spirit of Christian service."[48] The difference
may be coincidental, of course; but it is also symbolic of the era beginning in the late 40s and running all the way to the 1970s. From about
1948 on, halcyon days for hospitals, doctors, and even, to some extent,
patients, had arrived. The enormous advances in medical care and hospital equipment were coupled with significant relief in funding from
government sources.

All the early medical pioneers understood the hospital's role as the
first line of defense for dispensing drugs and treatment to the public in
the event of widespread communicable diseases such as typhoid and
TB. They also understood its increasing role as capable of saving or bet-
tering individual lives stricken by acute or chronic disease and injury.
Following World War II, the four pillars of modern medicine were now
complete and available to masses of humanity. Arriving to aid good
nursing and antisepsis, antibiotics and improved surgical techniques
were now vastly improving the morbidity statistics as well as altering the
types of diseases most commonly encountered. Innovators and surgeons such as Harold and Jim Griffith were now able to increase the
quality of care for individual conditions. This new focus happily coincided with new sources of funding for hospitals and, in Canada especially, with the stability of newly legislated government stipends.

The combination of safer anesthetics that enabled surgeons to
remove formerly fatal tumors or defects, along with drugs to manage
or cure cancers, diabetes, epilepsy, and more, elevated doctors and surgeons to dizzying heights of public esteem and admiration in the 1950s

and 60s. They, and the hospitals where they worked, were seen as nothing less than heroic: exciting, vitally useful, dazzlingly competent, innovative, and, that necessity of heroism, brave in the face of danger. It was natural that wealth, both public and private, was attracted to this social prestige, and both medical salaries and hospital budgets ballooned during this period.

In most respects, the Montreal Homeopathic faithfully reflected the demographic and medical changes that accompanied these Baby Boom years. Every year of the late forties and early fifties saw a record increase in the number of babies born in its wards.[49] By this time, most people were drawing their last as well as their first breaths in the hallowed and trusted halls of hospitals. The patience, understanding, and confidence invested in hospital care by the average patient was at an all-time high, although with hindsight, we should add that this trust was partially due to the ignorance of both patients and doctors about what was actually going on.

For example, in the same breath that Harold Griffith announced the continuing success of curare and praised new methods of using spinal anesthesia in delivering babies, he also applauded the use of X-rays for treating sinus infections and shoulder pain. Clinical trials were invented in the late 1940s, but regulations didn't require the kind of testing they now do. Beyond that, it wasn't the style to question a hospital – or heaven forbid, sue one – about what would now be considered experimenting with unproven treatments. Of course, it can be argued that the massive advantages represented by the development of curare and spinal anesthesia during those days seem in retrospect worth the losses incurred by the mistakes, even including the suffering caused by society's lavish use of X-rays throughout the 1950s and 60s. It can also be argued that many patients actually knew all this, at least intuitively, and entered into their treatments, especially for previously catastrophic conditions like cancer or diabetes, more as participants in medical progress than as victims of it. Many people embarked on these new and experimental procedures with their physicians in a spirit of mutual trust and gracefully accepted their fate if the miraculous new drug or procedure failed.

Eager drug and medical technology companies were a vital part of this scenario. They worked with individual doctors and hospitals to field new products – usually with even less safety research than we get today – for a public that could hardly wait to try out their wares. One of the only constraints on the growing influence of drug companies was the widely held ban on direct advertising to consumers, which today has been removed. Throughout this period, however, doctors remained the checkpoint for new treatments. By and large, they handled this responsibility well enough to at least preserve their patients' trust.

On top of the doctor/patient/drug company partnerships, new funding was flowing in from governments. Public taxes rapidly became the major source of medical funding in Canada, but at this period, their stipends were added to the still unabated help from charities, individuals, and the rock-solid Women's Auxiliaries. Such a situation provided unprecedented financial security and stability for hospitals and research centres. Private fees for what was still a two-tier system never attained their pre-war excesses because government money helped keep the hospitals from having to inflate fees, but these fees continued to contribute to the overall prosperity right up until Medicare. In short, just as natural organisms or ecosystems benefit from a rich variety of inputs and genetic or species variety, the Canadian medical system enjoyed a dynamic balance between these varied sources of knowledge, cooperation, and funding. Between World War II and the 1970s, hospitals enjoyed an unprecedented golden age.

So bright was the light of these days that the Homeopathic took the long-delayed and extremely symbolic step of re-naming itself. Homeopathy had been in decline since the 1920s and had continued to fade as the new methods of antisepsis and inoculation advanced. Now that antibiotics and curare were available to practitioners, few medical professionals wanted to be publicly associated with the old German theories. So in 1951, the Homeopathic Hospital of Montreal became the Queen Elizabeth Hospital of Montreal. The gala naming ceremony did not just attract professionals from McGill and all the local politicians. The Queen Mum herself, for whom the hospital was named, arrived to christen an institution that was being re-dedicated to the new medical values of science and the market.

This ideological change had been building steadily since the end of the War. In keeping with the new spirit of evidence-based scientific enquiry, Jim Griffith required his surgeons to start keeping records of the use of specific drugs before 1945, "so that the Hospital may be able to establish a technique ... and also in [what] conditions it was of most advantage."[50] Autopsy reports, which continued to be done in about 70 to 80 percent of hospital deaths, were now not afraid to list "unknown" rather than inventing Latin code words. And although staff responsibility for deaths, which was formerly openly discussed, was no longer publicly listed from this date, anesthetic overdoses were being clearly described as "too high a dose" rather than "the patient couldn't tolerate."[51]

The Hospital's first in-house psychiatrist was hired in February of 1947. This was followed quickly by its first alcoholism clinic in November of 1949, and a Neurology Clinic in December of 1951. Doctors were increasingly and officially being restricted to their own specialties, and doctors and nurses were sent on serious courses, some as much as a month long, on such topics as post-operative care, blood banks, and cytology. The Hospital also brought in presenters to teach staff about hepatitis, because of an epidemic in the 1950s, as well as on subjects such as blood coagulation, drugs for hypertension, and advances in tuberculosis treatments.[52] Although many of these procedures were and are routine for any hospital, it was during this period that they were refined. For example, in the 1950s numerous deaths resulted from contaminated donors to blood banks. Labs couldn't screen blood for hepatitis, which may explain the continuing epidemics of the period, and ambulance workers had not yet been taught to match for type.[53] Continued attention to blood banks brought results so that by the late 1960s there was no longer a problem.

Along with knowledge comes an opening of minds. Harold Griffith always worked to hire women physicians and proposed that the Hospital hire a Chinese woman doctor in November of 1949. The board voted against it but reversed their decision less than a month later. The Queen Elizabeth continued to exhibit its flair for innovation when a home-made defibrillator, hastily constructed from forks and other materials from the cafeteria, was used to shock an emergency patient back to life in the OR on 12 November 1951. Only a year later, in January of 1952, the hospital was the first in North America to use coloured dye to detect lung lesions[54] and one of the first to clinically connect smoking with cancer of the lung.[55] As well, Harold Griffith virtually invented the first Intensive Care Unit in Canada, which was opened on 3 July 1961. He believed this innovation saved even more lives than the use of curare, for which he was still so honored and respected, and he was probably right.

On the financial front, Blue Cross, the non-profit, physician-founded employment insurance plan, was paying a full 90 percent of all semi-private patient costs, "excluding x-rays and anesthetics," by 1951. However, the almost continuous acquisition of new gadgets between

October of 1953 and February of 1954, including such items as a camera, epidiascope, "skin therapy machine for the cancer clinic," new radiation machine, and an audiometer, explains the unending quest for more and more money that became the overriding feature of the halcyon days.

The educational and technological problems that were so daunting back when the Griffith family started their odyssey back in the late 1800s had to a great extent been solved. The old needs of hospitals to attract patients and to actually help make them well were history by the 1950s. What has remained is the problem each country concerned with maintaining public health has had to face in turn. That problem is simple: how to find the money to pay for and also to adequately distribute medical care. Both difficulties are more social and philosophical than they are economic. Many countries, such as Holland or Denmark, currently operate well-functioning and accessible hospital care systems even while other far richer countries, like the United States, do not. The challenge to continue to run good hospitals is always reappearing, but providing equitable hospital care has not proven to be impossible for modern societies. It's just that in North America in particular, we keep attacking the problem from the wrong direction.

SPENDING MONEY ON THE RIGHT THING

As the frequency of hospital births grew, ... so did evidence that
hospitalization did not reduce maternal and infant mortality and ...
probably exacerbated both before the 1940s.
                    David and Rosemary Gagan, *For Patients of Moderate Means* [56]

During the glory days for hospitals, that is, following World War II, innovators such as Harold Griffith were reaping the rewards of their devotion to science. In his case, as with most innovators back then, the rewards weren't monetary, as they might be today, but they were definitely personal and professional. Harold Griffith was, by all the evidence, a kind and well-intentioned man who was lucky in that the beginning of his career coincided with the rise of medical science. Those happy days lasted for most of his professional life; but towards the end, managerial disappointment and the same kind of financial destabilization that blighted his father's last years returned to haunt him and most of the rest of Canada's hospital administrators. There wasn't a worldwide economic depression to blame it on this time, but for hospitals, it was the same old problem. Medical expenses under a mostly private, partially public funding system, which was then very similar to the one still in place in the United States, were shooting beyond the control of hospital boards or the means of most patients. Already, by the beginning of the 1960s, it was becoming very clear that a new way to fund medical institutions had to be found, and quickly.

Because of increased public demand and an utter dependence upon profit-making suppliers, hospitalization costs had begun to accelerate in a worrisome manner as early as the late 1950s. There were a few other systemic problems to deal with, even during this halcyon time. Nurses were still poorly paid. As a result, they were in such scant supply that beds and even entire floors sometimes had to be closed; no one was there to provide daily care. Long waiting lists resulted from these bed shortages and that pressure led directly to the abuse of ER admissions, a problem that continues today. The East Wing of the Queen Elizabeth Hospital remained closed in June of 1961, even though there were 191 anxious patients on the waiting list. On 27 June 1962, the whole sixth floor joined the fifth and closed its doors because of nursing shortages. At the time, the hospital board was campaigning for funds for an extension to the building. Obviously, private systems can be just as mixed up about their funding priorities as public ones.

Labour problems increased in the 1960s primarily because the government, which had taken charge of salaries, was paying inadequate wages. Although the Queen Elizabeth was near the high end of Montreal hospital rates – $22.50, set by the Quebec government by 1961 – that was up from $3 only 20 years before and was simply not enough to cover costs.[57] As financial constraints frustrated acquisition of the apparently limitless new technologies and techniques, it's not surprising that the heretical concept of full Medicare was becoming more discussed in hospital circles even in the late 1950s, when Hospital-funded presentations were on such subjects as "Health Insurance in the Western Provinces."[58] Increasingly throughout this period, the hospital turned to the government for whatever it needed: increases in staff salaries, help with the new wing, purchases of equipment, or salaries for new specialists. Even though the government turned down these requests as often as not, it had clearly become health care's major funding source.

There will always be money problems when an institution tries to manage health care for large numbers of people, and thorns will mar the perfection of even the rosiest years. So despite the increased professionalism, better equipment, consumer enthusiasm, and rapidly expanding scientific knowledge, the newly named Queen Elizabeth Hospital still experienced some chronic internal difficulties in the 1950s and 60s. For example, its record-keeping was chaotic. This was largely because doctors were too busy to keep up with their files and almost no amount of disciplinary action helped, even withdrawal of privileges. Medical accreditation continued to be a headache for all small hospitals because it was annual, had to be obtained from a confusing array of separate organizations, and was linked to funding and other kinds of privileges. Accreditation bodies kept changing their criteria, often in order to gain some kind of control over the individual hospital, so achieving accreditation was not always worth the effort.

The exodus of newly trained doctors to the U.S. and abroad and the need to hire foreign staff had already begun by the mid-1950s. Hospital administrations were now beginning to be worried about litigation and malpractice, which explains the increase in secrecy in the Medical Board Minutes, especially about such things as surgical deaths.[59] For example, although the Infection Control Committee was established in 1959, they rarely admit in writing to the hospital's actually having had any infections. Similarly, the Tissue Committee, according to Medical Board researcher Ken Hechtman, "invariably reports either 'no irregularities' or, rarely, 'minor irregularities' throughout the decade. There was more honesty when there was less bureaucratic structure."

As for the treatment of the patients themselves, overall it was becoming very much better, at least for those patients who could afford all aspects of hospital care. However, statistics show that as the sixties began, fewer people could actually do so. Consequently, the exciting advances in medical treatment that were making doctors so happy are not as clearly reflected in such things as infant and adult mortality statistics as one would expect. Of course, even for people who could pay for lab tests, therapies, or operations, some conditions were undertreated. Then as now, doctors worried about the severe lack of cancer patient follow-up. Technically part of preventative care, this type of activity has yet to gain much clout in hospitals even today. Mysterious illnesses like chronic fatigue syndrome were already being reported. It was called "half-sick" syndrome at the time and was blamed on poor posture, in much the same way that many modern conditions might be misdiagnosed or badly treated today.[60]

Other illnesses were over-treated. In particular, births continued to be very much over-medicalized. In Ontario, even as late as the mid-

1930s, the Gagans report that "the hospital rate of maternal mortality ... was twice as high as the rate for home births."[61] Even more indicative of medical interference was the fact that "maternal mortality rates among those principally middle-class women whose labour was controlled or intervened in by a doctor was *four times higher* than for women in the hospital public and indigent wards who were left alone to experience natural labour."[62] There were also far too many appendectomies and tonsillectomies, the biggest surgical rages of the era. In a perfect demonstration of PID (Physician Induced Demand), like so many other Ear, Nose, and Throat specialists, Eli Katz, the Queen E's ENT man, had to fit in operations on Saturdays as well as all week. These procedures brought in a great many customers, caused the deaths of an unacceptable number of small children, and were, by the mid-1960s, discovered to be mostly unnecessary.[63] To the hospital's credit, once the research was in, tonsillectomies were rapidly phased out. However, physicians have jealously guarded their right to interfere in births and only a few provinces, such as Quebec, have state-sponsored midwife programs in place.

The happy partnership between the fledgling medical drug industry and medical care practitioners, still relatively balanced at this point, began to develop cracks that foreshadow the future. As we saw with the dark history of anesthetics, the human lust for magic potions tends to create many casualties and, as the profit motive became stronger, the casualties became both more numerous and more innocent. One example is Bonamine (meclizine hydrochloride), a thalidomide-like drug that causes birth defects and is now outlawed. It was regularly prescribed in the 1950s to relieve morning sickness. It's unlikely the victims' families ever knew why their children were so disabled or deformed because the connection between pre-parturition drug use and birth defects was not made public for another decade.

Although many new and potentially dangerous drugs were introduced in the 1950s and 60s, doctors were starting to get the picture. There were also more and more presentations on toxic reactions to local anesthesia[64] and belated concerns about safe radiation dosage for x-rays. There was even a guarded response to the powerful anti-inflammatory and, as they would later learn, carcinogenic steroid drug, cortisone. About this, Harold Griffith very wisely remarked, "One must be cautious in the evaluation of new drugs since all too frequently time erases the apparent advantages."[65] As recently as the 1930s and 40s most hospitals made their own drugs or got them from doctor-run cottage industries, as Harold did when he ordered his lisle catheters back in 1940. But by 1955, nearly every hospital Clinical Conference included a "new drug presentation," or what we would now call an "infomercial," presided over by highly enthusiastic and increasingly well-paid trade reps from growing companies like Merck Frosst and Squibb. Such activities increased and started to feature more than the free samples and nice lunches of the 50s and 60s, which medical committees increasingly counted on. Eventually there would be paid vacations, board memberships, cars, and prestigious job offers available to any physician willing to lend an ear, or a pen, to a sales pitch or a pre-researched set of clinical trials.

SHARING TO SURVIVE

Health is not a privilege but rather a basic right which should be open to all.

Justice Emmett Hall Royal, Commission on Health Services,
19 June 1964[66]

The Montreal Homeopathic's pride in the last years of A.R. Griffith's life regarding their increasing triumphs over tuberculosis, typhoid, and the other communicable diseases of urban poverty was verified by scientific statistics. By 1941, although far from eradicated, the incidence of tuberculosis, for example, had declined not just in Montreal but across the country. However, a conference held that year to investigate the idea of a federal health insurance plan revealed that Canada's venereal disease rate, at 70 cases per 10,000 people, was at least ten times that of countries like Sweden. Canadian maternal and child mortality rates also were higher than in comparable European countries where government medical care schemes were in effect.[67] Moreover, after the war when it became obvious that medical incomes were still not climbing back to their pre-Depression levels, even the profession began to show some "renewed enthusiasm for state action" to pay for all the new and proven advances in treatment.[68]

Over this period, disease demographics had shifted. As heart disease, stroke, and cancer began to replace tuberculosis and pneumonia as major killers, "An era of chronic – and expensive – diseases had arrived, and the costs of health services bore heavily on a larger proportion of the population." Many doctors, including Gordon S. Fahrni, CMA president in 1942, were disturbed to notice that wage-earners and salaried employees, the largest segment of medical consumers, were unable to afford operations and other expensive procedures. They frequently couldn't afford modest hospital or specialist consulting fees and sometimes couldn't even pay for lab tests ordered by their GP. "Only too often," he wrote, "this has resulted in inadequate investigation and inadequate treatment, much to the disappointment of the medical attendant."[69] This means that while researchers and hospitals may have been thrilled they could now put such a dazzling array of medical offerings in the shop window, fewer and fewer people were able to walk in and buy them.

Professional organizations such as the Ontario Medical Association OMA and CMA began to evince increasing interest in various forms of pre-paid medical insurance. The most obvious were the physician-founded Blue Cross indemnity insurance schemes and others similar to it. The old idea of municipal or institutional doctors for places such as colleges or logging camps was also revived but with bodies like the CMA overseeing to make sure fees did not drop below a minimum level. Because going to a company doctor can be just as disadvantageous for the consumer as shopping at the company store, the kind of employee group coverage that was most amenable to the profession was to have employers subsidize consultations through a fee-for-service plan with private practitioners with a reduced CMA fee schedule.

Various doctors' and professional groups, including the OMA, tried to set up their own pre-payment plans and clinics just as Dr Andreas had in Chicago a decade earlier. As a member doctor put it, "If we do not socialize ourselves and develop the proper technique of service, Government will be forced to try their hand."[70] At the same time, these plans assumed that their foundation efforts would eventually "be absorbed by a compulsory state health insurance plan." Because this eventually happened, it's important to understand why these private-sector arrangements didn't work out in Canada, and also why they continue to fail large segments of the population in the United States. C. David Naylor points out in *Private Practice, Public Payment: Canadian Medicine and the Politics of Health Insurance 1911–1966* that payment plans without professional support simply invite irregularities and even when they enjoy that support, they often let adherence to their own professional standards slip. Most of the unsatisfactory private health insurance schemes that emerged in Canada were very similar to the HMOs that are being used in the U.S. today and were subject to the same types of economic advantages to the funders but criticisms from the profession and consumers. Essentially, Canada tried and then rejected the system that the U.S. has embraced, back before the 1960s.

Anyone interested in the details of why Canada developed a single-payer, public system in the years following the Second World War while the United States solidified its two-tier, essentially private system, should read Terry Boychuk's dry but penetrating account of the process, *The Making and Meaning of Hospital Policy in the United States and Canada*, as well as *The Economic Evolution of American Health Care: From Marcus Welby to Managed Care*, by David Dranove. Simply stated, recounting the history of single-payer, non-profit, and for-profit private, provincial, state, or national health plans is a complex endeavour that can easily confuse (or bore) the non-specialist. However, it's still useful to boil down the many details and permutations of this history into a form fit for mass consumption, especially because Canadians are once again being presented with serious economic questions about their health care system.

In summary, early in the century, the medical profession in both the U.S. and Canada had brief flirtations with the idea of federal payments to help alleviate costs but came to oppose full governmental control over health plans and institutions. One needs to bear in mind, as Naylor says in *Private Practice, Public Payment*, that "the profession's enthusiasm for state intervention understandably tended to vary inversely with medical incomes and the percentage of accounts paid for services rendered."[71] This means that Canadian doctors begged for government help in the lean years of the teens and again during the Great Depression and fought it tooth and claw in the fat decades of the 1920s and the 1950s and 60s. In contrast, doctors in the U.S. generally remained opposed to it even during the Depression. In both countries, doctors and their associations at first succeeded in fending off full government involvement. But in Canada, doctors and their professional associations failed to prevent eventual government control over their work and institutions. This was largely due to the fact that, while the doctors were fighting to close the door to government funding, Canadian hospital administrators were busy opening it. It was not the medical profession itself but hospital administrations that were significantly more needy in Canada than they were in the U.S. Therefore, Canada's hospital administrators proved to be much more open to the idea of government funding. Ironically, as it has turned out, the U.S. doctors who succeeded in fending off government interference and are now working in for-profit HMOs have far less power on average over both the treatment of their patients and their fee structure than doctors working under the governments of Quebec or Britain, who have the advantage of being a very large union able to pressure the funding bureaucracy.

CONSUMERS VS. PROVIDERS, OR WHY WE GOT MEDICARE

> The lobbying activity of Canadian doctors has resembled that of the British Medical Association rather than the American Medical Association ... the CMA and its provincial divisions have consistently been more open minded than their American counterparts about the need for some degree of government involvement in prepayment of medical and hospital bills.
>
> C. David Naylor, *Private Practice, Public Payment*[72]

Eugene Vayda and Raisa Deber, in an article titled, "The Canadian Health-Care System,"[73] mention a famous law that failed to pass in 1945. It is interesting because it was the first Canadian proposal for a National Health System modeled on Britain's. It would have paid physicians on a capitation basis, that is, according to the profession's deeply desired fee-for-service method. Services would have been available in health centers, not offices, however, and the system would have been administered by a commission of consumers and professionals, not government bureaucrats. "Although the 1945 proposals were viewed favourably by the public and key professional groups, including the CMA, they failed to be enacted because they were viewed as federal incursions into provincial jurisdiction."[74]

The medical act therefore failed for jurisdictional reasons, but on the other hand, "hospital facilities were perceived to be insufficient in number, inadequate, and outdated, and government action was seen to be necessary." So in the case of hospitals, these difficulties of jurisdictional power-sharing had to be overcome, simply because the need was more desperate. "In lieu of a full health-insurance program, the federal government made grants available to the provinces for planning and hospital construction. This marked the first acceptance of the concept of federal-provincial cost-sharing for health services, a principle that has been the foundation of all subsequent health policy in Canada."[75] In other words, in Canada, the population and the general political will favoured the government as an overseer of public health, at least in hospitals. The economic reasons had to do, at this key moment, with generalized under-funding for hospitals within the community as well as a long tradition of finding money by appealing to higher, provincial rather than municipal, levels of government.

This tradition more or less paved the way for the involvement of these higher levels of government. To switch back to the specific example, every year from the 1920s and into the 50s, the administrators of the Homeopathic echoed A. W. Griffith's much earlier complaints about how seriously the Montreal Homeopathic was being taxed by its obligations to care for the indigent or those covered by the increasing number of government programs like Workmen's Compensation.[76] Although hospitals were obliged by the government to treat such cases, the state did not provide enough funds to actually cover their costs. Instead, they made the hospital add the difference to their deficits, much as they continue to do today. This forced hospitals to continue to beg wealthy citizens and organizations to help fill the gap, also as they continue to do today.

The president of the Montreal Homeopathic was typical in his entry for 1953 when he wrote, "As in the past, the Municipal, Provincial and Federal Governments have provided monies from the funds which have been set aside under the Quebec Public Charities Act, and for the patients suffering from diseases of a cancerous nature. However, these funds providing only a minimum benefit have not covered the total cost of our operation and so we have been forced once again to approach the public of Montreal for sustenance in terms of dollars and cents."[77] Such economic conditions influenced the adoption of single-payer, government-funded health care. However, historical and cultural elements were crucial additions to these more obvious financial incentives. The Canadian public's acceptance of the government as a reasonably trustworthy manager of public funding and public health – especially as compared to the American public's refusal to surrender basic personal powers to the government – harks back to fundamental constitutional and attitudinal differences between the two countries.

The late Pierre Berton's analysis of the War of 1812 claims that this was the moment that defined this split. Berton wrote that the "Canadian way of life ... significantly [differs] from the more individualistic American" from this time forward, in terms of that one clear choice – about whether to trust one's government or not. For example, like the Queen's power, which is largely ceremonial, Canada's governor general is still an appointed crown representative who is accepted in the

21st century as our head of state, a political feature which sustains Berton's point that Canadians came to feel that "certain sensitive positions are better filled by [government] appointments than by [popular] election." He mentioned other key attitudes: "that order imposed from above has advantages over grass-roots democracy...; [and] that a ruling elite often knows better than the body politic."[78] In short, the feeling developed and spread throughout Canada that government is a relatively benign, orderly, and trustworthy force in the lives of the people it represents. This is possibly because, as Terry Boychuk argues in *The Making and Meaning of Hospital Policy*, the British Crown had learned a lesson when it lost the American colonies and from the 1790s on ruled Canada with a far more inclusive and enlightened hand than it had the U.S. Moreover, people immigrated to the two countries for different reasons and with different expectations.

Boychuk's study compares the two countries and their health care systems and contends that although most hospitals in both countries started out exactly as the Montreal Homeopathic had done in 1894, as "voluntary" institutions that were privately funded, hospital administrations and the associations they formed in each country gradually revealed "differing ideological tendencies" that, in the end, frustrated or advanced the cause of national health insurance. Boychuk points to the fact that, "U.S. hospitals never wavered in their efforts to pre-empt government-sponsored hospital insurance for the gainfully employed." To counteract a popular trend towards public support, "U.S. hospitals demonstrated formidable skill in arranging a legal, administrative and economic basis for private hospital insurance." They were also successful at, of all things, "limiting the scope of publicly financed hospital benefits to the poor," and "in making [private] hospitals the beneficiaries of new sources of public funding for hospital care." On the other hand, Boychuk contends that, "By contrast, Canadian hospitals did not dispute the objective of universal hospital insurance," nor did they attempt to organize private hospital insurance on the same scale. In Canada, both hospital administrators and the public at large seem to have felt that "Canadian governments had the right and obligation to ensure universal access to hospital care." Moreover, they both believed that "mandatory hospital insurance was a practical necessity."[79]

Canada had had its share of poor houses and infirmaries for the dispossessed but, as previously discussed, they were either under-attended by a public that feared them or they were founded by religious groups and began to serve richer clients – travelers as well as the poor – early on. The later and more common hospices were so generously endowed and supported by their local communities that they easily translated into modern institutions around the turn of the century. In the U.S., on the other hand, Boychuk states that there were far more hospitals "uniquely built and maintained [just] for the poor." This led to a set perception in many cities and towns: the sights and sounds of the misery in the public institutions, that is, "the identification of government [publicly-funded] hospitals with the poverty-stricken, coupled with the dramatic growth of [private] hospitals attending to the self-supporting," deeply affected American thinking "about public and private responsibilities for financing and managing hospital care."

This led to a particularly American take on the situation that might be argued still affects U.S. attitudes towards health care: "The prevailing view held that *extending government sovereignty over hospital care, beyond that needed to provide for the poor, threatened private enterprise and initiative, jeopardized standards of care, and endangered scientific and technological progress.* U.S. hospital associations and state legislators remained loyal to these precepts and worked at cross-purposes with national advocates of universal health insurance. The U.S. Congress affirmed those understandings of the public interest in hospital care: government programs would specifically address the needs [only] of those excluded from the private economy of health care."[80]

Boychuk probably has a point when he says that the best way of gaining insight into the U.S. or Canada is to study the opposite country. Because they are so similar in so many ways, "the fewer the differences, the more likely they matter." In Canada, from the earliest days, the most progressive hospitals, that is, those that wished to gain reputations as "the best," operated as the Homeopathic did. They were open to all, which means they were open to all patients as well as to all doctors. This policy seems to have reflected the general attitude of the public because within the first decade of the twentieth century, "the provinces adopted laws that called for open admissions to all voluntary and municipal hospitals and that obliged provincial and local governments to compensate hospitals for the expense of caring for patients who could not afford all or part of the costs of their treatment."[81]

Even though the compensation was inadequate, the precedent had been set. In every annual report, first A.R. Griffith and then succeeding administrators complained that the fees given for public patients were not enough. Along with the rest of Canadian hospital professionals, however, none of them ever suggested that the province get out of hospital funding – merely that they do a better job. So instead of a perception that public funding would harm the level of care in hospitals, Boychuk says that in Canada, "These mandatory subsidies were perceived as a mechanism for *assisting local initiative, enforcing high standards of operation, encouraging patterns of hospital ownership that mirrored the social diversity of Canada* [i.e., French, English, Catholic, homeopathic, etc.], *stabilizing hospital budgets, and releasing hospitals from the constraints of revenues derived from fees and endowments.*" The provincial fee system fed into "the overriding value informing pre-World War II hospital policy in Canada: universal access to essential hospital services."[82]

Boychuk is actually a little too simplistic in this analysis. Although Canadian hospital administrators had welcomed the small and grudging amounts from governments that increased dramatically after the 1945 health care act mentioned above, they still regarded "socialized medicine" with deep suspicion. That lifelong defender of egalitarian values, Harold Griffith, was almost in despair when it was forcibly introduced into his hospital just before his retirement. In 1962 he wrote, "I hate to think of the bureaucracy of officials and accountants and clerks which will be built up," and added, in opposition to Boychuk's view, "Such plans promote neither efficiency nor economy, and I only hope that it will be possible to maintain the very high standards of medical care which have been developed in this country by private enterprise."[83] He and many other doctors, such as Bob and Wesley Bourne, deeply resented the implication made by the zealous social reformers of the time that Canadians were dying for lack of care, because they were proud of the fact that their hospital had never turned a patient away for lack of money. These doctors had freely donated their time and energy to the poor, working as hard for their welfare as for paying patients, and felt that, in the charitable sense, they'd done a good job.

And they had – for the very poor. There's a telling statement in the Annual Report of 1954 – during the financially turbulent years before Medicare was introduced. Hospital president L.B. Unwin states, "Admitting Office policy has been strengthened. Incoming patients or their relatives are being interviewed to ascertain which class of accommodation they can afford, so that the patient will not be burdened needlessly with a debt he will take years to pay. No patient has been refused admittance due to his financial status, but an appreciable reduction in bad debts has resulted through placing the patient in the appropriate accommodation."[84] Even at the charitable little Homeopathic, whose logo for two decades was a portrayal of their front portal with the slogan, "The Open Door," the "class" of accommodations differed enough to tempt people to go beyond their depth. No doubt most such people were both working and middle class, motivated by the desire to make sure they or their loved ones received the best care.

The system as it stood meant that even at the most compassionate community hospitals, when working people were hospitalized, they very often lost their savings and their future financial stability. Moreover, their increasing inability to pay weighed the hospitals down with unpaid debts. Doctors may have been experiencing their halcyon era in terms of scientific opportunities and social prestige, but in the years leading up to Medicare, both patients' and hospital budgets were cracking under the strain. In fact, in order to meet its increasing costs, the little hospital with the "Open Door" resorted to somewhat draconian methods to increase fees. In 1960, the Medical Board reversed their 1951 admitting policy of warning people in advance about costs and declared that, "all patients are to be assumed private or semi-private until the patient asserts he is unable to afford" that level of care. It's unlikely that many people knew they would be automatically placed in the more expensive rooms unless they objected, so this policy must have wracked up even more debts for the hospital and caused distress to patients or relatives who had been too ill, upset, or misinformed to appreciate what these on-the-spot choices would mean to their pocketbooks.

Researcher Ken Hechtman noted in a 2004 unpublished paper that, "the hospital didn't want to turn away patients who couldn't afford to pay but didn't want to give a free ride to those who could. The only strategy they had was trying to make people self-select." Only a year later, unbalanced budgets had gotten so bad that the Queen E proposed an actual by-law change: "No patient treated in hospital or out-patient department shall be exempt from professional fees unless he can prove he is an indigent."[85] And by 1965, still before Medicare was fully functional, the board demanded that, "all out-patients carrying the Provincial Welfare card [must] be billed by the doctors giving the service." Hectman remarks, "They pretty quickly went from making people assert they were indigent to making them prove they were, to billing them anyway, even if they were carrying cards that proved their inability to pay."[86]

During this period, when a two-tier system was still in effect and up to 700 people a year were waiting for beds, filling the need for more paying patients was made at the expense of caring for non-paying ones, just as it is in the U.S. today. In 1961, before Medicare, the Queen E

was making outpatients pay *in advance*, "to minimize the rather large
financial losses in the outpatient department"[87] and by 1962, it was trying to close its five-bed, or poor, wards and replace them with four-bed,
"semi-private" wards.[88] ER patients were a continuous problem because
they had to be treated for free unless they were admitted. As usual, the
Queen E started out with the most altruistic intentions: when their ER
was created in 1965, they decreed that, "an emergency patient is anyone who says he is." Only four years later, they were determining how to
screen and bill ER patients.

The Queen E had had an overloaded ER ever since it opened but continued to accept everyone who showed up. However, as early as 1966,
the Hospital hired a collection agent, on commission, to collect fees
from public – that is, poor – patients. As Ken Hectman put it in his
unpublished comments, "You can see the progression here. They're no
longer a charity, they're not yet a government department, so they're trying to reinvent themselves as a business. You have to wonder how far this
business-like progression might have gone, even at a hospital as idealistic
[as the] Queen Elizabeth, if Medicare hadn't been implemented."[89]

In addition to the difficulty of finding enough patients who could
actually pay for their treatment, hospitals at this period were also faced
with steadily increasing government and professional demands.
Accreditation via various college boards and government agencies was
a constant headache for all the smaller hospitals. As Hechtman puts it,
"It was still their hospital to run; but unless they wanted to be a private
clinic specializing in diseases of the rich (which a small faction did at
one time consider), they needed cheap labour. If they wanted cheap
labour, they needed interns. If they were to get interns, they had to be
accredited. If they wanted to be accredited, they had to follow the dic-
tates of the governing bodies of the accreditation organizations – and
these tend to be nothing less than thinly disguised extortion." What
Hechtman is referring to is administrative takeover. Close to the time
when Jim and Harold Griffith were about to retire, the government
and the established accreditation organizations, which operated
largely out of the universities, were preparing to seize internal administrative as well as budgetary control over small hospitals.

Full accreditation by the Canadian Committee of Medicine came for
the Queen Elizabeth Hospital of Montreal in October of 1963, but
Royal College accreditation in 1964 required giving McGill a veto over
department heads. Each head also had to have a teaching position at
McGill. "Within fifteen months," Hechtman writes, "the top ranks of

the Queen Elizabeth Hospital were completely purged and replaced with Royal College men." In a bitter speech given on Jim Griffith's retirement in 1964, Dr Lloyd-Smith told the assembled Medical Board, "No longer are men selected because of their special surgical aptitudes or because they are steeped in hospital traditions or because of their proven interest in the patient or the community – no longer are such men chosen to head a department."[90] The chief physician, chief surgeon, chief of obstetrics/gynecology, chief radiologist, and medical superintendent all retired the same year and were replaced by outsiders. The Griffith brothers were of retirement age, but the other three heads probably, as Hechtman puts it, "took a bullet for accreditation."

Although these debts and administrative changes were real problems for once-independent private hospitals, their patients' difficulties with financing their hospital care were obviously much more acute than any workplace distress felt by hospital administrators. The popularity of Medicare with the Canadian public contrasts very sharply with the resistance to it from administrators and doctors. Harold Griffith was so worried about the coming changes that he confessed in his 1961 report: "Sometimes I am glad I am coming near the end of my own professional career." Nonetheless, he was still fair and objective. He went on to admit, "the public demand for a comprehensive health insurance program is overwhelming."[91] For twenty years previously, in fact, polls had shown popular support levels for a national health program at 80 percent and higher.[92] So even as most citizens rejoiced over their new health care plan, the hospital administrators, faced with what amounted to a government takeover of the hitherto free management of their private hospitals, had real and grievous sorrows. And even as mortality statistics and the general health of the population improved through the 1980s and 1990s due to Medicare, the administrative and bureaucratic woes of hospital administrators in Canada kept multiplying. Which goes to prove that what's good for the consumers of goods is not always so good for the providers – and vice-versa.

RECOVERING FROM SHOCK

There is an excellent possibility that the [medical] profession's independence has been guaranteed in many respects by the very implementation of the national medical ... insurance plans [that they so feared]

C. David Naylor, *Canadian Health Care and the State* [93]

Reading the Annual Reports of the Homeopathic and other privately funded hospitals between the 1890s and the late 1950s is like listening to a familiar song. They are filled with proud recitals of accomplishments and breakthroughs; pleasure mixed with shock and some consternation concerning the continuously increasing demand for hospital services; pleas for more funding for expansion and equipment; and gratitude to volunteers and donors. Suddenly, in the early 1960s, even in the most official internal reports, this soothing litany is interrupted by an outpouring of anguish. For the next decade, as fledgling Medicare programs were being solidified – and in Quebec, as Bill 64, demanding full proficiency in French, was also coming into effect – hospital administrators abandoned their professional masks and expressed personal and emotional shock.

Hospital Board President A.H. Marden was not a doctor but a professional administrator. In 1970, in contrast to the claim Terry Boychuk makes that Canadian hospitals easily accepted state-sponsored medical care, Marden filled his Annual Report with a litany of criticisms and complaints, many of which will sound familiar to anyone living in Canada today. "When the Medicare program was first rumoured we strongly opposed it, firstly, *because of its universal coverage,* and secondly, because of its timing and cost ... Virtually forced upon the Provinces by the Federal Government, it has contributed not only to the inflationary cycle in Canada, but also to the current difficulties confronting our hospitals." With the benefit of hindsight, Marden's complaints can be interpreted as any established institution's teething period when faced with a new system, but this temporary destabilization also had the effect of causing many doctors and nurses to flee both the province and the country. So many left that he asserted, "In the long run ... better that these men and women seek their future elsewhere than that they remain in Quebec, frustrated and perhaps bitter, unable or unwilling to contribute to the success of the health care system of this Province." He added, rather wistfully, "In any event, Medicare is now with us, and those who think in terms of its possible repeal are simply dreaming."[94]

Some of this criticism, of course, goes beyond adjustment shock and pinpoints continuing problems with government-controlled health care plans in Canada. Many provincial initiatives, including early Medicare management plans, hospital closures in the 1990s, the sudden decision to expand CLSCs (Centre local de services communautaires), or other provincial clinics, the centralization of care in "super-hospitals," are still vulnerable to Marden's 1970 complaint. "It seems only sensible that such major programs should be more carefully planned, that costs should be more accurately assessed, and that they should not be put into effect until the necessary organization is completed and until all those involved have a thorough understanding of the program."[95]

Still, by 1974, many of the teething problems seem to have been ironed out and there was a new mindset as well as a new administrative staff. Reports began to sing a more soothing song again. The old hospital somehow retained its values and its team spirit and by its 80th year had adjusted to the most sweeping change of its lifetime thus far. J.R. Houton, the new president, wrote ebulliently, "During the year we have worked closely with the ministry of Social Affairs. Thanks to the efforts of our Executive Director, I can report that we have excellent and close relationships with appropriate authorities at Quebec. This of course is very important since the Provincial Government has the responsibility for funding the growing needs of basic health care." There was even sympathy and understanding for the enormity of the government's job, as Houton went on to explain delays in certain decisions. "They are faced with the need to improve standards of care in many areas of the Province, and to determine priorities among the great number of projects and requirements put to them by the many institutions."[96]

As mentioned in chapter 1, nurses and doctors who reminisced about the culture that made the Queen Elizabeth such a good place to work described how the hospital itself – its traditions and history – seemed to inexplicably convert very different kinds of personalities. People who didn't at first fit in rapidly became more egalitarian, fun-loving, and open to new ideas, miraculously developing fierce loyalties to the institution. Following its greatest rupture in tradition – the loss of the last of its founding family when Jim and Harold Griffith retired in 1966, together with having to adjust to new department chiefs coming from outside the institution – the Queen Elizabeth was still able to work its magic. In 1972, faced with the new government Bill 65 that threatened the autonomy of small hospitals, the Medical Board Minutes from all its chiefs of staff advised that everyone "exhibit some masterful inactivity as far as recommending any sweeping changes in our mechanisms of self-government, which have kept our hospital community on a true and steady course for many years."[97] "In terms of protecting the Queen E from any outside interference, this is great stuff!" Ken Hechtman remarks. "You'd never know it was written by the same

McGill/Royal College clique that had mounted a hostile takeover only six years before."

In fact, throughout the 1970s, hospital reports revert to talking about the latest expansion, their pride in the quality of their service, and their gratitude to their staff and donors – the only difference being that some of that gratitude is now going to the government. Albert Nixon, the popular new general director and a nephew-in-law of Harold Griffith's, sang in key, adding, "I am happy to report that our relations with the Ministry of Social Affairs have been most cordial. We have received the utmost cooperation from the different Services of the ministry."[98] Indeed, under Albert Nixon's reign, there was a dizzying expansion of services that rivaled any of the changes that had come before. Besides having renovated and expanded the building almost two-fold in the early 1970s, the Queen E began to increase the type of services it offered with, as Albert Nixon describes, "a big psychiatry department under Drs Neiman and Subak. Under Duplessis, we were getting federal money for mental health. We bought duplexes on Marlowe for a Department of Psychiatry. We had people rotated between us, the Children's and the Douglas (Montreal's largest psychiatric hospital). We had thirty beds always full, a big outpatients' department. It was really needed." Albert was certainly correct in that assessment. The Queen E's catchment area of 250,000 people included Verdun and Ville St. Pierre, two working-class neighbourhoods with many residents suffering from the ills of poverty and despair.

It was also the Queen E's "hey-day of cardiology," as Nixon puts it. Although advanced technologies now require that cardiac cases be sent to the biggest teaching hospitals, the optimal treatments of the day could be dispensed in small hospitals. "We had stopped doing pediatrics," Albert says, "so in the late 1970s we made a progressive cardiac unit that took the patient from the ICU to the last bed. Back in 1973, we had opened the first Family Medicine unit in the McGill group. Although we had had to close obstetrics, we started a day surgical clinic, doing orthopedics, orthoscopies, that kind of thing, as well as Ear, Nose and Throat. We had four anesthetists at any given time, and our clinic had its own separate OR. That was a first – we were ahead of the General. In fact, we were often on the leading edge; Laval University came to see that OR, it was so well done. And after our Day Surgery, we set up a Vascular Lab and an Oncology Centre. We also had a gastro-enterology lab set-up, with an examining and treatment room; we even offered plastic surgery." In the 1970s, the Queen E also instituted something that's considered cutting-edge today: a polyclinic for specialists. "We renovated it with our own money; it could handle 5,000 people. You'd come in, be referred and see the appropriate doctor very rapidly, who'd be paid by Medicare."

So, despite the radical fiscal and managerial changes brought by Medicare, the halcyon days under Harold Griffith of steady advances clearly continued after his retirement. These are exemplified by the Queen E's use of pre-operative antibiotics, a first for Canada, and its breakthroughs in laproscopic and laser surgery. In fact, innovation and expansion of services didn't slacken from the 1970s right up until the hospital's busy creativity was suddenly cut off in 1995. So the fears the old administrators expressed of a loss of quality of care or service under Medicare gradually evaporated over the 1960s and 70s. A large majority of the doctors who entered the profession about this time or later continued to laud the creation of Medicare right through the 1980s and into the 1990s. It is only with the real and measurable erosion of hospital services that became acute after the hospital closures in the middle 1990s that the old idea of two-tier care has once again begun to have some appeal to a few of them.

Today, an even more significant number of Canadian physicians, surgeons, and patients are frustrated by waiting lines, overwork, micromanagement by strapped politicians, and serious under-funding. So far, however, hospital boards are still not clamouring for privatization. Even so, the big U.S-based health and HMO corporations are already knocking on the door, offering their services. For a price, of course.

MEANWHILE, BACK IN THE U.S.A.

Publicly funded health care has its problems, as any Canadian or Briton knows. But like democracy, it's the best answer we've come up with so far.

Doug Pibel, Managing Editor, *Yes! Magazine*[99]

If we want to see where our current situation might be headed, we have only to look at what was happening during this same period south of the border. From the 1930s on, the Americans also tried to alleviate health care gaps through increased use of pre-paid employment insurance plans. They encouraged professionally led private hospital insurance plans like Blue Cross and for-profit insurance plans. The difference is that, as the decades went by, the nation's health care planners never seem to have looked at the international statistics that show that such funding inevitably leads to poorer public health.

In virtually all of the rest of the industrialized world, including many developing countries such as Mexico, it has been viscerally understood that, as Terry Boychuk puts it, "private insurance would [never be able to] cover all necessary hospital procedures and services; and that even minimal protection [is] beyond the reach of the poor, the working poor, and those with the most serious health problems."[100] To anyone looking at health care statistics worldwide today, this seems to be an unavoidable fact, particularly applicable to the working poor and the seriously ill. How many lower-middle or even middle-middle class citizens, even if fully employed in privileged North America, are so fully covered by hospital insurance that they need not fear losing their houses, education, or savings to a catastrophic illness? In fact, over half the family bankruptcies registered every year in the wealthiest country in the world, the United States, directly follow a health crisis.[101]

The majority of researchers agree that the most efficient way to provide health-care funding for large populations is summed up by the axiom "Universal coverage spreads the risk." That is, publicly funded plans such as U.S. Medicare and Medicaid, as well as the provincially administered, single-payer Canadian plans, use their pool of funding to insure people who are young and healthy as well as people who are old or infirm. That means that at any given time relatively few of the pool of payers will need the medical services they're paying for. Those who are old or ill and thus unable to contribute through pre-paid employment plans, for example, can be carried by the much larger number of their neighbours who remain healthy. Christine Cassel, president of the Internal Medicine Association in the U.S., argues in her most recent book, *Medicare Matters*, that in a for-profit system, it is very much in the interests of the private insurer not to serve a deep pool of customers reflecting the actual population with all its diverse needs but rather to have a shallow pool of people who will rarely need any medical services at all.

This is to say that in the case of publicly funded insurance, the goal of the coverage provider is to *protect as many people as possible* for the least amount of money. In the case of private, for-profit insurance, the coverage provider's goal is to *avoid paying benefits* so that reliable profits can continue to go to shareholders. That's why people with existing conditions cannot get insurance at affordable rates and people who develop serious medical conditions so often find themselves unable to renew their policies. In order to create profits, for-profit insurance companies must get monthly payments from people who are at very low risk of ever needing the services for which they are pre-paying. It's similar to the bad old days of the 19th and early 20th century when the working poor, the old, and the sick – that is, those who most need health care – are able to get only limited care and little or no protective coverage. Today in the United States, more than 40 million people, that is, well over the entire population of Canada, are in that position.[102]

There are theoretically fewer problems with non-profit health insurance plans such as Blue Cross. However, the same financial squeeze that makes government-funded hospitals tight-fisted with various expensive procedures has an even greater effect on these plans, simply because their access to funding is so much more limited. In fact, a key problem with all forms of private insurance is that when a person takes out a personal policy, she's not just gambling on staying well. She's also gambling that if she does need access to medical services, her illness will not be really serious. That's because once a private policy-holder experiences a serious or long-term health crisis, insurance coverage from private sources, even non-profits like Blue Cross, tends to disappear or become unaffordable.

Given the problems caused by government-funded and managed health care, the idea of "public/private partnerships," in which part of the population is insured privately and the rest publicly, seems to make a lot of sense. In theory, it should take some of the burden off the public system, leaving more money available for poorer people. Because of this, it is becoming discussed as a possible option in Canada and is already functioning to a limited (and possibly illegal) extent in Quebec and Alberta. As we shall see in more detail in chapter 6, "The Queen Must Die," the public/private balancing act has been accomplished in a few countries, such as France and Germany, but it requires rigourous state control and delicate handling, with well-enforced legislation, to block the many opportunities for corruption. Serious expense and access problems arise when those rigorous criteria are not met. In Australia and Scotland, for example, both of which have been experimenting with the latest in public/private systems, these problems include serious diminutions of access to care that actually costs significantly more than did their formerly all-public systems.[103]

It is a matter of great importance for any society to maintain its population's health. A healthy citizenry is the basis for everything that follows: economics, culture, security, prestige, and well-being. Even if many of their members may believe in the Darwinian survival of the fittest, no society can afford to take care of its population in needlessly expensive ways that leave significant numbers without adequate care. It is a simple physical fact of life that *every* person in any society will get sick or injured, occasionally or eventually, and need care; no one can predict how extensive that need will be. A society that permits a large number of sick people to remain without health care will incur greater health risks for all its members, however rich or hidden in gated communities they may be, and that societal risk has been increasing in the past few decades. And even Americans know that: a majority of them already support a universal health care system over their current one.[104]

Not long ago, countries thought they could ignore the catastrophically ill and poor because most of the illnesses they had to worry about in their middle-class populations – cancer, diabetes, hypertension – were not catching. But today, as we all know, the great scourges of the 21st century may well turn out to be either new viral diseases, such as Ebola, bird flu, or SARs, or communicable diseases such as *C. difficile* and tuberculosis, which do not respond to antibiotics. With the diminishing power of antibiotics, that is, with the gradual loss of one of the four major pillars of modern medicine, governments and the public are finding themselves in what any medical historian will recognize as a very familiar position. In A.R. Griffith's day, contaminated water and poor food were primary destroyers of the public health. In the 21st century, these problems are resurfacing. In addition to the risks – especially on Canadian native reserves and increasingly industrialized rural areas – of becoming contaminated with materials such as raw sewage and sludge used as fertilizer or being exposed to infectious agents like tuberculosis, our food and water today are often full of carcinogens and other chemical toxins that erode health more slowly.[105] The widespread contamination of fresh water across the world by industry, especially industrial farming, combined with the increase in processed food loaded with heart-clogging fats and diabetes-inciting carbohydrates is once again filling hospitals with large numbers of people suffering from widespread but avoidable illnesses. For example, 1 in every 31 teenaged American boys now has clogged coronary arteries.[106] It could be said that the mass public health dangers that led to the establishment of publicly funded, universal health care in the first place, from contaminated food and water to ineffective medications, are lining up once again to challenge us – just as we start to think that public health care systems are too expensive to maintain.

Currently, a really useful analysis of our most pressing problem, that is, how to fund both individual and public health care in an age of endless technological development, continues to be influenced and even sidetracked by culture and politics instead of being shaped by hard economic and morbidity statistics. As we see ahead, there is ample statistical proof that single-payer health plans such as Canada's, even if frustratingly complicated, bureaucratic, and stretched, still remain the most efficient and least expensive method of caring for the public health that humans have yet been able to devise. These statistics also demonstrate that despite the popularity of mixed systems with politicians and in the media, using private insurance and private clinics to try to improve public health care systems adds significant increases in cost while often disappointly decreasing efficacy of treatment.

PRIVATE'S BETTER! NO, PUBLIC!

Undoubtedly the most germane information is the substantial empirical support for the proposition that for-profit hospitals are lower-cost than government hospitals.

The Fraser Institute[107]

According to the Center for Health Program Studies at Harvard Medical School ... administration costs in the private US system are four times what they are in Canada under the public system.

Nancy MacBeth, MP, Alberta, Question Period,
Alberta Legislature, 1 Dec. 1999.[108]

At the risk of getting into the game of I'll show you your study; you show me my study, there are studies going back and forth.

Premier Ralph Klein, Question Period,
Alberta Legislature, 1 Dec. 1999[109]

In trying to decide which argument is supported by reality, the United States is a very useful standard for comparison. As most people know, it's the only industrialized democracy in the world that doesn't have a largely state-supported medical system. However, as most people also know, the U.S. spends far more per capita on health care than does any comparable country. In fact, the gap is so enormous that a recent study by the University of California's James Kahn estimates that the U.S. would save over $161 *billion* dollars every year, *in paperwork alone*, if it switched to a single-payer system.[110] These billions of dollars are not abstract amounts deducted from government budgets. They come directly out of the pockets of people who need medical care.

The year 2000 marks a crucial period when international trade rules, economic theory, and political will, especially in the United States but to some degree throughout the whole world, had begun to fully implement a belief in the efficiency of private, as opposed to public, management of almost any kind of system. By this year, the U.S. health care system had been fully taken over by what has been called "the HMO (Health Management Organization) Revolution." Within only five years, by 2005, U.S. citizens were paying more than twice as much for their medical care as they had in 2000 – before they got the HMOs.[111]

For-profit medical plans – which is what most HMOs are – support the importance of evidence-based medicine when trying to decide what services and procedures are profitable to offer to their clients. If we apply the same standards of evidence-based medicine to judging not just treatments but also different types of hospital systems, there are two criteria that could be expected to demonstrate the merit of any country's health care plan. The first would be its overall success in creating and sustaining health in the population. The second would be its ability to keep costs as low as possible while doing so. Such studies have been undertaken in recent years, and one of the largest meta-analyses of these studies compares the mortality rates in private, for-profit U.S. hospitals with those in non-profit U.S. hospitals. This very large epidemiological and biostatistical investigation found that death rates in for-profit hospitals are significantly higher than in non-profit hospitals. An enormous cohort of 38 million adult patients in 26,000 U.S. hospitals revealed that the increased death rates were clearly linked to "the corners that for-profit hospitals must cut in order to achieve a profit margin for investors, as well as to pay high salaries for administrators."[112]

P.J. Devereaux, a cardiologist at McMaster University and the lead researcher, wrote, "to ease cost pressures, administrators tend to hire less highly skilled personnel, including doctors, nurses, and pharmacists ... The U.S. statistics clearly show that when the need for profits drives hospital decision-making, more patients die." The same study revealed that people receiving care in a for-profit hospital also have a 2 percent higher chance of dying there or within thirty days of discharge than those receiving care in a non-profit. At that rate, if we Canadians switched to a private system, 2,000 more of us would die every year. The report warns that "the very same for-profit hospital chains in the U.S. that were the subject of this study would be purchasing hospitals in Canada" if the public system continues to be weakened.[113]

Historically and around the world, income inequality has been associated with unyielding higher rates of both illness and mortality. It's one of the cruelest aspects of income distribution: poor people not only experience material want all their lives, they also suffer more illnesses and die younger. Yet, *in Canada, there is very little statistical association between income inequality and mortality rates.* In the early 1990s, Statistics Canada analyzed income and mortality census data from all Canadian provinces and all U.S. states as well as 53 Canadian and 282 American metropolitan areas. This unusually massive study by McGill professor Nancy Ross concluded that, "the relation between income inequality and mortality is not universal but instead depends on social and political characteristics specific to place." In other words, government health policies have an effect. "Income inequality is strongly associated with mortality in the United States and in North America as a whole, but there is no relation within Canada at either the province or metropolitan area level ... between income inequality and mortality." The same study revealed that among the poorest people in the United States, even a 1 percent increase in income resulted in a decline in mortality of nearly 22 out of 100,000.[114]

Fairness demands mention of the poorer health experienced by Native groups in Canada, where both infant and adult mortality rates are substantially higher than in the white population. Mortality rates in northern Ontario, for example, are 20 percent higher than in the population in the southern part of the province. The infant mortality rate, at 11 deaths per thousand, is at levels that are up to 60 and even 100 percent higher than in the rest of Canadian society. And life expectancy for Native men and women is 68.2 and 75.9. In contrast, it's 75.7 and 81.5 for their white counterparts. Our natives also suffer higher rates of diabetes, respiratory and infectious diseases like TB, anemia, gall bladder disease, and many other disorders than do the rest of the population. Their lower life expectancy is also related to the high death toll taken by accidents, alcohol, and violence. A truly inclusive health system should be more aggressively tackling such things as the ongoing water contamination on reserves, poor health education, fewer doctors and nurses per capita, and the difficulty of providing hospital care over the wide, depopulated areas of the far north. The other factors strongly influencing native health are social and political and are closely tied to their lack of ready access to land, jobs, housing, and education.[115] Canadian Indigenous peoples are considerably better off than natives in many other countries, such as Aboriginals in Australia, but Canada has still been rebuked by UN Human Rights Committees and Working Groups for its record.

What makes Professor Ross's study, which concentrated on the general population, particularly interesting is not the simple fact that income is generally not a factor in mortality in this country. Instead, it's that Canada used to have statistics that mirrored those in the United States. In 1970, for example, U.S. and Canadian mortality rates calculated along income lines were virtually identical. But 1970 also marked the introduction of full Medicare in Canada – universal, single-payer coverage. So the simple reason nearly all of Canada's citizens, regardless of income, have become equally healthy most likely lies in the fact that Canada has a publicly funded, single-payer health system and that the control group, the United States, doesn't. Even Canadian Natives, relatively speaking, have shown enormous gains in health and longevity that date from the early 1970s. In general, Native groups were already experiencing steady downturns in child, infant, and adult mortality and disease rates between 1951 and 1971 but the consistent improvement of their general health since Medicare mirrors the rapidly escalating drops in mortality as other Canadians have experienced. French-speaking groups, especially during the 1950s and early 60s, had intermediate levels of longevity and health, while British and other ethnic groups had the best. Frank Trovato of the University of Alberta notes in one study that, "the roots of inequalities in survival probabilities are [in fact] partly a result of social and economic disparities ... [However], over time the general pattern is one of declining mortality [for all groups], with some narrowing of the differences."[116]

Public Health and Preventative Medicine in Canada, a widely used Canadian public health text book by Chandrakant Shah, gives graphs of trends for mortality rates per 1,000 in Canada between 1958 and 1998. While the 1950s and 60s were halcyon days for doctors, the present era looks more like the halcyon period for patients. Although rates were more level for older people, the graphs are startling in what they reveal across the spectrum of age and sex. Most mortality rates steadily decreased during this period, but even so, the effects of Medicare are clear. Infant mortality rates are considered to be one of the most reli-

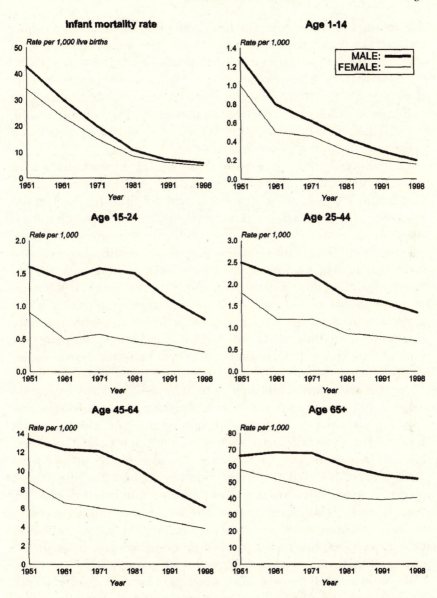

Figure 1   Trends in Age- and Sex-Specific Mortality rates per 1,000
Population in Canada, 1951–1998

SOURCE: Adapted from Health Field Indicators, Health and Welfare Canada, 1986, and Statistics Canada.
Shah, Public Health and Preventative Medicine in Canada, 139.

able statistics for measuring the health of a population. For example, in Canada in 1951, out of every 1000 births, between 35 and 45 infants of both sexes died at birth or before reaching one year of age. That's comparable to Peru's rate of about 43 today, but better than Afghanistan's 150. At that time, about 20 percent more male than female infants died, which also reflects world norms. But by 1996, the sex differential in Canada had almost disappeared, to less than 1 percent, and an average of only 6.5 infants was dying.

Infant mortality today is down to about 4.7. That puts Canada 23rd in the world, in the highest quarter of 225 countries assessed, right after Japan, Finland, Norway, Sweden, and South Korea, and in the company of the Netherlands, Luxembourg, Australia, and Denmark. These are all countries with extensive public health care and hospital access systems. The United States, despite its wealth and technical advancement, is at 43rd place and barely makes the top half of world nations. Its infant mortality comes in at 7.1 per 1,000, by far the highest in the industrialized world, and its immediate neighbours in this survey are Croatia and Lithuania.[117] U.S. infant mortality rates are equal to or above those of Taiwan and Cuba and are higher than even some of the poorer states in India. Note that these last two countries have public health systems in place, at least for mothers and infants.

The countries with death rates as high as the U.S. have little to do with the G8 powerhouses with whom Americans normally associate. They all have private or public/private systems, or like Cuba and Kerala, India, have public systems but are extremely poor. The closest industrialized country to the U.S. rate is Italy, with 5.83 infants dying per thousand, but that's still five countries higher. The number of infants dying at birth or in their first year does not reflect rates of disease, of course. It measures the health of the mother and her access to pre-natal and immediate post-natal care. Among the inner-city poor in the United States, this access rate is even more abysmal; more than 8 percent of mothers never see a doctor before giving birth.[118]

We would naturally expect steady decreases in overall death rates per thousand people in the mid-20th century simply because so many new drugs and procedures were becoming available. But the general mortality rate did not descend as expected in Canada. In fact, *it leveled off for an entire decade,* throughout the 1960s, at about 2.4 for the youngest group and a very high 12.5 for people aged between 45 and 64. It even rose slightly for the elderly from around 66 per 1,000 in 1951 to about 68 throughout the sixties. Despite the halcyon days of physician and hospital prestige, this was also the period we have just reviewed in which two-tier care was intensifying in Canadian hospitals and many people couldn't afford the new treatments being offered. For every age bracket, including the ages 25 to 65, the graphs detailing pre- and post-Medicare mortality rates tell a clear story of how health care systems affect survival. Looking like a broken branch starting in 1971, the same year that Medicare was fully applied, the graphs in *Public Health and Preventative Medicine in Canada* show mortality rates in Canada plunging downward and maintaining a steep downward angle to its present rates of 0.7 for young adults aged 15 to 24 and only *1.2 deaths per thousand for adults from 25 to 64*. For that last group, mortality rates declined to 10.4 percent of their former rate, from 12.5 per thousand down to 1.2 per thousand! Although death rates were beginning to level off for elderly Canadians by 1998, children aged 1 to 14 fared the very best over this period, with death rates beginning at 1.17 per thousand in 1951 and dropping to less than 0.4 for both sexes by 1998.[119]

In the U.S. during the same period, overall mortality rates also dropped, reflecting the same medical advances, but not nearly so precipitately and not in a rush in 1971. Today, given that the U.S. is the richest country on earth, overall mortality rates are shockingly high at 8.4 per thousand deaths, compared to Canada's 6.5. Young adults from 15 to 24, who ought to be the healthiest members of their population, die at a rate of 1.65 per thousand in the U.S., that is, at the same rate young Canadians died 35 years ago, which is more than *four times* the Canadian rate today. It's worse for every age; people aged 45 to 64 can expect to die at a rate of slightly less than 6 per thousand in Canada but almost twice as many – 10.65 – Americans in the same age group will die.[120]

There are some difficulties in comparing Canadian and American statistics because U.S. stats are more often arranged by race or ethnicity than by income. Canada, along with many other countries, has carefully measured the effect of income levels on health over the last twenty or thirty years, but the U.S. has only been doing so relatively recently. Over this period, many papers and studies have been published that compare *racial* health differences in the United States. Typical U.S. health studies show that in 2001 infants born of black mothers were dying at the rate of 14.2 per thousand, which is getting close to Russia's level of 17 per thousand. In comparison, white babies had a rate of only 5.7 deaths. These studies have given rise to the popular misconception that black babies suffer higher rates of mortality because their mothers are "culturally" less likely to breastfeed them or eat properly during pregnancy. It has also led to studies drawing the conclusion that, for example, black males are somehow – because of diet, culture, or genetics – more susceptible to high blood pressure, heart attacks, and cancer, especially fatal prostate cancers, than whites are.[121]

These days, however, we have learned that cultural conceptions of "racial" differences have almost no basis in human genetics. So Americans have also begun to drop race separation in favour of measuring in terms of income. Like so many other researchers around the world, they have discovered that black men with prostate cancer, the classic example given for racial differences in disease rates in the old U.S. statistics, have the same rates as white men in the same income bracket. A recent article in *Cancer*, reviewed by Robert Jasmer, a medical professor at the University of California at San Francisco, makes the situation clear in its title: "Poverty May Outweigh Race in Excess Prostate Cancer Deaths."[122] When more than 61,000 black, Hispanic, and white men – the racial terms used in the study – who were over 65 and had prostate cancer were followed for up to 11 years, "those in the lowest quartile of socioeconomic status had a 31 percent higher risk of dying from all causes than those in the highest income brackets." That means that if ten men were suffering with such a cancer, no one would die if they were all rich, but three would die if they were all poor. It is simply a factor of socioeconomic status that in the United States, more of those dead men would be black, or as the researchers put it, "differences in mortality between African American and Caucasian men were substantially reduced (after adjusting for poverty or income or composite socioeconomic variable) ... This indicates that socioeconomic differences are one of the major barriers to achieving equal outcomes for men with prostate carcinoma."

A typical American study of "Breastfeeding Rates, by Race/Ethnicity, 2001" and another, "Very Low Birth Weight among Infants, by Race/Ethnicity 1985–2001" makes the "racial," or what others might consider the "income," differential, even clearer. Over the 16 years between the mid-eighties and 2001, a period of unparalleled prosperity and technological advancement in the United States, the death rates for all American infants, including white ones, did not decline – they *rose*. The mortality rate for black babies also rose, so much so that showing its climb required an extended graph. It went up from 2.5 to 3.0 in those 16 years. Mortality rates for all other "races/ethnicities" also rose, from a low of about 0.8 per thousand in 1985 up to a current high of 1.3 babies dying per thousand in 2001.[123]

Most medical researchers in the world would interpret these statistics as illustrating the results of the mothers' inability to access adequate pre- and post-natal care and not as an outcome of "racial," that is to say genetic, differences. In fact, from newborn babies to old men, statistical evidence shows that mortality rates that put the United States in very embarrassing company are due to a lack of egalitarian health care. This demonstrates that the poor suffer more under privately funded systems. Most remarkably, however, the latest data is showing that the overall health of a society, which is most often attained through publicly funded systems, translates to better health for even its rich members – the group one would assume to be the main beneficiary of a private system. If we look at the 5.7 per thousand mortality rate of just the – presumably richer – white babies in the U.S., while lower than the average rate of 8.3, Canada still does better at 4.7. Canada's figure is lower by 1 percent, even though it includes all ethnic groups and all income levels, not just the supposedly advantaged white group's statistics. A 1 percent difference may not sound like much, but when measuring mortality, it's huge. In fact, in countries such as the U.S. or in the Third World, where there are large inequalities of income and health care opportunities within the population, even the richest people are more unhealthy than the poor people in countries such as Canada where health care is available to all. Evidence from the United Nations Human Development Report also shows that poor people in Britain receiving social assistance (but with access to universal health care) also live up to four years longer than the richest Americans.[124]

If we continue to look only at statistical evidence, we are forced to conclude that, for all its many, many problems and inefficiencies, publicly funded health care not only saves more people's lives and makes all citizens healthier overall, it's cheaper. Once again, the U.S. makes a perfect control group for studies. In 1971, Canadian health care costs were 7.4 percent of our GDP, compared to a very similar 7.6 percent in the U.S. But by 2002, the Americans' health care share of the GDP had almost doubled, to more than 14 percent, while Canada's remained relatively stable at 9 percent. This fact has also made Canada more competitive internationally. It's axiomatic that Americans pay more for their health care than people in any other industrialized country. Health insurance premiums paid by American employers amount to 8.2 percent of the gross annual pay, while Canadian employers are paying less than an eighth of that. Among many other such statistics, a recent study by Stewart MacKay of KPMG rated competitive advantages

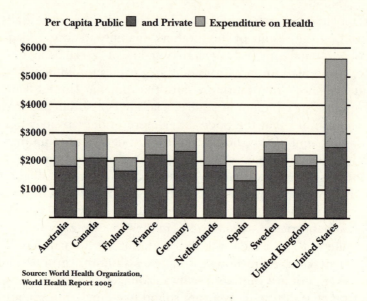

Per Capita Public ■ and Private ■ Expenditure on Health

Source: World Health Organization,
World Health Report 2005

Figure 2 Comparison of public and privage per capita spending on health
U.S. public per capita spending, which covers 26% of the population, is
higher than public spending for universal health care in Europe, Canada,

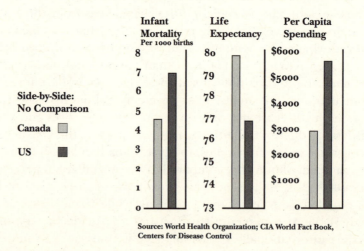

Source: World Health Organization; CIA World Fact Book,
Centers for Disease Control

Figure 3 Comparison of US and Canada for infant mortality, life expectancy,
and per capita spending.
Canada and the U.S. used to be twins on public-health measurements. Here's
how it looks after 35 years of Canadian universal health care.

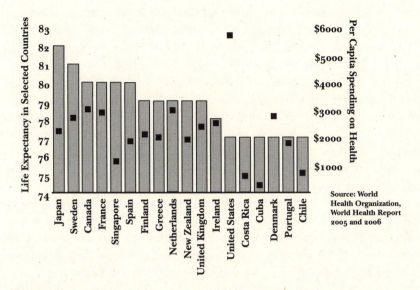

Figure 4 Comparison of life expectancy and per capita spending on health

Dressel, "Has Canada Got the Cure?" *Yes! Magazine* www.yesmagazine.org (fall 2006): 29

based on comparative wage and benefit costs, taxes, transportation, and utilities for companies based in North America, Europe, and Japan, "KPMG reported that Canada has a 14.5 percent cost advantage over the United States. The company cited Canada's health benefits as the single biggest factor in this difference."[125] The reason for the demise of the economic power of huge U.S. corporations, such as Chrysler, is that they have to bear so much of the cost of health care through pre-paid employee insurance. It's this aspect of health care, not worrying about more people dying, that currently fuels the greatest enthusiasm for public health plans in the U.S.

It ought to be of some comfort to Canadians that our health and hospital care system is statistically more effective and less expensive than that of many other countries. Nonetheless, most of us still feel that hospital care is deteriorating in Canada, at least in comparison to what it was in the recent past, and the chunk that health costs take out of government budgets grows more alarming every year. This has led many Canadians to support the idea that public plans have gone as far as they can and must be buttressed with private options. In fact, on 9 July 2007 the polling firm Leger Marketing released results claiming that two-thirds of Québecers wanted more privatization in the medical system.

Pressed for further details, the pollster admitted that respondents wanted such clinics or doctors under the control of the province, in other words, the French system, and they did not want any out-of-pocket expenses. Moreover, their reasons for wanting more private surgical and x-ray clinics and so forth were not based on the famous "wait times" for these services but on their difficulties in finding family doctors. It is this kind of report that fuels the increasing beliefs that private payment will somehow solve problems caused by factors that are not directly linked to payment methods.[126]

Resistance to allowing governments sole power over social planning is now affecting more countries than just the U.S. and Canada: U.S. economic and cultural attitudes towards health care are increasingly influencing public health systems in countries such as Britain, France, and Australia. This is largely due to two factors. Publicly funded health care systems are buckling under increasing medical and especially drug costs that are fed by public expectations that grow more extravagant with every medical breakthrough. Secondly, because of these burgeoning costs, the claims that private, competitive, for-profit insurance plans and clinics will bring greater efficiency for less cost are gaining credence, even in Europe. These private systems offer spectacular care for the very rich – private rooms, luxurious extras, shorter waiting times, rapid treatment for elective surgery and non-critical illnesses – which is unavailable in a public system. But the real reasons for the apparent collapse of many public health systems are not widely discussed.

Eugene Veda and Raisa Deber, in their seminal article, "The Canadian Health-Care System," sum up the situation. "Not surprisingly," they write, "the universal health plan has encountered both difficulty and conflict. Government began by paying bills. With rising costs, government paymasters took on an increased role. *They chose to use the blunt instrument of cost-containment rather than the more difficult step of modifying the organization and management of the system.* As a result, providers now complain that the system is under-funded while governments see only what they perceive as the insatiable financial appetite of the health- care system. Both charge that the system is in crisis."[127] Certainly our hospitals are stretched almost as far as they can go. Confusingly, however, in terms of hard statistics, the morbidity and life expectancy rates continue to show how well the whole system still works. And if you ask fellow Canadians who have had to go into the hospital for a broken arm, to have a baby, or to get an operation or a diagnosis, the great majority will confirm the statistics and tell you that they were cared for in a reasonably timely fashion *and at no out-of-pocket cost.* However, even if their personal experience was distressing and seemed to reveal serious problems with the health system, it is important to compare such problems statistically with those which can also be encountered in a private system.

It turns out that, statistically, the risks of such common difficulties as unnecessary wait times, misdiagnoses, surgical complications, errors, and even hospital-borne illnesses such as *C. difficile* are not only equal in private systems (with the exception of wait times for elective procedures), they are sometimes significantly greater than in a publicly funded system. We have to add to that distressing fact the even more upsetting idea that many citizens can't afford to get any medical care at all in a private system. In short, fixing our hospital and medical care system in Canada is not going to be as easy as we might hope. It is probably not possible to get out of the current financial bind by simply throwing out one kind of funding system for a stylish new one.

This is not to say that Canadians should just accept the many problems in their system as all they're going to get. That's a sure recipe for further slippage in services, more pressure and demands on doctors and other medical personnel, and a gradual but inexorable erosion of care. And, as we shall see ahead, there are bureaucratic methodologies in the government management of Canadian public care that are both enraging and have injurious consequences; they must be changed. Doctors and nurses must be increased in number and they need Canadians to pay attention when they complain of the pressures and demands that mitigate against their ability to take real care of their patients. However, problems in Medicare are still dwarfed by the frightening systemic problems that privatization would bring back to the practice of medicine in Canada. It's worth remembering that every country, including our own, experimented with private funding for the first fifty or sixty years of modern medical care and then rejected it – for very good reasons.

BALANCING THE EQUATION

Just a decade previously, it had been hospitals that drove [medical costs] ... At the dawn of the twenty-first century, pharmaceuticals [are] the new engine of health care inflation.

Laurie Garrett, *Betrayal of Trust*[128]

To sum up, from the very beginnings of the halcyon years of technical and professional development in medical care in Canada and indeed around the world, i.e., from the late 1940s into the 60s, most industrialized countries were beginning to experience problems financing their hospital and health care systems. Their desire to keep up technologically ran up against their experience, hard-won during the Depression, that charity and fees from rich patients were not enough to fund hospital operations or the larger public health care system. In the late 1960s and early 70s, the populations of almost every developed country on earth that hadn't already done so turned to their federal governments to demand national health plans completely or largely supported by taxes. A few countries, such as Germany and Great Britain, had long since instituted such programs. The U.S. was the exception, but even it created some government plans, notably Medicare and Medicaid, which provide very limited coverage when compared to the public/private systems of France or Germany. In Canada, Europe, Australia, and around the developed world, these programs gave a few decades of high-quality, state-sponsored, and almost totally inclusive health care. Statistics clearly demonstrate that during this period, life expectancy steadily increased and mortality decreased most strongly in countries with public health care systems.

In Canada, our particular economic, cultural, historical, and political situation led first to single-payer, universal insurance for hospital care, which began to be established right after the Depression. However, the method of providing federal funding to hospitals introduced in 1945 led inexorably to the establishment of universal medical care, mandated by Canadian law in 1961 and fully extended throughout the country by 1971. As we saw with the Queen Elizabeth Hospital, many doctors, even in Canada, fought this tendency, but most adjusted to the new regime when they saw that the quality of care did not suffer. Since then, the biggest problems in Canadian health care, which are still unfolding today, have much less to do with the social justice issues that animate the Medicare debate than with skyrocketing expenses. Technological, pharmaceutical, and private care innovations are reaching greater heights than ever before because of global economic, trade, political, and especially philosophical factors. This means that in the 21st century, the same problem of uncontrolled health expenses faces virtually every country, regardless of level of development or type of payment system.

Looking at the entire history of hospitals allows us to isolate and recognize recurrent trends. When we do so, it seems that approximately
every thirty years, intractable funding problems resurface. Introducing
single-payer plans helped control the crisis of funding public health
care in the generation following the biggest crises in the 1940s. But the
underlying reasons for these constantly reappearing financial crises in
every kind of modern hospital system, whether private or public, have
never been dealt with or even identified until quite recently.

The real problem is that no matter whether the health system is
mostly private or mostly public, *paying* for increasingly expensive and
complicated hospital care has been left to taxpayers in most countries
and individuals in the United States and much of the undeveloped
world. In all cases, however, the other side of the financial equation,
controlling the rising costs of hospitalization and general medical care
has been left entirely to the very entities that stand to gain most from
every price hike – that is, the private, for-profit corporations that produce medical drugs and technologies as well as the private insurance
companies and chains of health care management facilities.

Given this situation, it's not surprising that the irresistible force of
rising pharmaceutical, surgical, insurance, and medical supply costs
are overwhelming the immovable financial limits of sick people,
whether those people are publicly or privately insured. Instead of
attacking the systemic reasons for this problem, however, hospital planners, governments, and public health experts continue to tinker with
only one side of the equation, much as they did back in the thirties
before mass public funding brought hospitals a few decades' reprieve.

Moreover, as we will see ahead, when the health care funding crisis
that has been a regular feature of the history of modern hospitals
returned in the 1980s and 90s, it was due more to global than to
national forces. This resulted in a fatal outcome for the Queen Elizabeth Hospital of Montreal and many other productive and altruistic
institutions like it. Systemic problems with funding public health care
that are actually caused by national and international economic priorities have simmered beneath the surface of every generation's solutions
so far. Whether charging all health expenses to richer patients, as
Canadian hospitals did in the 1920s, or expecting taxes to keep up with
the endless avarice of for-profit corporations, as they have done since
the 1970s, the underlying necessity of trying to make health care work
like a business has never been properly addressed.

The very big questions – Is public health care really a business? Should it have to respond to and satisfy market forces? Is there any way it can partially avoid such forces? – have not been asked either internally, by hospital administrators, or externally, on the political level. The final two chapters of this book will explore the reasons why so many of our hospitals, especially the smaller ones that served their communities so well, have been closed. Why health services, in both public and private systems, are becoming poorer. Where public health dollars really need to be concentrated. And what systemic changes might enable our increasingly challenged governments to help us provide stable health protection for our children and grandchildren for the rest of this century. In short, if we want the answers to the local issues, like who killed all our hospitals, we are forced to ask the big questions. By the end of the book, some big answers may begin to emerge.

5

The Queen Must Die

During 1973, at the direction of the Ministry of Social Affairs, our
Department of Obstetrics was closed, as were those of a number of other
hospitals. We were sorry to see this ... but it must be admitted that our
facilities were being under-utilized. The phase-out was accomplished
smoothly.

> Report of the President, The Queen Elizabeth
> Hospital of Montreal, 1973[1]

The Queen Elizabeth, like every other old private hospital in Canada,
adjusted with as much grace as possible to the new regime of all-public
funding that began in the 1970s. It is to its credit that its pleasure in
continuing to be of service was at least equal to its grief over the loss of
its autonomy and many of its traditions. Throughout the 1970s, as previously mentioned, that grief is clearly expressed in internal documents. In 1969, medical staff, that is, orderlies, nurses, and other
hospital workers, were unionized to become employees of the state,
official civil servants, which came as a deep blow to the 19th century
dream of independent medical professionals functioning as equals or
superiors to any funding body. From then on, each province determined the rate of pay as well as the length and type of training, especially for any staff below the rank of physician. Moreover, hospitals
could no longer alter their budgets in order to respond to special
needs of their own or their employees. For the next two decades, bud-

get constraints, along with advances in medicine that permitted shorter stays, brought about the first sustained experience that required hospitals to retract, instead of expand, their services. These constraints also demonstrated that what we have seen as being good for the health of patients, i.e., universal, single-payer care, is not always equally welcomed in terms of the continuing economic and technological expansion of the profession and its care-giving institutions.

As an illustration, in the late 1960s the Queen Elizabeth Hospital had begun one of its periodic construction expansions in order to meet growing public demand for beds and services. The now all-powerful Quebec Health minister stopped the work in June of 1970; no reasons were given in the hospital minutes that describe this action. The Queen E must have resisted because two months later it received a formal letter from Quebec ordering it to "drop its expansion plan." In fact, although the hospital was renovated over the coming years, it was never again allowed a construction expansion: it was restricted to interiour design changes like the new ER.

Many people have also noted that in Quebec in particular, the government seems to have rapidly adopted an antagonistic role towards the hospitals and medical service personnel it now had to fund – a bit like a parent bird getting angry with its nestlings for constantly demanding more worms. As for the province's gift for the art of administration, as heart specialist Derek Mapole has said, "We all know there are two ways to manage people: with carrots and sticks. Quebec never seems to have heard of the carrot." For example, many Quebec doctors felt so strongly about the new government interference, represented in 1970 by Medicare (Bill 41 in Quebec), that they organized walkouts. The province reacted to this very quickly in a draconian way. Doctors who spoke out publicly against Medicare, the Medical Board minutes warned its staff, risked "jail sentences of up to a year and fines of up to $50,000 a day"[2] No government carrots were mentioned.

Still, a year later, it was clear that both sides were capable of compromise. For instance, Quebec promised to allow at least the desperately necessary expansion of the Queen E's lab facilities.[3] But as early as 1972 and 1973, these disturbances and resentments quieted down, and services began to hum along again as usual. A quick reading of the Medical Boards makes most of the Hospital's daily round of business sound much as it had before Medicare arrived. The concerns are not administrative or budgetary, but professional: infections in the OR, new drugs, accreditation, expansion of psychiatric services, new procedures such as tumor rounds, and new equipment. There are a few budget cuts and mention of the old problem of too many chronic care patients, but in general, nothing ominous for the historian except for the creeping closure of beds due to nursing shortages, which started getting serious attention in 1974.[4]

Because the government now set salaries and decided how many people of each skill an institution could hire, hospitals like the Queen E had lost most of their power to make sure their staffs were both adequate to their standards and reasonably happy. The nursing shortage that became serious in the mid-1970s mushroomed in the 1980s, for several reasons. In 1972, all the private schools of nursing in Canada, including the Queen E's beloved Philip's School, were closed. From that time on in Canada, nurses have been educated in CEGEPs, colleges, or universities, where academic standards could be more directly controlled by the government. One stated reason for these pedagogical changes was to attract more nursing students: their numbers had begun declining as far back as the early 1960s. But despite these more modern training approaches, the downward trend in nursing enrollments continued. Relatively low pay combined with government refusals to budge on long hours of rotating shift work were disincentives, especially because women had many more options in the workforce by the 1970s. Despite the shortages, throughout this period there were disturbing rumours that the government was rejecting qualified nurses or discouraging them from applying; no one could say why.

Provincial authorities must have been stunned in those early years by the enormity of the fiscal and organizational responsibilities that Medicare had suddenly thrust upon them. One can only surmise that they were scurrying around trying to save money wherever they could. Staff salaries, until just a few years ago when they were bypassed by drug costs, had always been the largest single item in a hospital budget. Many analysts have noted that chronic shortages of nurses and, later on, of doctors, are the direct result of crude ploys by governments whose only object was to get a budget down quickly. Of course, it's the health of the citizens that suffers when the professional shortages hit some years later. In 1979, for example, there was a serious surplus of trained doctors. The Queen E had 180 applications for only 14 intern openings and 110 for the 6 available family medicine positions.[5] Typically, however, the government and the College of Physicians and Surgeons both overreacted and took the opportunity to limit medical school and especially family medicine enrollments so drastically that by the 1980s, there were shortages again, especially of GPs, who by the late 1990s had become as rare as hen's teeth.

This is a recurring problem when governments manage medical training because elected entities are more concerned with the political effect of balanced budgets each fiscal year than with the eventual lack of professionals a decade down the line – the typical time it takes for cutbacks to become apparent. One way of dealing with it would be to make health ministries much more autonomous, as they often are in Europe. John Hughes mentions that as soon as the supply of doctors became even slightly stabilized, by the late 1980s, then-Finance Minister Paul Martin "shut down the medical schools in 1992; it was just to save money that particular year. The deans screamed for a decade: 'You can't do this! The baby boomers are hitting old age, we won't have enough doctors!' Lo and behold, in November of 2002, Allan Rock stands up and announces that Canada doesn't have enough doctors! The demographics show that for yet another decade, until 2012 – and that's the best-case scenario – we're stuck with a serious doctor shortage in Canada."

With nurses, after the glut that lasted from about 1920 up to World War II, there have never been enough, although the situation in Quebec is no longer critical except at night. One typically odd, counterproductive government regulation that added to the frustration at the Queen E during this period was that the government granted the hospital only first and second year nurses, not final, third-year trainees, which made it harder for the hospital to recruit students on graduation. In 1974, the Queen Elizabeth reacted by hiring more foreign nurses, especially Filipinos. This ended up working very well for both hospitals and the nurses. One such nurse, Eleanor Fajardo, who had come over from the Philippines, "intending to stay for two years," was still there at closing more than twenty years later. "I fell in love with the hospital," she said later. "It was so small, so friendly."[6] When it closed, she finally packed up and went back home.

Starting as early as 1975, the Corporation of Physicians and Surgeons warned Medical Boards in an official letter that, "Medical records and committee minutes must be kept confidential" from provincial Social Affairs bureaucrats.[7] This was ostensibly in the interests of patient privacy, but it also illustrates the growing lack of trust between the two bodies. But by far the most upsetting thing to happen in these years was the government's decision to close the obstetrics unit of the hospital. The Queen Elizabeth had been birthing babies for its entire existence, but the province counted the numbers of beds devoted to maternal care and awarded obstetrics, for the English population anyway, to another small community hospital, the Catherine Booth. Albert Nixon, the ever-creative director general between 1971 and 1987, immediately remodeled the maternity ward into a day surgery unit.

Scandals surrounding unlicensed nursing homes in Quebec around this time put pressure on community hospitals to take on more chronic care patients and on provinces to fund their care. Throughout the 1970s and 80s and right through to this day, no provincial government has ever been able to bring itself to allocate enough money to adequately finance chronic care. They have kept hospital bureaucracies humming with memos, restrictions, and unenforceable bed requirements, which probably reflects multiplying government departments operating without any kind of master plan. For example, in 1977, the Quebec government *forbade separate care units* for chronic patients, likely in an effort to block acute care hospitals from admitting such patients. Three years later, in 1980, the province put out a directive demanding that *hospitals create separate chronic care units*[8] but that demand wasn't formalized until 1982, which created a lot of confusion.[9]

A new system of government forms, called EROs, was required by 1983. But these forms were so confusing and complicated that the Medical Board expressed fears that they prevented needy chronic care patients from being admitted.[10] Quite a few must have made it in, however, because by 1988, all small hospitals, including the Queen E, were living in fear of being declared "chronic care only" because of a government directive that forbade them to close any chronic care beds. That meant that in the increasing cases of budget shortfalls, they could only close acute care beds. And, if acute care beds fell below a certain level, they would lose their teaching accreditation and status. By 1988, the hospital was forced to turn patients away even in the ICU because of "long-term ICU patients," and had begun to suspect the government of consciously trying to close them to acute care.[11] Yet, only a couple years later, they were ebullient about the government funding expensive acute care renovations and equipment, including a new ER and equipment.

By the late 1980s, bureaucratic government management had naturally become focused on the fundamentally political concerns of containing skyrocketing medical costs. Whether they were located in a distant provincial capital or a nearby Regie regionale, government civil

servants entrusted with health care management were issuing regulations that became increasingly contradictory, confusing, and debilitating to many small hospitals all across Canada. In their defence, the
bureaucrats were fighting a losing battle with continuous rises in costs
and public expectations. The crisis mentality that has come to characterize Canadian medical care had officially begun.

The late Eli Katz, whose career overlapped both systems, spoke with
enthusiasm about the lack of bureaucracy when dealing with professional needs in the halcyon days under Harold Griffith. Eli remembered, "Dr Harold always got what we needed as each specialty
changed, like a microscope which could look at a bone a half a millime-
ter long. I explained why we needed such a thing in the ENT department, and he said, 'Go ahead!' They raised the money I needed for it.
After, the government took on this burden. When Griffith was in
charge, I may have had to wait a little bit, but I got what I needed. With
the government, I may have gotten it eventually, but we had to wait so
long and fight so hard!"

In early 1974, under government management, the Queen E
decided it wanted to become the first non-smoking hospital in Canada.
Almost two years later, in July of 1976, only the elevators and part of
the cafeteria were smoke-free zones. Medical Board researcher Ken
Hechtman remarks, "This isn't the best example, but it does make
clear how things had changed. In the old days, if you had an idea, you
sold it to Dr Harold. Harold said, 'Make it so,' and it got done. Compare the turnaround time of less than two months to create an entire
cancer department in the 1940s with this non-smoking policy. The
essence of bureaucracy is that there are a dozen different people who
can say 'no' and not one who can say 'yes' and overrule all the others."
The problem with a government-managed system is parsimony, bureaucracy, and medically dangerous delays. But in a completely doctor-
managed system, physicians would constantly be agitating for new toys
and equipment (not to mention higher salaries) until the public could
no longer afford health care costs. Obviously, some kind of power sharing, which always characterizes the most successful systems, like Germany's, would be the best way to go. In Canada's case, however, the
powers went mostly to government. The infamous Regies regionales
discussed earlier were introduced in 1977, putting yet another level of
bureaucracy between hospitals and the government.[12]

These problems of increasing bureaucracy and lack of funding are
ominous only in hindsight. On the surface, the general tenor of hospi-

tal life through most of the 1970s was pretty peaceable and optimistic. Of course, clouds were gathering. Since its foundation, the Queen Elizabeth, like most community hospitals, had always run deficits, and Albert Nixon was very much of the old culture. The Quebec government was not amused by the deficits he accepted and, when they got up to $30,000 a month in November of 1976, instituted serious cost-cutting, demanding that the hospital close some of its clinics. The Catch–22 in all this is that about 80 percent of the cost-overruns the Queen E and other such hospitals were experiencing were because of the government's negotiation of higher salaries for union workers, whom the hospitals were not permitted to lay off.

By January of 1977, the hospital's deficit was running at about $50,000 a month. Only three months later, it nearly doubled to $98,000 a month, again primarily because of government-negotiated salary increases to union employees.[13] The same kind of situation continues today, with hospitals cited and punished for deficits that are beyond their control. These deficits are largely caused by provincial governments that knowingly grant inadequate budgets for political reasons and then heroically bail out the hospitals with special allocations. This dance kept the Queen E spinning. In March of 1979, their spiraling budget was miraculously balanced at $13.9 million, by means of attrition cuts in staff and consolidating the accumulated deficit in another column of the accounts book.[14] Such last-minute saves happened again and again. They gave hospitals the continuing hope of bail-outs and also provided governments with the disingenuous excuse for closing many of the small hospitals they administered "for budgetary reasons."

Mario Larivière, the Queen E's director general at the time of closure, says that on top of the government-engineered staff and nursing shortages, hospitals all across Canada aren't given enough control over their budgets to allow them to respond to their particular situations. As DG at St-Eustache, he said, "I'm simply not allowed to help my employees in any way." If he wants to adjust his budget to local needs, such as hiring more nurses on weekends, for example, "The government auditor prevents me from giving people any benefits or incentives whatsoever to work overtime. They are expected to just keep on working anyway, under absolutely miserable conditions. I administer $60 million annually, but I'm not allowed to use any of it to alleviate the particular problems my employees come to me with. That's because the Ministry of Health is micro-managing our hospitals, making decisions to save political face, not decisions that benefit patients. The only way we can get out of this bind, that causes real suffering to the staff and to the public, is to go back to community decision-making."

Larivière's frustration goes back to the most fundamental problems that every public institution has to address but that are not discussed today because of the current emphasis on the central problems of economics and political expediency. Larivière says that, due in part to the famous closure of seven hospitals in 1996, "this hospital went from serving 50 percent of the local population to serving 74 percent – that is, 225,000 people. Closures contributed, but in-migration to the area at a rate of 10 percent a year is also to blame, as well as the fact that St Eustache has a good reputation for equipment and patient-centred care. Our budgets, however, have never been raised in amounts appropriate to the number of people now being served, so St Eustache has the largest deficit in Quebec. We're running with a deficit as large as Sacre Coeur's, even though we're one-third the size."

Although a far smaller deficit got the Queen E in trouble, Larivière says his hospital is not being punished for this, "because they know perfectly well why we're in deficit. The budget is raised by only 2 percent every year even though demand is going up by five times that – so although we're in deficit, we're deemed to be so efficient that the province awarded the hospital $650,000 in extra grants – even though there are no larger allocations in the official budget!" Clearly, this is a political paper game. Larivière says that because of it, "Hospitals in deficit have to ask for loans and grants and spend all their time proving their every request is genuine, even though both the ministry and I know this is simply a budgetary short-fall problem. So we're always under stress – my directors, my board, my staff, the whole institution. The government is, in fact, very proud of our efforts, as we see through the extra grants, but they're not comfortable working in a deficit." The obvious response in a democracy would be for hospitals to go public with these problems and demand higher official budgets. "Haut-Richelieu did that," says Larivière, "and they got a higher budget, but at the cost of their director general and the entire board. We are not ready to leave in our case. We think we're still doing a good job for this community."

So what does it mean when a hospital is in deficit and doesn't have enough money to operate optimally? "Without adequate funding," Larivière says, "we're forced to make choices between this thing and that. Should we reduce surgeries or beds? Which services should be curtailed? The government imposed a surgical quota on us; they reduced our activity level. But because of demand, I have to increase it again. And every year, there's never enough. If you go public with your problems, you're put into trusteeship. I was a trustee for several hospitals, L'enfant Jesu and St. Sacrement in Quebec City, for example. That means that the hospital's board, all the people who know and care about the place, lose control. The trustee replaces them. The trustee gives control back when they leave, but usually that entails naming a new board, breaking in new people with maybe very different attitudes and goals. That can help in a few cases, but can be terribly destructive in others. In short, it's a drastic measure that shouldn't be resorted to very often."

Although a director general is supposed to act rather like an insurance adjustor by balancing the needs of both government and institution, back in the 1970s and 80s, Albert Nixon's loyalties definitely favoured the hospital side of the equation. The government, which typically has the same person in charge of a dossier for no more than a few years and often for only a few months, was, to the recently un-privatized Queen E, an adversary to be manipulated, not an ally to consult. Moreover, the government's contradictory rules that demanded creative, red-ink accounting and then rewarded fiscal acrobatics with life-saving grants and debt forgiveness mitigated against a feeling of partnership. Nixon was at the cusp of change, so the old variety of private funding options remained intact with the handy addition of new, confusing, but relatively stable public stipends.

When asked how his little hospital, which at that point was funded by panic-stricken and still rather disorganized government bureaucrats, could find the money for a major expansion and all the new services that came to be offered in the 1970s, Nixon says, "Our donors gave us the money for all this." He is referring to the same community of donors the hospital had always had, which enabled them to raise the money for their new clinics. "A.H. Marden, our old president, was a professional fund-raiser. I'd tell him we needed, say, $60,000 for a new machine. Three months later, we'd buy it; we didn't even bother to tell the government. Marden was so good at raising money that Alex Paterson, another proponent of the Queen E, liked to say that, 'people used to cross the street when they saw him coming!' These funds made possible the latest in cardiac and anesthetic equipment; we had it all well before the Montreal General. In that twenty years (the 1970s and 80s), we did so many things!"

The Queen E, like many community hospitals, was managing somehow to survive and expand despite tight government budgets. In the
1970s, the bureaucrats who were new to the health management game
didn't really interfere. Nixon says, "During my time, there was little
trouble with the government. That came towards the end, when they
would harangue me to cut beds." He did so, but in at least one
instance, he forgot to inform the government officially and was
accused of running the hospital inefficiently. By the time he left, however, inexorable rising costs meant that even the extra revenues from
charity weren't enough. "We reduced our 272 beds to 100 and cut surgeries. During that period, I'd work so late so often that I had a suite in
the hospital to sleep in."

Nixon maintains that the way the Queen Elizabeth managers
retained their standards in the early age of public funding had to do
with their low overhead and continuing ability to solicit private charity.
"The Queen E was kept up with private donations. We were small, so we
could get the money we needed for new departments and technologies
without big committee meetings. We'd get the money to serve Christmas dinner to the staff every year, to have all those lunches and parties.
Marden and Aspinall would go out to donors such as D.W.
MacConnell, the Molsons, and the Women's Auxilliary! They were
always there. They gave us over a million dollars over the time I was
there, at $30,000 to $40,000 a shot. And, they knew exactly what they
got for their money. I had no assistants – no bureaucracy. The Neuro
today also has a big volunteer base and young people to help, like we
did. So do other successful hospitals, like the Jewish."

THE 1980S

Bed closings due to nurse shortages also impacted our operation,
especially during weekends and holidays ... [but] the Queen Elizabeth
Hospital did not get the media's attention with pictures of patients lying
outside emergency rooms ... thanks to a very dedicated and co-operative
group. We have here, I believe, a unique system of efficiently handling
emergencies.

Ian D. Mair, President's Report, Annual Report of the
Queen Elizabeth Hospital, 1988[15]

By the early 1980s, despite a more experienced and organized provincial health care bureaucracy, demand for services and subsequent med-

ical costs were once again catching up with the fiscal juggling that had managed to keep them at bay during the previous decade. In 1983, Albert Nixon succinctly reported to the board that the reason Quebec was threatening trusteeship over their once again unbalanced budget was that, "Supplies cost more, hospital activity has increased, prosthetic devices are charged to global funds, but the budget has not been increased to match these increased costs."[16] The ER, the Queen E's pride and joy, was submitted to periodic ambulance bans as early as 1982 in an effort by government to curtail costs. Whether such methods served urgent public need is obviously a separate subject, and detailed studies of mortalities caused by overcrowded or closed ERs during this or any other period are very hard to come by. In another bid to save money, nurses began working four-day weeks in the early 1980s and the new, specialized clinics were closed on Fridays.[17]

Duties such as opening IVs, taking blood, performing cardiac resuscitation, and treating anaphylactic shock, that were once the prerogative of doctors alone, were steadily delegated downward from doctors to nurses and subsequently from nurses to nurses' assistants. Starting IVs, suctioning, and removing sutures, tasks recently granted to RNs, were being done by nurses' assistants by 1989. These "designated acts" move ever downward, from nurses assistants to nurses' aides, and from there, in the U.S. these days, sometimes even to general HMO employees who are almost completely untrained in any medical procedure. In the 1980s and 90s, the practice of using the highest-paid staff as minimally as possible and delegating tasks to increasingly unskilled and untrained people was recognized as a fast way to control costs and has since only escalated.[18]

By the late 1980s, at the Queen E, despite being entrusted with specialized medical practices only recently considered too dangerous to be performed by anyone without a medical degree, nurses found themselves working the 12-hour shifts they had fought so hard to eliminate 50 years before. At the same time, they were required to do onerous and dangerous tasks, such as recapping dirty needles by hand, because the hospital couldn't afford the foam blocks that do a much safer job. This means their situation was reminiscent of the dangerous scut work that characterized nursing in its earliest years.[19] The Queen E's intern and resident quotas were also cut in 1987, saving the government a lot of money.

Medical tests had become more controlled, with the Medical Committee emphasizing that no test could be considered "daily" or "routine." Ken Hechtman notes that this illustrates an increasing tendency "for doctors to be caught between the fiscal pressure to cut costs by doing fewer tests and the new legal pressure to practice defensive medicine by doing more tests." Things got bad enough for Quebec nurses that they went out on strike in 1982. Although an overwhelming majority of the public supported the nurses, Quebec legislated them back to work with Bill 160 – which mandated penalties of $10,000 and a year of seniority lost for every day out on strike. The strike was in fact broken by government legislation, although these unprecedented penalties were quietly reversed a few years later.[20]

The nurses didn't get the pay raise they struck for in the first place. Instead, their salaries were cut back by 20 percent, an enormous amount never surpassed before or since. It took three years for Quebec nurses' incomes to inch back up to what they had been before the strike. Nurses and other hospital staff were permanently demoralized by this experience. They realized that because their employers had the power to enact anti-strike legislation, more or less at the drop of a hat, they would never be able function like a real union. That is, they could never use the withdrawal of services as an effective negotiating tactic. Much of the story of Canadian health care policy can be told through the confrontations between nurses and provincial governments. Nurses are exposed to the worst aspects of the economic antagonism between hospitals and governments largely because of the oppositional framework of unions versus management. There is no politically expedient way to batter down doctors, to say nothing of powerful drug and technology producers. Nurses and other staff end up paying for the whole system.

On May 7, 1985, the Queen Elizabeth Hospital's last personal link to their first 100 years was severed when Dr Harold Griffith died of Parkinson's Disease at the age of ninety-one. Although he'd been away from it for more than twenty years, the hospital had remained recognizably the same, in both negative and positive senses, largely because, even after his death, his protégé and family friend, Deirdre Gillies, continued to rule the chiefs of staff through the still-powerful Anesthesiology Department. Even with the government in charge, John Hughes remembers that, "She maintained a very forceful input from the doctors of the hospital. There was no way the board or the management could upstage the positions taken by the chiefs of staffs, which she chaired. This situation is very different today. It may have had some downsides, but I believe it also helped maintain an equilibrium between government concerns about budgets and human resources and the needs of the profession, which hopefully also included the needs of the patients."

The Queen E continued to dance on a financial tight-rope, however, as it always had. In a throw-back to the 1930s, deficits had become so severe that in 1984 the hospital had to raise a million dollars in private funds just to remain open. But, as in the Griffiths' days, even as fiscal challenges mounted, science-based medicine also continued to ascend. During the same financially desperate period, the medical staff decided to start doing expensive regular audits on heart attacks, urethritis, appendectomies, and acute psychosis. These audits resulted, within only three months, in concrete changes in tests and treatment.[21] In May of 1989, the Queen Elizabeth introduced what is thought to be the first accredited mammography service in Canada.[22] In June of 1990, it got $35,000 worth of equipment to do laparoscopy, another first in Canada.[23] And the same year, the hospital started agitating for its own CT scan, a machine in great demand in the Montreal area at the time.[24]

This is the real Catch–22 of health care management. Hospitals cannot resist, and are expected by the public to provide, the latest medical advances. But their budgets simply can't keep up with the pace of modern, business-based technological offerings. For example, throughout this whole period there were steady acquisitions of very expensive equipment, such as a choleo-nephrofiberscope and two double-channel gastroscopes in 1984, new vascular lab and ultrasound machines the same year, and more library research materials in 1985, all paid for by private funds. But a six-page open letter sent on 6 March 1984 by Queen E doctors to their Board of Directors testifies to how alarming these technological costs were becoming.

In this letter, the signing doctors were trying to alert their board to their helplessness before the fiscal monster they were all facing. "There are miraculous but very expensive advances in modern medicine we want the money to provide," they wrote. "Synthetic lenses for cataracts, for example, arterial replacements, new antibiotics for hospital-caused infections, but" as the letter went on to say, antibiotics alone had cost the hospital a total of $49,000 in 1978, a cost that had risen to $399,000 only five years later, in 1983. Needless to say, budgets had not gone up by 800 percent in that time. These occasional alerts via open letters to the board in the 1960s and 70s about the need for new ways to recruit nurses, to figure out how to fund chronic care, or provide more preventative medicine or about the alarming escalation in technological offerings in the 1980s, surface from time to time above the sea of hospital business, trying, like drowning victims, to signal for help. They are, however, subsumed in the day-to-day crises and bustle of hospital life.

Although governments also sporadically tried to design a future for medical care, most of the time the people involved in providing health care all across Canada have been too busy putting out daily fires to take time to plan long-term fiscal or medical strategies. This is a very real problem; medical staffs neither have the time nor are trained for economic analysis. Provincial governments cynically take advantage of this when they negotiate with medically trained people. The only other people interested are vested interests like private hospital or drug corporations. Canada only very recently acquired a Public Health supervisor on the federal level. In theory, such an office will encourage the practice of giving long-term planning and analytic power to disinterested judicial bodies; in practice, as we shall see ahead, Canada's public health departments are fragmented, isolated, and far too secretive.

In part as a response to all these disturbing issues, many hospitals, including the Queen E, devoted part of the late 1980s and early 90s to composing Vision and Mission Statements, holding "Quality Assurance" seminars, and distributing patient satisfaction questionnaires. This was part of a general worldwide effort by medical professionals to find some way to measure the quality of heath care. The effort is ongoing, but still largely eludes most analysts. And, as usual, these attempts at cost- and quality analysis dealt only with the demand side of the hospital economic equation. They never tried to gain any control over the supply side.

John Hughes explains that one reason for such a high level of concern about quality in the 1980s was the fact that this period was one of the hospital's most difficult. "We were trying to come up to speed and were modernizing. By about 1990, we realized there had been some stagnation in terms of development of facilities; various departments were learning about innovations and wanted them for the Queen E, too. Oncology, for example, crusaded for ambulatory care for their chemotherapy services. The ER staff desperately wanted their facility to be redesigned. In fact, the accreditation reports show that there weren't just staffing deals to work out with McGill – our ER and some other departments were not up to spec. That's normal for small hospitals like ours, of course. As the medical norm rises across the country, community hospitals often find themselves falling behind."

At this period, younger doctors and chiefs of staff realized that even the patient's bedrooms needed upgrading. The hospital was also short of certain kinds of complex equipment and needed more functional designs to properly use what they had. Hughes says, "The hospital hadn't participated in this kind of infrastructure change in the 1980s. In a way, this was Albert Nixon's issue, because he'd tried to concentrate on just keeping us going piecemeal. But when he was gone, frankly, we stumbled in terms of who we got to run the place. The vision and mission statements were our way of trying to figure out what we wanted to be and setting our sights on a goal."

An even more crucial concern was another provincial budgetary requirement: "per forma" occupancy rates. These are easily measurable but not so easily interpreted measurement figures, and government bureaucrats have had a good time playing with them for the past four decades. In 1979, an occupancy rate of 90 percent, i.e., a hospital with only 10 percent of its beds empty, was considered "dangerously high." To allow for the possibility of a serious flu event or a large accident like an urban gas explosion, hospitals were still trying to have no more than 80 percent of their beds full at any given time throughout the 1950s. But by the late 1960s, the perfect occupancy rate went up to 85 percent, and by 1988, the provincial government punished the Queen E for having an occupancy rate slightly below the golden number of 90 percent, which was by then considered highly desirable and no longer dangerous.

Obviously, economic considerations influence how a government interprets occupancy rates. As previously discussed, diseases and even accidents are organic, cyclic occurrences, not unlike the weather. So even though a 90 percent occupancy rate looks good on paper, keeping a hospital that full guarantees overcrowding, closed ERs, and beds in the hall about 50 percent of the time.

Many health professionals insist that quantitative measurements like this not only endanger the patients that end up on gurneys in hallways but can also hurt the hospital's administrative position. Although the Queen E was normally forced to close beds to keep out potential patients, it happened to have 50 empty beds, on top of 30 closed ones, on the day in 1990 that Quebec demanded occupancy rates on which to base its yearly efficiency ratings. The kind of unrepresentative bad timing that goes with one-time quantitative measurements continues to haunt relationships between hospitals and governments, providing the latter with even more ammunition for controlling the former.

Ongoing accreditation problems also caused regular mini-crises for board members, who must have reacted to them much as an individual does when hearing from the taxman; even if the Ministry of Finance can be proven to be wrong about disallowing your deduction, the event is upsetting. So, although nearly always averted at the last minute, throughout the 1980s and continuing in hospitals to this day, these bureaucratic exercises in accreditation or standardization represent constant threats to small hospitals. In October of 1989, for example, the Medical Board was put on the alert because a Quebec Health Ministry report had listed the Queen E as a "non-teaching hospital." If it had been even erroneously classified that way, it would have automatically lost its Board of Directors![25] Such paper crises provoke flurries of secretarial activity, internal stress, and wasted man-hours. Even if they are resolved, they don't endear provincial bureaucracies to hospital boards or vice-versa. They also, as we shall see ahead, became so common that boards and director generals began to regard them as normal problems that weren't really serious.

THE 1990S

The roof that once was safely set above our heads has been blown away. Gone. Our home is not what it was, not what we intended, not what we created and shared. The arsonists have come, and – God knows why – we seem to be powerless to prevent their fires.

Timothy Findley, *Writing Home*[26]

In 1989, following the retirement of Albert Nixon, the last of the administrative leaders to come from within the family, the Queen Elizabeth lost its way to some extent. Their first two director generals from outside the fold had various problems with the doctors, the board, and with the administration and were asked to resign after only a few months' tenure – and an important official also left under a cloud due to problems with a faulty computer system that cost the hospital a great deal of money. Even if these administrators seemed inadequate to the job, the Queen E probably wasn't a very easy place to administrate, given its strong traditions and demands for special autonomy as well as taste for parties, good food, and other perks. Although soon to retire, Dierdre Gillies, still the heir apparent of both Harold and Jim, ruled the OR with an iron hand, and there were turf wars between various other strong personalities in departments, such as orthopedics and psychiatry. Although such problems are common in small hospitals, they seem to have been sensed by the world at large. Family medicine interns had fought for residencies at the Queen E previously, but by 1990, as the Queen E Board Minutes ruefully admit, St. Mary's had become their first choice because of "better facilities and instruction in obstetrics and psychiatry."[27]

Throughout the late 1980s and early 1990s, minor fiscal problems seemed to cry out for a stronger, or at least a more cunning, economic hand. For example, although Quebec was deducting the money from the budget it "assumed" that the Queen E was charging for private rooms, the hospital didn't always actually charge for such rooms. The hospital was also in trouble over a low occupancy rate, because in an effort to save money the Admitting Office placed many patients in day surgery. However, the bed count had to be done at midnight after those patients had gone home. At the end of 1990, the Queen E was applying to become a Trauma Centre because that seemed to be the safest way to prevent closure of their ER.

The worst blow of all, after years of fighting to retain teaching status, was a new Quebec Health Act, Bill 120, which declared that the Queen E "does not qualify as either a university hospital or a university institution." St. Mary's and two French hospitals lost their university status only a month later, so this looks suspiciously like some sort of bureaucratic finagling that somehow was going to save the government money.[28] In a real irony for the birthplace of modern anesthesia, there was also a critical shortage of qualified anesthetists in Quebec throughout the mid-1990s, caused directly by fiscal government policies that were attempting to save money by limiting medical school enrollments. As so often happens when cutting budgets is concerned, the accountants miscalculated. The Quebec Health Ministry had been limiting medical training positions since the 1980s and the resulting lack of doctors began to be felt by 1992–94. The lack was most keen for anesthesiologists and other specialists, which are never in sufficient supply. This is still true today, especially outside of urban centres.

"This was a real problem at the Queen E," John Hughes remembers, "[there was] also a lack of pathologists. But you can wait for a pathology report longer than you can for an airway specialist! We had qualified candidates applying to come to us but because they were post-fellowship foreign students, Quebec wouldn't give them a license. That's still a serious, ongoing problem here." The lack of anesthesiologists increased survival problems not just for patients but for the Queen E itself and many other small hospitals. Surgical patients had to be turned away, which meant admitting more medical patients, many of whom were chronic cases. This would eventually doom the hospital's university status and attractiveness to interns.

The Quebec government's oddly schizophrenic attitude towards young doctors – alternatively giving them financial aid to study and then passing laws to discourage them from practicing in the province – had gone into high gear by this time. In 1991, at the same time it was denying licenses to foreign anesthesiologists, it issued a directive that all new specialists had to complete a one-year fellowship *outside* Quebec before they could join a university hospital in the province. Eight months later, this directive was rescinded because virtually no specialist would cooperate with it. But it was definitely a forerunner of the future disincentives the provincial government was prone to apply to young doctors. Beds were still being closed because of nurse shortages and there were increasing signs of professional strains in the 1990s, with much discussion in the minutes of morale problems involving both doctors and nurses.[29]

The Queen E had its own particular difficulties during this period because of increasingly dangerous psychiatric in- and out-patients, the perhaps predictable result of trying to apply a general hospital's mimimal security standards to serious psychiatric care. Despite warnings, which included having guards walk staff members to their cars at night, a nurse was attacked just outside the hospital in February of 1992.[30] And in a move that foreshadowed today's ongoing orthopedic crises, the Queen E's popular hip- and knee-replacement facilities were so swamped with patients needing these very expensive prostheses that they began to refuse some of the work.[31]

Yet, even among these difficulties, the future still looked pretty bright: construction on a new ER, which was doctor and nurse-designed and emerged as one of the best in the country, was approved by the Regie regionale in 1991. Moreover, an exciting new CT scan, the latest in prestigious equipment, was dangled before the board's eyes as a definite possibility.[32] Cost overruns on the ER started almost immediately but didn't dampen the enthusiasm for yet another expansion, this time to the tune of $12 million, which was supposed to be built between 1996 and 1998. The outcry from all the hospitals that lost their university status must have been considerable because only a few months after taking it away, the government started to talk about tabling a new article to the Health Act that would have granted the dean of the

McGill Medical School, rather than the government, the power to des-
ignate university-affiliated hospitals.[33] The Queen E opened a new Palliative Care Unit in 1992, and the new methods of measuring hospital
performance, Patient Satisfaction Surveys, gave the Queen Elizabeth
extremely high marks: 88 percent satisfaction overall, with 91 percent
confidence in doctors and nurses and 84 percent satisfaction with hospital services.[34] The board did notice, with some trepidation, that it was
not included in McGill's nascent plan for a new "super-hospital," when
those plans first became public in November of 1993.

In August of 1993, the Queen E's latest director of professional services, Anne Duffy, was suspended and soon after, Mario Larivière, the
hospital's last director general, was hired – to general acclaim. As their
first francophone head administrator, with remarkable credentials,
contacts, and experience, he signaled, as John Hughes put it, "a whole
new era for the Queen E." They were finally letting go of some of the
last of their stubbornly held internal control and were trying to open
up and join the Quebec mainstream. Larivière inherited something of
a mess, with deficits beginning to overwhelm a brief period of surpluses. But he also had a very loyal team: as recently as the year before,
in a show of remarkable institutional solidarity, Queen Elizabeth doctors made up a third of the hospital's $548,000 deficit out of their own
pockets, and they did so only three months after it was announced.[35]

There were increased instances in the mid-1990s of the hospital having to close beds or even the ER and of having to send "very sick
patients" away. The board noted that, "In comparison with a group of
hospitals of comparable size, it seems that our total budget is appropriate, but our costs are higher in some areas." These were the "big heart"
costs mentioned earlier: chronic care and orthopedics. The board's
agreement with this assessment of the reasons for their cost overruns
was honest, if a little self-aggrandizing: "the QEH has many good orthopedic surgeons, they do more complicated and expensive work, with
more expensive prostheses, than anyone else."[36] When Larivière
arrived, one of the first things he did was to begin cutting costs. In
1994–95 alone, these cuts, referred to as "reviews," added up to $3.6
million and were primarily gained through cancelled overtime and
attrition. Larivière also reorganized departments in a bid to break up
some of the traditional fiefdoms and make the place less idiosyncratic
and more functional.

The general worldwide trend in hospital care towards more home,
community, and day therapy was obvious by the mid 1990s and

reflected in a March 1995 Queen E Board motion to reduce the average length of stay from ten days to seven. In the 1950s, the average stay
had been over two weeks. Although governments often claim it is
under six days today, that figure isn't reflected in recent studies, which
still peg it closer to eight.[37] And although there were heady plans for
construction and expansion, the new areas were to be devoted to special facilities, not beds. There had been a proposal the year before that
the hospital's 272 beds be cut to 244 permanently, in order to maintain
the much sought-after 90 percent occupancy rate, and also to reflect
shortened stays and the hospital's success with day surgery. This came
out of a belief that government funding was based on activities performed, not bed count; the Queen E figured if they closed beds and
stepped up day surgery, they would come out ahead. Of course, when
closure actually threatened, the government chose to concentrate not
on activities but on the closed beds.[38]

The lack of anesthetists continued, with ICU patient numbers curtailed and very often no airway management available in the ER on
weekends. Today, this serious situation has spread across the province.
Everyone agreed that more specialists had to be hired, but no one
wanted the salaries to come out of their budgets, so there was much
discussion between the OR, the nurses, and the hospital. Clearly, the
government wasn't helping out; the tendency to regard trained anesthesiologists as expendable in times of budgetary crisis recalls the early
days of the profession. It became so critical that "inhalation therapists,"
respiratory technologists who deal with ventilators, oxygen masks, and
also work with physiotherapists, were being trained to intubate, even
though that difficult act had *not* been legally delegated away from doctors. And the frighteningly long waiting times that have become a feature of big-city ERs in Canada were just beginning. In January of 1995,
the Queen E Board of Directors was scandalized by a report of people
waiting in their ER for more than 24 hours. The board was also alarmed
by more obscure talk from McGill about "Centres of Excellence," i.e.,
offshoots of the super-hospital, which again seemed to leave the Queen
E out of the picture.[39]

By spring of 1995, just a few months after their exciting Centennial
celebrations which had netted them over half a million dollars in gifts
from grateful patients, the board could no longer ignore the negative
change in the air. The minutes become almost paranoid, noting, "It is
unclear what the plans of the Regie regionale are regarding the future
of the QEH ... The Regie is presently quite secretive." And then, almost

a month to the day before its closure was announced, the board became exultant: "For the year ending March 21, we achieved another balanced budget; last year's budget was also balanced, although [only] two years ago we had a $2 million deficit."[40]

On 6 June 1995, right on the heels of this achievement, they received their totally unexpected death sentence. From then on, board minutes go into crisis mode, reflecting disbelief, counterproposals, committee suggestions for resistance, lawsuits, and, eventually, numb compliance. The hospital's first counter-proposal, hammered out the same day closure was announced, was to meet Quebec halfway by increasing the chronic-care beds the province needed so badly, decreasing acute-care beds, and having doctors rent private offices.[41] Less than two weeks later, they were inaugurating the CT scan unit that they had believed was a symbol of the government's commitment to their ongoing survival. Costing nearly a million dollars, even now it seems an odd thing for the government to have given them at this time.

In the background, patrons, patients, doctors, nurses, and the entire staff, from workers in the cafeteria to the parking lot, went into high gear organizing committees, fundraisers, demonstrations, and candle-light vigils. Patient Linda Vincelli, who was born at the Queen E, found out about the closing when she brought in her sick husband, Armand, for care. Her testimonial was typical: "They don't just throw you in a corner and forget about you the way you hear about in the big hospitals. It's an English family hospital, and there aren't many of those in Montreal ... I really dread to see it close."[42]

As bed and institutional closures spread across the entire country, people anguished over why their institution was being punished. Was it geography? Language? Provincial party loyalty? Insider influence? The super-hospital? The strength or weakness of their resistance? Three hundred supporters from Lachine staged noisy demonstrations at their City Hall and many wept when doom came anyway a few months later. One hospital in Edmonton miraculously escaped closure, although no amount of fighting was able to save equally beloved hospitals in Calgary. Joan O'Brien, like many others in the Queen E's local community of Notre-Dame-de-Grace, had raised thousands of dollars, in this case for a family room in the new palliative-care facility. O'Brien wanted to know how the government could destroy her work and sacrifice with the stroke of a pen. Remembering Hollis Marden, Albert Nixon's indefatigable fund-raiser, Queen E board member Alex Paterson told *The Gazette*, "He must be ricocheting in his grave just now."[43]

Not just the Queen E, but all the doomed community hospitals, including those in BC, Saskatchewan, Ontario, and Alberta, were founded and survived through gifts and support from thousands of individuals over many generations. Susan McGuire, a patient on the Queen E's action committee, said, "Nobody realizes that each of these hospitals has a loyal following. For each following, it's a terrible thing; it's a sociological affront." Stephen Laudi, president of the Community Council in the Queen E's borough, said many people who depended on and had personally supported the hospital felt betrayed by the government. They understood that medical practices change, but, "They don't accept that their hospital will be shut down without impact studies, a transition plan or community involvement ... They've lived and worked in the area all their lives. They've paid their taxes and contributed to these hospitals. Now they need them and they feel ripped off."[44]

A NEW KIND OF HOSPITAL

It's not a catastrophe. It's not cutting services to the people. It's developing more adequate services.

Quebec health minister Jean Rochon, 1995[45]

Throughout the traumatic year of 1995, the board minutes contained news of lawsuits and replacement schemes and also reflected the board's legal obligation to prepare for what even they knew might be inevitable. As early as July 1995 members were creating plans to divert "complex cases to other institutions," and trying to make sure there would be no orphans. "Pipelines to other hospitals must be set up so that a hospital cannot refuse to take a patient."[46] The board also had to try to find new homes for its own staff. This was easy for the anesthesiologists who were already in such short supply but more difficult for the radiologists and the Queen E's unusually well-trained, specialist nurses. There was great concern that people would be thrown out of work. If closing eight hospitals across the city was really being done to save money, the board worried that, "Since 80 percent of the budget goes on salaries, [how will] the government save money unless it dishonors contract provisions?"[47] Conrad Sauvé, the head of the regional health board's administrative council, told the papers he was aware of worker concerns, but "we've already told them, there won't be any job losses."[48]

The Queen E board minutes had at first eschewed gossip, but by the fall of 1995 had become distraught enough to report rumours such as, "Dr Lewis believes that any general surgeon moving to another hospital should expect a 30–50 percent cut in income."[49] Doctors and surgeons were also being aggressively wooed by recruiting firms from the United States within weeks of the death announcement in May. Agents came to Montreal to headhunt, running ads and sending letters. "We aren't trying to kidnap doctors and bring them down to the States," one said. "We're just running a service here." A total of seventy doctors had already left Alberta in 1994, but it's hard to know exactly how many fled Canada as a whole because of the closures all across the country. The fact that the whole country still suffers from a shortage of physicians does point towards a drain from out-migration on top of the ill-planned training quotas.[50]

In Quebec at least, the Regional Health Board assured everyone there would be jobs. But they meant any kind of medical jobs, not the ones people had trained for and loved. Michael Moss, one of the Queen E's most involved doctors, wrote in *The Montreal Gazette*, "Has any thought been given to what will happen to a 50-year old specialist emergency-room nurse who cannot or will not be accommodated in another emergency room? Can you imagine how traumatic it will be for him or her to have to work in, for example, chronic care, spoon-feeding demented patients? It seems the most appalling waste of our resources to reorient such people to alternative-nursing care." In fact, as related earlier, these nightmares came true for many nurses, especially the younger ones. Operating Room and ER specialists were reduced to doling out shots at CLSCs or were forced by bureaucratic employers to re-take lifesaving courses they were capable of teaching. Most such experts were lost to the medical system forever, taking early retirement, like ER specialist Pat Titterton, or leaving the province for other work.

By September, the board was unable to remain unbiased. The minutes were discussing the various action committees' work, and members of the board were having meetings with Pierre Marsan, the opposition Liberal health critic. The inauguration of the new CT scan was now to become a rallying point to protest closure. The board used first $140,000 and then $250,000 of its Griffith Foundation money for action committee lawsuits and activities, even though it wasn't sure if this was legal. No doubt the Griffiths, at any rate, would have approved. Two lawsuits were launched, one with Ogilvie Renault, representing the hospital, and another, by the doctors, with the famous Canadian lawyer Julius Grey. The time period during which all this was happening was very short – only a few months.

It was, in fact, a devastating time for the whole country, because so many hospital beds and so many ERs were simultaneously closing. Moreover, once closure was public news, only desperate people showed up for care at the various doomed hospitals. The board minutes noted, "The quality of practice is already diminishing by the patient type being brought here. Patients do not want to go to a hospital perceived as closing."[51] The social effects that were never scientifically measured were nonetheless clear to practitioners. By October, the board recorded, "The waiting period to see specialists [in all hospitals] has increased and this in turn increases morbidity of patients."[52] Like closing one road to traffic, simultaneously closing eight hospitals resulted in tremendous back-up. By January, 1996, Urgence-Sante, Quebec's ambulance service, "went to the Regional Council to tell them there is a crisis situation in Montreal in that so many ERs are closed to ambulances because the hospitals have no beds."[53]

The Health Ministry's response to the hospitals' pleas for at least more time to negotiate patient transfer and care was a terse demand that each hospital "complete a detailed questionnaire on current existing waiting times." As Ken Hechtman remarks, "that's like asking for daily progress reports explaining why you're so far behind schedule." So as the staff drained away – doctors first, but even Mario Larivière by January, 1996 – there was less money to be had and the remaining staff had to cope with a vast increase in bureaucratic work. Lists of doctors, consolidation of patient's charts, union and other employee lists, fiscal reports – all had to be compiled and sent to the government on the appropriate forms, although as government statistics quoted ahead illustrate, staffs were so overwhelmed, this was often not done. These grueling demands on demoralized people made taking care of the remaining patients even more difficult. The same day Larivière left, the minutes noted, rather desperately, "We have appealed to the Royal Victoria Hospital, St. Mary's, the Jewish General, and Sacre-Coeur for manpower and so far they have not assisted us in any way. The Reddy Memorial [also being closed] however, has been very helpful."[54]

Slowly, all seven of the other Montreal hospitals being closed shut their doors. In May of 1996, the Queen Elizabeth board noted, "Layoff notices are being sent to staff and all temporary and availability positions will disappear."[55] "No patients will be seen in Emergency after midnight on May 31."[56] The full text of one of the board's very last entries, for 7 May 1996, reads: "By July 1, inpatients should be either convalescent, chronic or palliative care." From the receipt of the government closure notice to the last day of recorded board minutes, the destruction or diminishing of so many thriving medical careers, not to mention the annihilation of the old hospital's 101 years of work and struggle, took exactly eleven months and one day. The Queen was dead.

LOOKING FOR THE KILLERS

I accuse the federal government of undermining Canada's ... health care system by imposing drastic reductions in transfer payments to provincial governments.

Dr Samuel Levy, chief of biochemistry, QEH, letter to *The Monitor*[57]

There's a strong case to be made for diverting scarce resources away from expensive hospitals into home care and CLSCs. But ... the regional board has no such idea.

Mark Abley, *The Montreal Gazette*[58]

Ralph Klein's spending cuts left health care particularly disrupted in Calgary ... Despite Calgary's mushrooming population, the Calgary Regional Health Authority decided to shut down the Grace Hospital and sell the Holy Cross to for-profit investors ... [and] in October 1998, demolished the ... Calgary General with a spectacular explosion.

Kevin Taft and Gillian Steward[59]

In chapter 1, we noted that 20 percent of hospital beds and scores of thriving health care institutions were closed in Canada in the mid-1990s. Some closures may have simply been a sign of the times, but in the case of the Calgary General, it seems very odd that Alberta's provincial government would remove its largest city's only ER. It also seems strange that Ontario would reconfigure several of the province's most popular and well-used hospitals, effectively destroying their autonomy, for no apparent fault of budget or use. And of course, why was the innovative, finally-in-the-black Queen Elizabeth, widely considered to be the best community hospital in the entire province, so summarily closed? In most places, people were promised more ambulatory care, specialty centers, and 24-hour a day community medical clinics, like

Quebec's CLSCs, staffed with both nurses and doctors. Ten years later, it seems reasonable to ask if they actually got these services, and if they did, are they getting better care? Even the question of whether present services have turned out to save money has never been posed, much less answered. There are no studies available that even graze any of these questions.

In both Alberta and Quebec, health care workers were assured of appropriate jobs. We do know that thousands left the field, causing shortages of beds, physicians, nurses, and ER services that persist to this day. Because closures were supposed to be based on budgets, perhaps the most important question of all has to do with money. Did losing so many services save the provincial (and federal) governments substantial amounts of money when all the new out-patient costs, changes in equipment and facilities, early retirement packages, and job retraining efforts are tallied up?

In Alberta, many people focused their anger on Premier Ralph Klein, accusing him of engineering a fiasco in order to discredit public health and encourage privatization. They no doubt have a point. But the fact is that dozens of hospitals were closed and downsized across the board in Canada during this period, and, once the death sentence was announced, almost none were spared, no matter whether the provincial governments in question were Liberal, Conservative, NDP, or even Parti Quebecois.

Premier Klein may have closed Alberta's hospitals with particular vigour and enthusiasm, and as noted below, apparently took advantage of the situation to permit several government insiders to reap financial benefits. But hindsight has proven that it's unlikely that even such baffling choices for closure as the Queen Elizabeth and the Calgary General would have survived any other premier's attentions, regardless of party affiliations. *In all cases,* each province's stated reasons for closing – the unbearably high cost of keeping hospitals open, along with the obsession with budgetary deficit controls that were the political hallmark of the era – are demonstrated by subsequent statistics to be largely illusory.

In their book, *Clear Answers,* Kevin Taft and Gillian Steward charge that, "Hospitals, schools, seniors, roads, and other public programs were blamed for something that wasn't particularly their fault: the growing provincial deficit[s]." They point out that in Alberta, only a month after gaining office, Premier Klein, "singled out health, education and social services as areas of great concern ... he didn't tell his audience that spending in these areas had been curtailed for years, and that the fat had already been removed. The bigger culprits causing Alberta's fiscal problems were enormous private-sector subsidies, which consumed two to three billion dollars of Alberta's public wealth every single year from 1983 to 1990."[60]

Industrial farms, and especially the oil industry received enormous infusions of money over these years, as much as half a billion at a time. The same situation holds true, varying only in degree and type of industry, in every other province of the country. In Quebec, an indignant Alex Paterson, interviewed by the *Montreal Gazette*, pointed out that the province's decision to close hospitals "is being driven by budgets, not community values ... The only ideology forcing the government to board up hospitals and expand CLSCs instead of, say, shutting down Quebec delegations or cutting out 15 percent of the Quebec bureaucracy, is political choice."[61] In Nova Scotia, a Tory win in the election of 1999 was partly attributed to their success in blaming the Liberals for choosing to close hospitals in Halifax in order to support the failing provincial and Crown-owned Sysco steel mill in Cape Breton, the same one implicated in the worst toxic waste dump scandal in Canadian history, the Sydney Tar Ponds. Opposition groups claimed that the Tories, in their turn, would quickly jettison election promises to increase social spending and would end up "slashing health and other public services ... so as to satisfy Nova Scotia's creditors."[62]

The key to judging the good faith behind the claims all these provincial governments made a decade ago would be studies on whether the health care system really is more "streamlined" and efficient now than it was before. Health Minister for the PQ government, medical doctor Jean Rochon, claimed that "the objective of this transformation is not closing down hospitals – it's the development of the kind of services and resources that we need. And we need more home care, long-term care and more ambulatory care." But Liberal health critic Pierre Marsan suggested that before any hospital beds were closed, "the government should reduce waiting lists for surgery, relieve crowded emergency wards and improve hospital support for people who'll have to leave hospitals early," all precautions that emergency room and crowding statistics of the subsequent years largely prove were never done. Even in 1995, Dr Paul Landry of the Quebec Hospitals Association pointed out the real catch that increased his suspicions that Rochon's assertion only applied to a purely economic objective. "We think it's a bit technocratic to start from a ratio of beds per resident rather than starting from the needs of the population and deciding how to meet those needs." *Montreal Gazette* columnist Peggy Curran remarked, "There's something alarming about the scope of the cuts and the fact that medium-sized, community-based hospitals will carry the load."[63]

The government's method of dividing the number of potential patients in a city by the number of beds available and then developing a one-size-fits-all ideal bed-ratio is very popular with financial institutions and budgetary think-tanks, to say nothing of banks. This was especially true in the 1990s, although the tendency persists to this day. Bed ratios may be convenient for number-crunchers, but they don't take into account many critical factors, such as higher than average disease or accident rates in a city core or even normal hospital-use habits in areas like Montreal, Winnipeg, and Calgary, where many patients using the services are coming in from suburban and distant rural areas. It also doesn't include any unique services, such as the Queen Elizabeth's psychiatric department, the only one in that part of Montreal and one of the few in the city available to English-speaking patients and to sexual abuse victims. In short, determining demands on a system is not as simple as counting heads in the neighbourhood. Subsequent studies show that bed cuts ended up affecting many more people than the accountants in Ottawa or provincial capitals ever imagined.[64]

Journalist Peggy Curran's concerns, which were the burden placed on community hospitals and the slow and steady elimination of general practitioners, continue to radically affect accessibility of health care today, as we will investigate in chapter 6. Community hospitals were formerly often run by GPs, and as doctors Richard May and Robert Weinman wrote in that fateful month of May 1995, "all operate under a model based on continuity of care. Family physicians (GPs) play an extremely active role in providing care in these hospitals. These same doctors care for patients in the emergency room, in the intensive-care unit, and on the hospital wards. They also provide health care to these patients in their offices in the community and in chronic-care facilities. *The resulting continuity is unique and essential to ensure appropriate cost-effective care.* Health-care experts in Quebec and throughout North America recognize that a health-care system co-ordinated by family doctors is best suited to the delivery of quality medical services at the lowest cost ... the cooperation between family physicians and specialists within the hospital and other community resources ... prevents needless duplication of procedures and examinations often seen in larger, more specialized institutions."[65] Hindsight lets us realize how supurb an economic as well as professional analysis that was. We have also learned in recent years that hospital beds – termed "hotel costs" – were not at all the most expensive part of hospital management. They were merely the most vulnerable.

Today, several years into the 21st century, this picture of family physician–coordinated community hospital care is being re-emphasized as vital by a raft of new books and proven by evidence-based studies centred on geriatrics, whose clients are the heaviest users of any health care system. Unfortunately, this type of hospital care has also completely disappeared in much of Canada because general practitioners were thrown out of hospitals in reforms in the late 1990s. As John Hughes remembers it, "This was an American concept which, again, was thought to reduce the length of stay and thereby save the system some money. The idea was that if your patient was admitted to hospital, she would be looked after by the doctor on duty on that ward; you could consult on the case but you were no longer physically present and your opinion was not sought in terms of treatment. Maybe this does reduce the length of stay. I don't know." In fact, today, family doctors have no contact with their patients once they enter a hospital, and hospitals have little information about the whole patient beyond their immediate acute symptoms.

As we'll see later, the lack of continuity in patient care in our current health system costs far more money than we can begin to imagine. A patient with a history of rectal bleeding known only to her GP, for example, would be more carefully monitored for serious bowel disease if that doctor were consulted by hospital staff, even if the patient had come in for another problem, say a digestive upset. This foresight would save money on future acute problems and expensive surgery, to say nothing of preserving the patient's life. However, despite their long-proven efficacy in terms of health care delivery, community hospitals continue to take the brunt of budgetary constraints while specialty teaching hospitals and centres of excellence, which both tend to deal with rare diseases and ground-breaking treatments that have little or no impact on the general public health, continue to be expanded.

Rafts of studies, beginning as early as the 1980s and therefore readily available to provincial health care managers well before the mass closures, have shown that investing in small hospitals is a superior tactic from both an economic and a public health point of view. That evidence gets only stronger with time. Knowing this, it's difficult to avoid the conclusion that the central concern of Canada's mass hospital closures in the mid-1990s was not health reform. It was, surprisingly, apparently not even greater economic efficiency. Even within the constraints of what was known about hospital care at the time, these closures make the most sense if they instead represent a rapid, coerced reaction to some urgent and very powerful economic demand.

Such suspicions may seem fairly obvious now, but at the time such ideas were mostly lost in the heat of local politicking and local blame. In 1996, the year after all the hospitals closed, analysts such as Graeme Hamilton at *The Gazette* were still trying to give the governments' arguments their due. "What some observers find troubling is that the health-care overhaul is being driven by budget cuts imposed by the province ... [but] the numbers show clearly that Montreal has an excess of acute-care beds per capita when compared to other provinces. Why not put some of the money spent on hospital beds – which are very expensive to maintain – into home-care services that can be provided by CLSCs, the network of community health clinics?" There was a lot of talk about money being taken out of one place and "pumped into" another. But today's statistics show that very little new funding ended up providing any kind of health services – municipal, provincial, or federal. Moreover, money does not seem to have been moved from one provincial area to another. It seems to have disappeared. Mostly it was the speed of the reforms that confused those people who really were trying to believe the governments' stories. Concerning Quebec's plan to expand home and community care, one of the regional health board's medical advisors, Dr Marie-France Raynault, remarked at the time, "This can be done very well. It is feasible. But the objective is so obviously economic, things are happening so rapidly with a cascade of closings, that I don't get the feeling people have been trained or that CLSCs are ready."[66]

Even much later media stories continued to quote health reform and super-hospital enthusiasts, such as Montreal's Nicolas Steinmetz, or studies that do support the idea of the evolution of medical care away from long hospital visits. An early super-hospital story in the *Montreal Gazette* claimed, "Gone are the days when most patients spent weeks lying in a hospital bed ... The average length of stay in hospitals across Canada and the United States has been on the decline in the last decade, and many experts predict the trend will continue." Most media writers hammered this theme home for many years, and although sympathetic to the distress of workers and patients cast out of their hospitals, few seriously questioned the government's assertions. To be fair, the studies we now have showing that hospital stays were not nearly as expensive as closure proponents had claimed and that they did not drop as quickly as the governments optimistically predicted were not yet widely available, at least to the public and the average journalist. When the studies did come in and inspire questions, it was too late for many hospitals and even too late to contain the move towards further bed closures and a super-hospital.[67]

Throughout the 1990s, politicians were spreading the same message – that hospital beds weren't really needed and that costs had "mushroomed." Alberta Health Minister Shirley McClellan wrote in 1994 that health care costs had "doubled" in the twelve previous years, but Taft and Steward point out that, "spending on health care by the Alberta government was $1,183 per person in 1982 and, correcting for inflation, only $1,325 in 1993." As this statistic shows, health expenditures per capita at the time were remarkably stable, increasing on average by about 1 percent a year or 12 to 15 percent in twelve years. But in Alberta and elsewhere, they were most often characterized by politicians and the press as "skyrocketing" or "spiraling." So, between 1992 and 1995, Alberta cut its health care funding not by 3 per cent, the rate by which it was going up, but by a full 18 percent. Close to 15,000 hospital and other health-care workers lost their jobs, lab services were reduced and privatized, and "thousands of [other] health care jobs around the province were downgraded to part-time and lesser-skilled staff." As for hospitals themselves, as we now realize, a full 21 percent of the beds available to Canadians in hospitals vanished. As at the Queen Elizabeth in the late 80s and early 90s, doctors in Alberta and all over the country were also angry and frustrated, nurses threatened strikes, hospital workers disrupted services, and perhaps most ominously of all, "public confidence in the health-care system [began to be] eroded."[68] Because Canada's health care system has long been a major source of pride for its citizens, this was a significant political and social development. Serious criticism of the Medicare system starts from this time forward.

EVIDENCE-BASED CHAOS

The period during the mid-1990s, when hospital expenditures
decreased, was a period of *significant change in the Canadian health care
system*, as provincial governments restrained expenditure growth in most
programs *in order to balance budgets*.

Hospital Trends in Canada 2005[69]

Evidence-based medicine applies to more than everyday decisions about patient treatment: it also affects macro-decisions such as how to fund health care or when to cut hospital beds. *Hospital Trends in Canada 2005* is a national database report covering the past twenty-seven years, published by a branch of the federal government and partner of Statistics Canada, the Canadian Institute for Health Information. It states that, "the total number of hospital beds [in Canada] was relatively stable until the mid-1980s, but began to decline somewhat after 1986." It adds, "The average length of stay for hospital inpatients remained stable during the 1980s." This particular statistic contradicts what Quebec and other provinces told their constituencies when the cutbacks were going on; they claimed it had been steadily decreasing.[70]

Although "a considerable amount of hospital care and financial resources have been shifted from inpatient settings to ambulatory (outpatient) clinics," it's clear from the statistics that the biggest impact arrived a few years later, when, "Hospital beds and inpatient utilization fell rapidly during the period of cost restraint and reorganization in the 1990s." The mid-1990s was over a decade ago, but the report adds, "Trends *appear* to be stabilizing at present." These are strong statements for a statistical report and reveal that in Canada, hospital accessibility became seriously unstable following the intense national reorganization of the mid-1990s. They also illustrate that this accessibility is only now, after more than ten years, beginning to show some signs of recovery. The statement quoted above uses some of the strongest language such documents ever employ and, coming from the government itself, amounts to a belated admission of the scope of changes that were, in fact, nationwide at the time. Few citizens are aware that, as the report sums up, "The period during the mid-1990s, when hospital expenditures decreased, was a period of *significant change in the Canadian health care system,* as provincial governments restrained expenditure growth in most programs *in order to balance budgets.*"[71]

The charts that illustrate this same report show a visible crash in the mid-1990s in availability of hospital beds in Canada, a drop that reflects the mass hospital closures. Beginning in the mid-1970s, the graph showing available beds per fiscal year is remarkably smooth for over seventeen years, despite large increases in the population. It shows only slight variants between totals of about 170,000 and 180,000 over all that time. Then the line breaks suddenly and dramatically downward in 1993 to a low of only 115,000 that doesn't begin to level out until 2000. The report summarizes the results: hospital beds, that

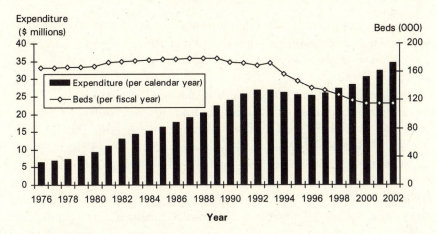

Figure 5 Trends in hospital beds, Canada, 1976 to 2002
SOURCES: Canadian Institute for Health Information and Statistics Canada.

is, availability of hospital rooms, whether the institution was closed or downsized, plummeted by nearly 21 percent in only three years, between 1993–94 and 1996–97, the same years the Calgary General and the Queen E were closed.[72]

Nowhere is there a list of the names of the actual hospitals closed or downsized, or even which institutions' beds and medical functions were transformed from acute to "residential" care. Nor do the rare studies or statistics currently available include the names of successful hospitals serving small communities, such as Wellesley in Toronto or Riverside in Ottawa, whose names sometimes persist but which were merged either physically or administratively with other institutions.[73] It's clear that even this large number of 21 per cent of beds lost to the acute-care system does not adequately reflect the level of disruption in the health system as a whole.

Besides the dramatic physical loss of buildings and beds, we would have to add to this picture an as yet uncalculated loss of medical team-work, community cooperation, funding sources, protocols, referrals, and methodologies. Probably the most surprising of all the implications of the statistics is that although the loss of beds was nearly cata-strophic, the economic savings that these closures may have brought to the system are barely visible. In 1994 to 1996, the graph dips from an annual hospital-bed expenditure high of about $27 billion to a low of $25 billion in 1996 – that is, a savings, Canada-wide, of around $2 bil-lion, which is only the same amount that Mike Harris cut from Ontario health services in 1995. Even that minimal savings doesn't last for long, and by 1997, the graph resumes the steady upward trend it had established since 1976, ending at about $34 billion in 2003, the last measured year.

This nearly uninterrupted climb in national health care expenses, regardless of bed closures, reflects the findings of a 2006 international study on the economic results of such closures conducted by the Health Evidence Network (HEN), a division of the World Health Organization's Regional Office for Europe. The study concentrated on North American and Canadian hospitals, largely because these two areas had experienced many bed closures in the recent past. "The most important source of information, from a European perspective," it states, "is *Canada, a country that has experienced major reductions in hospital capacity,* but where, uniquely, those changes have been studied in ... detail." This meta-study states further on, in the summary of its findings, "Many countries have decided to reduce the number of hospital beds ... Some have succeeded by making a sustained investment in alternative facilities, but some have been so successful that they now face shortages, meaning growing waiting lists and difficulties in admitting acutely ill patients."[74]

By these criteria, Canada seems to have achieved a very high rate of success. The study points out that it is possible to cut back beds by the various means sought by Canadian provinces beginning in the early and mid-nineties. These included such things as "shifting from inpatient to ambulatory interventions; facilitating earlier discharges ... directing patients to more appropriate facilities and coordinating disease management programs." The whole point, as we have seen, was to save money, either because the system was perceived as wasteful and too expensive, or as we'll see ahead, because debt-ridden governments chose closing hospitals as a way to pay back international bank loans. But either way, the study has determined that "there is ... contradictory evidence suggesting that *both reduced admissions and reduced length of stay may lead to increased cost per patient, and that many of the anticipated cost savings arising from bed closures may not be realized* because of the cost of alternative modes of care."[75]

This shows that, in the end, Canadian governments didn't benefit very much, if at all. The Queen Elizabeth and the Calgary General and other such institutions were destroyed and their workforces scattered, so they certainly didn't benefit. And even in the hospitals that were spared, the study points out that, "There is extensive evidence that

reductions in hospital capacity adversely affect the remaining staff –
especially those transferred to other facilities – mainly because of poor
communication and increased workload." As for what bed closures are
proven to do to patients, it all depends on whether the system really did
have too many beds, and "specifically on the availability of spare capacity or alternative facilities. There is limited evidence that where there is
spare capacity, a relatively modest reduction in hospital beds may not
adversely affect either quality of care or the health status of the population."[76]

Knowing exactly how much "spare capacity" you have is the key here.
The HEN authors state, "*where capacity is already constrained, major bed
reductions may substantially reduce the ability to admit acutely ill patients in
emergencies.* There is also limited evidence suggesting that a dramatic
reduction in hospital beds will substantially reduce the length of stay
for patients at the end of their lives, thus significantly increasing the
number of patients who die away from the hospital." If authorities do
want to cut back their number of hospital beds and do not want to
adversely affect their population's health, HEN strongly suggests they
take into account the following criteria: "*sustained investment in alternative facilities*; carefully planned transfer of staff to other facilities; and
mechanisms to reduce inappropriate admissions and facilitate more
rapid discharge."[77] Although many of the studies that led to HEN's
recent conclusions were available to serious health planning organizations before the mass closings in the mid-1990s, these criteria clearly
could not have been applied, even with the best will, in the hectic
period of weeks or months between the very sudden closure announce-
ments and the loss of beds.

To sum up these conclusions, it's clear that established hospital beds
did not cost as much as governments assumed. Closing them, while
causing the destruction of the institutions and anguish to professionals
and the population, did not really save the government money. This is
because the procedures surrounding the patient's arrival at the hospital account for the major expenses; keeping them in a hospital bed
during treatment is not to blame. As Dr John Hughes says, "To hear
that closing beds doesn't save money doesn't surprise me. The first
encounter is what's expensive, those first few hours or days that a
patient is receiving diagnosis, tests, therapy. To actually save money,
you have to avoid encounters in the first place, not actual admissions.
And that would mean paying more attention to prevention! It's usually
the neglect and flare-up of chronic disease problems – the managing of

cataract to avoid surgery, weight to avoid strokes and heart attacks, kidney failure to avoid dialysis – those are the places where you can save money. Chronic problems are sucking up the bucks. When you're dealing with end-of-life care, you're going to have the same costs; you can't save there unless you just don't provide the care. Broken legs, pneumonia, gall bladder, all of those kinds of things have their consistent costs no matter how you manage your system; that is, whether the patient is in or out of a hospital bed."[78]

The HEN study puts the same concept very well. Policies to "reduce inappropriate admissions, improve the efficiency of inpatient care provision, and facilitate more rapid discharge ... will often require the development of alternative facilities and services and while beds may be reduced, *the overall cost to the health system may not fall.*" They know this because they looked primarily at the statistics in Canada. The HEN meta-study, as well as more specific studies, explains that while reducing inappropriate use of ERs by using, for example, medical observation units to redirect patients is useful, "the most gains come from earlier discharge."

Earlier discharge "requires the creation of a wide range of alternatives to hospital care, including nursing homes and intensive intervention in the patient's home." However, "most interventions intended as alternatives to hospital care actually complement it, so *the total volume of activity increases.* Furthermore, *many interventions designed to support patients in the community are as expensive, or more so, than hospital care.*" This Alice-in-Wonderland fact hides a cruel reality. For any kind of health care system, costs that are offloaded onto the community, especially the women in that community, do not go away; they simply do not show up in the hospital books. That's also the great appeal of attacking LOS, Length of Stay. In the final analysis, we have to make specific demands that our system allocate funds to make certain that care such as counseling and follow-up actually are available. Although they are less expensive and more effective, this kind of preventative care is "unproductive" in terms of a profit-oriented economy, which is why they always tend to be ignored and under-funded in our societies. And as we'll also see later, technologized diagnoses and expensive pharmaceutical or surgical treatments are not necessarily as helpful to the sick as they are to our economies.

HEN goes directly to the period being discussed, pointing out that between 1991 and 1993, "almost 10 percent of the acute hospital beds in Winnipeg, Manitoba, were closed." They cite a study by Roos and

Shapiro published in *Medical Care*[79] that claimed that neither access to hospital nor quality of care was affected by these closures, at least according to their mortality and readmission rates. However, a follow-up study in 1995–1996 did show "*a large increase in numbers of common procedures, including cardiac surgery and cataract extraction.*" While people may not have been dying at appreciably higher rates, they were suffering, and the proof is that chronic conditions such as heart and eye diseases worsened to the acute stage, at which point they would have become far more expensive to the system as well as dangerous to the patient. Moreover, this alarming increase happened because of a mere 10 percent loss of beds, not twice that, which is what Canada as a whole experienced a few years later.

Other studies, such as one on a whopping 30 percent reduction of "short-stay" unit beds in British Columbia in 1986 and 1993 did not find such dramatic changes, at least in the elderly patients studied. In this case, there may actually have been too many hospital beds per capita in the area. The situation, however, only goes to show how important it is to develop a way to accurately measure needed bed capacity *before* cuts are made. In a particular case in England, HEN notes, "a relatively small number" of medical and surgical bed closures led "to an immediate increase in the possibility that the hospital would be unable to admit acutely ill patients." The reason why a modest closing had such dangerous effects goes back to the demand that hospitals maintain 90 percent occupancy rates. "One reason why the United Kingdom has been especially vulnerable," the authors of the HEN report wrote, "is the long-standing pursuit of 'efficiency,' interpreted as achieving bed occupancy rates of 90 percent or more, *even though mathematical modeling demonstrates that occupancy rates of over 85 percent greatly increase the risk of periodic bed crises, leading to failure to admit acutely ill patients.*"[80]

Part of the HEN report should be required reading for all government bureaucrats charged with funding health services. It reads: "Research from the United Kingdom during the 1980s suggested that *only about 20 percent of the cost-savings anticipated from bed closures were actually realized*, because of the cost of alternative modes of care.[81] Worse, several studies from North America have found that, contrary to expectations, reductions in hospital capacity *increased* the cost of hospital care. These studies showed that instead of being treated in small, community hospitals, patients had no choice but to go to more expensive teaching hospitals. In California, an 11 percent reduction in admissions was associated with a 22 percent increase in cost per case – in short, costs doubled. This naturally results in a net loss in both services and savings.[82]

HEN backs up the anecdotal assessments of hospital staff, saying, "these studies highlight an important point: *in many cases the first few days of admission are the most resource-intensive, after which costs per day are often small.* Consequently, reductions in lengths of stay due to faster discharge often yield only minor savings ... they do, however, have a substantial effect on the mix of patients that remain, so that *staff workloads increase* as a higher proportion of their patients are in the immediate, more resource-intensive, post-admission period." The loss of no less than 52 small rural hospitals in Saskatchewan in the mid-1990s, according to a 2001 article in *Social Science and Medicine,* did not result in increased health care problems over all, despite the long distances patients now had to travel. The HEN authors did say that communities had to become very "creative." Only those with "strong community leadership" were able to develop "acceptable alternative services" and "innovative solutions."[83]

Other rural communities suffer from hospital closures, as similar studies from the United States show. And closure creates other concerns, which hark back to the earliest days of hospital establishment.[84] Hospitals unite communities. They provide economic stimulus and a clear focus of civic pride and also attract a professional class of workers that might not otherwise live in a given town. The HEN study found that "more than 75 percent of the mayors" of American towns that had experienced hospital closures "felt that access to medical care had deteriorated in their communities ... with a disproportionate impact on the elderly and poor." Finally, "more than 90 percent felt that closure had substantially impaired the local economy."[85]

MUDDY WATERS

There's a culture in public health to withhold information they feel the public "can't handle." Manipulating statistics to some extent is part of that ... some of it's calculated, some isn't, but it's engrained to be fragmented and difficult to interpret.

Public health employee[86]

In order to see what has happened to health care as a result of the hospital bed closings, we have to leave international studies and go back to internal data. The Canadian Institute for Health Information reveals that Canadian hospital admissions were stable for the seventeen years previous to the changes. That is, from 1976 to 1992, they barely fluctuated, from about 4.0 to 4.2 million admissions a year. This is surprising, given the governments' claim that fewer and fewer Canadians needed hospitalization, but perhaps some of this number were being "inappropriately" admitted. Admissions did begin to decline slightly in 1992–93, to between 3.7 and 3.8 million. Then came the closures and admissions suddenly dropped precipitously, down to a low of slightly under 3 million, which re-stabilized in about 2000 and came back up to about 3.1 million, where it has remained ever since. Because every Canadian knows how hard it is to get a hospital bed for even a serious illness, much less for painful, degenerative conditions requiring "elective" surgery such as hip replacements or angioplasty, it is certainly debatable whether this drop in more than a million beds reflects the natural tendency towards more outpatient care cited by government, or whether it could point to either the accidental or intentional creation of an inadequate number of hospital beds available to service the public need.

The average number of days that patients spent in hospitals, despite government claims that hospital stays were steadily declining, is again belied by the statistics. Average inpatient time in hospital hovers between about 12 and 14 days for the entire 17-year period preceding downsizing. In 1990–91, there is a very significant dip, down to about 12 days, that is, slightly below the average of 1976, which no doubt is a good part of the reason for the government's claims. But following a black hole in the charts when no statistics were reported at all, between 1994–95, the chart becomes erratic, moving from an average stay of 11 days in 1996 up to 12 in 1997, back down below 11 in 2000, up again to 11 in 2001, and back down again to a low of 10 in 2002–03. These actual numbers have never come close to the supposed "average" of 6 days often mentioned by governments. With only 2 years at the same rate of 10 days, at this point it is still too early to say if these fluctuations, which do not reflect the slow, steady behaviour of the statistics up to 1990, have finally stabilized or what they mean in terms of patient care.

Moreover, no large Canadian studies seem to have measured mortality rates as they relate to the possible unavailability of hospital beds. The closest statistic to work with is termed "hospital separations." Hospital "separations" includes both the number of patients that are dis-

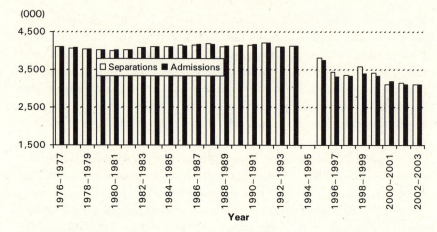

Figure 6 Hospital separations and admissions, Canada, 1976–1977 to 2002–2003

charged as cured and those who are discharged as dead, so there aren't any clear mortality statistics as such. Despite this rather significant difference, the statistics are interesting. Hospital "separations" reflect the same level numbers visible in hospital admissions from 1976 until 1993 and more or less mirror the same amounts. They then drop to a sudden low of about 3,500,000 in 1997–98. The interesting thing about this chart is not just that "separations," i.e., possible mortalities, generally rise or fall in step with admissions. Instead, it is the sudden, unprecedented discrepancy between hospital admissions, shown on the chart in black, and "separations," visible in white. While completely even for all the preceding years, in 1996, for the first time, *separations rise visibly higher than admissions,* with a high of about 3,600,000 separations in 1998–99, compared to only 3,400,000 admissions. It is impossible to tell if these figures represent more deaths or more discharges, of course. However, unlike the rest of the charts, they do not level off to normal levels in about 2000. It isn't until 2002–03 that separations do not visibly exceed admissions. The CIHI report makes no comment on this unprecedented gap between admissions and separations during this period, other than to note that these differences "possibly reflect greater variability due to lower response rates [from the institutions]."[87] Apparently the hospitals had the time to respond concerning admissions, but not separations.

It is worth noting that every one of these charts does not simply reflect "under-reporting," but exhibits actual blank holes for the year

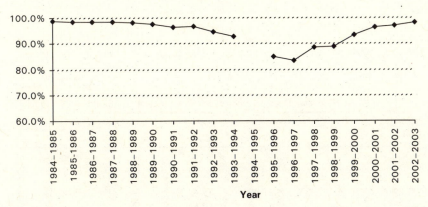

Figure 7 Response rates in Annual return of health care facilities (HS-1 and HS-2 and Canadian mis database (CMDB), 1984–85 to 2002–2003
SOURCES: Canadian Institute for Health Information and Statistics Canada.

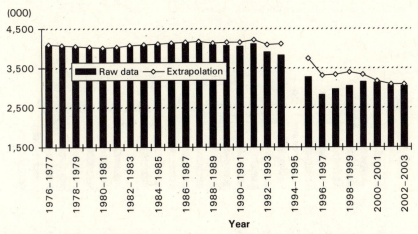

Figure 8 Hospital admissions, Canada, 1976–1977 to 2002–2003
SOURCES: Canadian Institute for Health Information and Statistics Canada.

the Queen Elizabeth closed: 1994–95. The Federal government of Canada has *no statistics* for that year, neither for admissions nor for separations. It has no statistics whatsoever for average inpatient days or response rates, either. The report explains these remarkable gaps occur because "health care institutions did not report" their numbers that year. That is rather striking, given that these institutions submitted reports for each of the previous 17 years and all of the following 10. Because of what we now know about the extent of hospital closures and their ripple effects on every hospital in the country, it is possible to

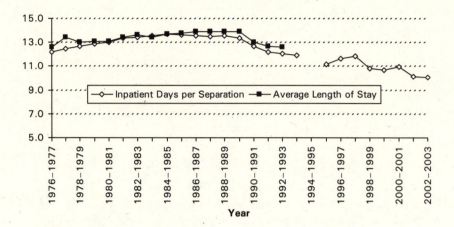

Figure 9   Average inpatient days, Canada, 1976–1977 to 2002–2003
SOURCES: Canadian Institute for Health Information and Statistics Canada.

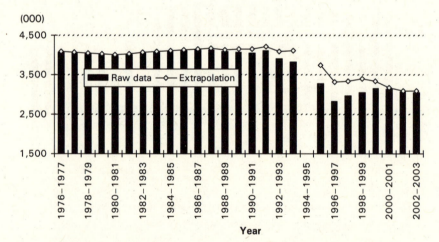

Figure 10   Share of hospital expenditure by selected functional centres, reporting hospitals, Canada, 1976–77 to 2002–03
SOURCES: Canadian Institute for Health Information and Statistics Canada.

interpret this statistical black hole as reflecting a state of near collapse that affected most of the hospitals in the country. Hospitals that were not being downsized, reconfigured, or closed were having to cope with the overflow from all the others. In short, the system nearly melted down. As in a war, epidemic, or other type of attack, important clerical activities, such as data gathering and submissions to government deadlines, were being ignored by a staff that most likely was finding it almost impossible to cope even with daily responsibilities.

This point, more than any other, suggests that all the separate provinces or the federal government as a whole made a serious tactical error in health care planning for the population in the years between 1993–97, an error that has never been adequately studied, assessed, or even recognized. This is partly because Canadian citizens believe that provincial, not Federal, governments control health care, and that each group's hospital closures were not directly related to those happening elsewhere in the country. Journalists, activists, and citizens' groups, to say nothing of hospital staff and patients, have largely studied each set of hospital closures as local phenomena and have energetically analyzed provincial and municipal budgets, policies, and personalities in their search for a clear understanding of the situation. As illustrated in the context of the Queen Elizabeth, this methodology has not enabled the people studying the phenomenon to agree upon a reasonable explanation for their loss. Therefore, the protagonists' anger and grief have not been relieved by understanding. With the benefit of hindsight, however, the statistics now being compiled suggest explanations other than simply "the evolution of medicine," or local political maneuvering – namely, that all across Canada, powerful external pressures were adding weight to the normal, steady, but nonetheless very slow medical trend of using fewer beds for shorter periods. The latter phenomenon has largely taken the fall for this disruption in Canadian public hospital care, but the former, external pressure, is much more likely to be the real explanation. And, the biggest hint is the report's reference to "balancing budgets."

STRUCTURAL ADJUSTMENT

Our governments are withdrawing from us, leaving us as refugees are
left, abandoned. Homeless. The very young and the greatly old, the sick
and the needy have been the first to suffer.
                                        Timothy Findley, *Writing Home*[88]

Elizabeth Kubler-Ross's famous five stages of grief all have one thing in common; they require time. The sheer speed of the loss of these large and vital institutions may be one reason why their mourners have taken so long to recover. Denial, bargaining, anger, despair, and acceptance are all in evidence in embryonic form in the necessarily formal board

minutes that are one of the few physical objects remaining from the
Queen Elizabeth Hospital of Montreal. But the same emotions have
been played out in ensuing years on the personal level, as evidenced in
this book's interviews with what might be called hospital survivors.
These people, whether in Montreal, Winnipeg, Toronto, rural Saskatchewan, Halifax, or Calgary, still have a lot of questions. Few of
these questions have been adequately answered by official explanations or even by the march of history. The questions for larger numbers
of Canadians who were not intimately involved in these institutions are
less emotional, but they are also important for reasons that are significant to our society at large. Even the most objective and uninvolved
observer, being told this story, would have to ask one key question: Why
were all these governments in such a hurry?

The first question that occurs to an outsider is what one might call
the macro-economic picture. That is, what were the budgetary forces
operating outside the affected municipalities and provinces? It is now
becoming clearer that international concerns had a strong effect on
the decision to downsize the national hospital system. Both Dr John
Hughes and Owen Ness, an active member of the Queen Elizabeth
Board of Directors, assert that one reason given to them by provincial
officials at the time of closure was "Quebec's financial standing in New
York. Standard & Poors, the financial rating company, was putting pressure on Lucien Bouchard [the province's current premier] to cut
costs." Indeed, as previously discussed, only six years before, a similar
situation – that is, the threat of Quebec's losing its "preferred" lending
status on the international economic stage – was one reason given for
the government's ruthlessness in breaking the nurses' strike and cutting their pay by 20 percent. The health system did not recover from
that budgetary decision for more than a decade. George Subak, Queen
Elizabeth Hospital psychiatrist, names the local personalities involved,
the ministers and premier, saying, "Dr Lazure, Parizeau, Rochon ... I
don't think they'll ever publish honest memoirs and let us know what
really happened."

He's probably right. The details of what may have happened on the
macro-economic level are by definition unavailable to the public.
Financial arrangements with stock lenders on Wall Street as well as the
World Bank and other high-level financial institutions do not have to
be made public to citizens in the countries or provinces affected. Negotiations that bind Canada to trade agreements and financial treaties
with primarily financial and trade entities, such as NAFTA and the WTO,

are also not open to the public. The parties to them – even the ones that represent Canada, such as Pierre Pettigrew and now Jim Flaherty, are not elected to the position but appointed. The public has no input or response strategy to enable it to deal with international agreements that also take years to unfold and make their effects felt. And the biggest problem is that Canadians do not realize that decisions made on these faraway international levels actually do have something to do with the cost of their child's college tuition, the budgetary problems of the CBC, or their difficulties in finding a family doctor.

Jean Chretien's campaign promise to withdraw from NAFTA (North American Free Trade Agreement) is one of the major reasons he was elected in 1999; that promise was subsequently broken. Since then, no party of record has made its positions on international trade and global financial negotiations part of its election campaign, nor, once elected, has any party informed the electorate about the details of its trade activities nor offered options concerning matters of debate. The first time the subject came up again was eight years later, in 2007, when the opposition NDP belatedly took a position against Stephen Harper's deals with "harmonizing" Canadian and U.S. laws and even foreign policy via trade deals like TILMA (Trade, Investment, and Labor Mobility Agreement) and the SPP (Security and Prosperity Partnership). Given this continued lack of transparency and public documentation, it isn't possible to prove beyond any shadow of doubt that macro-, rather than micro-, economic pressures played a part in the closure of Canadian hospitals at this period. Based on what hard evidence does exist, however, it is certainly possible to harbour suspicions.

Here are the facts. Throughout the 1980s, various "economic service organizations," from Standard & Poor's to international banks and the World Bank, encouraged national, provincial, and even large municipal governments to borrow large amounts of cash to pursue domestic development and support programs of every kind, from infrastructure construction to industrial incentives. The encouragement to borrow was especially tempting to poor and developing countries, but many economically powerful G8 nations, including Canada and France, succumbed as well. Ultimately, the billions of dollars that supported such programs came from financial giants like the World Bank and corporate entities such as major lending banks around the world. These organizations urged governments to invest in roads, modernize their industrial facilities, and get ready to serve new markets. It sounded like a great plan, and most of the countries in the world, from the poorest to the richest, borrowed increasingly large amounts. By the end of the 1980s, however, the promised revenues and business stimulation that would have enabled the borrowers to repay or even service these debts had not materialized. All over the world, the big financial institutions, led by the biggest of all, the IMF (International Monetary Fund) began to foreclose. That is the simplest explanation of why the subject of "debt reduction," "the deficit" (whether provincial or federal), and "balancing budgets" became a mantra for the early 1990s, in Canada and elsewhere.

The IMF, like the World Bank and many other international funding institutions, was set up following World War II for the best of reasons. Initially, it received a pooled fund from several nations. Its function was to stabilize the rate of exchange for member countries so they wouldn't be subject to the inflation and currency devaluations that created financial crises during the Depression and that are thought to have contributed to the start of World War II. But over the years, the IMF changed. By the late 1970s, the World Bank in particular was using the IMF to police debtor nations that weren't able to pay back their loans fast enough. Economist David Korten explains that the IMF, "more or less representing the interests of the creditors," meets with each government and offers to help "reschedule" their debt. This help, however, comes with a price; to get debt relief, reduction, or increased time to pay, governments have to agree to certain *internal economic reforms*, referred to as "*structural adjustment*" or "*economic rationalization*."[89]

To put it crudely, "structural adjustment" means a government has now agreed to get fast cash anywhere it can, generally in a manner suggested by the IMF. In a micro-economy, if an individual hasn't got the money in some liquid form to pay even the interest on her mortgage, much less the principal, she'll have to sell off her possessions one by one, just as is happening in the current real estate crisis in the United States. If she doesn't have enough possessions, she may lose the house. In a nation's situation, that is analogous to control over her territory. In the macro-economy, governments begin by either downsizing or privatizing public corporations and other possessions – the railroads, the airlines, oil companies, television stations, and any other industries they have invested in. After that, the only things governments have left to sell are the actual government services paid for by taxes: educational and public health programs and institutions, communications networks, farm and food subsidy systems, and consumer and environmental protection agencies. Because most such services are not for-profit, governments are required by their creditors to get out of the business of providing funds to them.

Besides the paper savings, private enterprises, often from other countries, then turn up to pay small amounts for liquidated buildings or supplies or to take over each program. This is how Via Rail, large numbers of public water testing services and Air Canada were handed over to the private sector. Poor countries with the most crippling debts – Yugoslavia, Russia, Somalia, Bolivia, and Rwanda, for example – have had to dismantle so many of their government services to feed the demands of international financial creditors that wars, famines, and general collapse have sometimes resulted. Some of the greatest tragedies of the early 1990s – the genocide in Rwanda, the collapse of Somalia and Yugoslavia – have been partially blamed by a growing number of economists on the demands of structural adjustment.[90] And, although many Canadians are aware of the effects of such actions on poor countries, largely through the many anti-globalization protests against NAFTA, the FTAA (Free Trade Area of the Americas), the IMF, or the World Bank that have occurred since the 21st century began, few realize that Canada is also a victim of structural readjustment.

Of course, debt reduction is not the only reason hospitals were closed or that the Canadian health care system is being downsized. Both the evolution of health care and technology and increasing pressures towards privatization are important. All the same, people who are wondering why Canadians no longer have enough doctors, hospital beds, ERs, and operating rooms available to them or question why a country as rich as Canada seems to be losing ground in areas such as post-secondary education, national transportation, communication networks, and viable programs for First Nations peoples can learn something by reviewing the country's global financial position in the early 1990s.

THE IMF PROGRAMME FOR CANADA

In the mission's view, it would be appropriate for the Government to aim to reduce the budget deficit to about 1–2 percent of the GDP in 1997–98 and to about 1 percent of the GDP in 1998–99 ... In certain areas, such as unemployment insurance, the tax system, and pension benefits, further action is required, not only to strength the fiscal position, but also to bring about structural reform.

Point 5 from *Consultation with Canada, International Monetary Fund*[91]

In 1995, the Liberal Party came to office in Canada in a left-leaning landslide so complete that it virtually wiped the Progressive Conservative Party off the map. Jean Chrétien had promised to return to the values of social equality and justice pioneered by his mentor, Pierre Elliot Trudeau. He also promised to withdraw Canada from NAFTA and abolish the new general income tax on goods and services, the GST. Despite one of the clearest policy mandates from the electorate a Canadian party had ever received, not one of these promises was delivered. Voters were first stunned and then demoralized to discover that there were very few differences between the social and economic policies of the new Liberals and those of the Conservatives they had so energetically destroyed. Partly to find out if international pressures were to blame for this situation, several Canadian NGOs (Non-Governmental Organizations), notably the Halifax Coalition and the Sierra Club of Canada, fought for years to get IMF documents released under the Access to Information Act. They succeeded in September of 1999.

The Canadian government at both the federal and provincial levels was a creature of its time. Both levels of government had taken the advice of the financial service organizations throughout the 1980s and had borrowed to develop their economies and satisfy their electorates. By the early 1990s, Canada had discovered it was in so much debt it could hardly pay the interest, much less the principal, so the IMF turned up to help reschedule the debt. The IMF, as most politicians tell their constituents, "has no power to make demands" on a sovereign government but "can only make suggestions." In accordance with this power, or stated lack of it, the IMF issued official – but secret – papers entitled "Statements of the IMF Missions 93/ 94/ and 95," including correspondence related to "Article IV, Reviews and Consultations with Canada." Many pages are still blacked out and marked "secret" in the version finally released to the public through Access to Information, but a great deal of interesting reading remains.[92]

The haste with which health policies were changed and hospitals decimated in Canada in 1994–95 can be better understood in the context of Part 4 of the *Article IV Consultation with Canada.* Although not made official until December of 1995, the policies it outlines had been ongoing for at least five years previously and officials responsible for federal government spending in Canada had to know all about them. The IMF states, "The large size and relatively short maturity of the federal debt ... make the budget highly vulnerable to interest rate shocks. The recent period has shown that market confidence in Canada's longer-term prospects is tenuous and can be easily shaken by domestic political events ... or financial crises outside Canada. In this context, *a faster pace of fiscal adjustment with a more rapid reduction in the debt/GDP ratio* would enhance the credibility of the fiscal program and lessen the risk that the adjustment process could be derailed by an economic downturn or other shocks."

In plain language, the last sentence says that if the government accelerates the liquidation of its remaining assets to service its debt, the "adjustment process," that is, paying the big banks back and re-structuring social and financial programs across the country, will reassure the financiers that they will get their money back quickly, before anything untoward, such as political reactions or an "economic downturn," threatens their investment. What this restructuring does to the Canadian public and their services is not the IMF's concern. The situation does explain the sudden political concern with balancing budgets, however.

In a communication from December 1994 titled "Article IV: Consultation Discussions, Statement by the Fund Mission to the Minister of Finance," the IMF's implicit threats are even less veiled. "The current economic situation presents both favorable elements and serious risks ... However, there is no room for complacency ... It is critical that fiscal policy takes the lead in meeting these challenges." Rather than the usual method of setting yearly interim targets of a 1 to 3 percent budget reduction, the article states, in extremely strong terms for such a document, "A more *fundamental correction of the fiscal situation is needed ... it is critical to seize the moment and put in place a front-loaded package* of fiscal adjustment measures *leading rapidly* toward federal budget balance." By "fiscal adjustment measures," the IMF means serious cuts in government spending. The IMF consultation statement even includes handy suggestions on where and even how to make such cuts: "The mission has prepared a detailed list of the measures that could be considered to achieve fiscal adjustment ... *Virtually no area of federal spending has been left untouched in this list.*"[93]

Considering that this document comes from an international financial organization without any political or democratic legitimacy, it uses extraordinary phraseology when suggesting that fundamental policy changes should be made by a supposedly sovereign, elected government. The phraseology makes the subordinate position of the governments very clear. "The mission would support efforts to harmonize the Goods and Services Tax with provincial sales taxes," the IMF notes, "but, if such efforts failed, *would advise against eliminating the GST.*" This state-ment alone may explain why Jean Chretien reneged on that particular campaign promise a matter of months later. The IMF generously left the government a tiny bit of room in which to govern. "The measures in the list add up to an amount somewhat larger than the desired size of the adjustment package, *thus permitting some choice* between them."

One typical suggestion that will enable the lending banks to get their money back quickly reads: "There may be scope for *reducing net outlays to veterans* by removing the tax exemption of benefits, and for *slowing the growth of transfers to Indians and Inuit* by rationalizing the delivery of transfers or *by tightening access to benefits.*" These documents also help explain the reckless speed of the health cuts and certainly leave no doubt that both Paul Martin and Michael Wilson, the Finance minister under Brian Mulroney, had to know exactly where Canada's debts left their promises and policies. The fact that service cuts spread across the country, even within services that Canadians believe are the responsi-bility of the provinces, may be explained by other paragraphs in the adjustment document. "*Fiscal adjustment also is needed beyond the federal government,*" the IMF notes on paragraph 13 of the secret document, which no doubt was eventually revealed to every provincial premier. "While most provinces have begun to adjust, [that is, to cut services], considerable additional action is still required, particularly in Ontario and Quebec."[94]

One of the hottest issues in Canadian politics is the accusation that the Federal government withholds a great deal of wealth from the prov-inces, despite having downloaded on them most of the services that governments typically provide. This situation is generally referred to as "the imbalance of transfer payments." On page 16 of its list of Revenue and Expenditure Adjustment Options, the IMF points out, "There is a concern that the current system of federal-provincial transfers has led to inefficient provincial spending programs, an over dependence on Federal transfers, and reduced incentives to develop provincial reve-nue bases." Again, the IMF provides a helpful list showing where trans-fer payments can be cut to the provinces; it includes social welfare programs, old age benefits, *health care,* equalization payments, support of territorial governments, and educational subsidies.

The section on education even states that Canada has too many edu-cated people: "Canada's spending on post-secondary education as a share of GDP is the highest among OECD [Organization for Economic Cooperation and Development] countries, and enrollment also appears to be among the highest. *In this light, federal transfers could be reduced* in order to encourage a more efficient use of education resources." This was done within the year, wrapped up in Paul Martin's first budget. The IMF again helped out by encouraging post-secondary funding through "interest-bearing student loans," rather than the formerly more prevalent bursaries. This has become the common situation today, one that is very familiar to every student and parent. Even allowing students to go into debt to the government is a worrisome expense, according to the IMF, which urges on page 16 that, while desirable in general, "it would be important to avoid the creation of a new entitlement." Although the IMF applauds the way human resource subsidies provide "small grants to local efforts to assist the unemployed through training, education upgrades and other services" and are not simply "passive income support programs," it has a good idea about how to deal with them. "There may be merit in shifting the responsibility for the funding and the implementation of such programs to the provinces."[95]

Because some of the institutions listed below have virtually disappeared from the Canadian scene, it's important to remember that they were all still very functional in the 1980s and early 90s – that is, until the IMF wrote that, "Subsidies to Crown corporations are large, and may be difficult to justify on efficiency or other grounds. Cuts could involve *eliminating regional programming and other television services by the CBC; eliminating transfers to VIA Rail and the CMHC [Canadian Mortgage and Housing Corporation], the National Film Board,* and the Canadian Film Development Corporation." Other than the continuously threatened CBC, most of these entities are no longer really viable in Canadian society today. People are aware that the condition of Canadian farmers has become increasingly economically untenable, and that Native and Inuit Affairs, Fisheries, and other resource agencies, as well as scores of scientific research departments, have disappeared or become starved for funding. In other suggestions to the Canadian government, the IMF wrote: "In many areas, there may be a limited need for an extensive federal regulatory or supervisory presence. Such areas include agricultural policy ... natural resource policy, Indian and Inuit affairs, social policies, fisheries and industry. In addition, federal funding for research is extensive ... there would seem to be scope for *rationalizing these services with a view to increasing the private sector's responsibility for such activity.*" In short, they suggested privatizing any government service possible.[96]

In fact, many formerly government-funded research services, such as chemical and water testing, have subsequently been awarded to private oversight and private industry, with occasional disastrous effects on the public health, notably the many deaths and disabilities caused by the lack of proper testing in Walkerton, Ontario.[97] The suggestion to farm out government water testing services to private individuals and labs, duly implemented in the 1995 budget and enthusiastically embraced by many provincial governments, has had direct impacts on water quality and testing programs as well as on food and product safety all across the country. The IMF suggestion directly affecting national health policies as a whole is particularly revealing. "While total Canadian outlays for health are well below those in the United States as a share of GDP, they exceed spending levels in other OECD countries. *Cuts in EPF-Health transfers to the provinces could encourage greater efficiencies or cost recovery in the health sector.*"

Besides debt reduction, other very specific social policies, such as the privatization of all government services including hospital and health services, has been an integral goal of most international financial bodies over the last ten to twenty years. This attitude stems from a belief in the efficacy of private over public management, variously termed "the Washington consensus," "the New World Order," or just "economic globalization." Bodies such as the IMF, the World Bank, and related trade organizations such as NAFTA, the FTAA, and the WTO (World Trade Organization) make their enthusiastic pursuit of the full privatization of government services clear in a section directed to the government of Canada in the same *1994–1995 Structural Adjustment Programme.* One would think that part 4, the list showing exactly how various government services could be cut back in order to pay back the debt, would be sufficient meddling in Canada's internal affairs. However, there is a separate section of the programme, part 11, which suggests how Canada's *external* affairs policies should be handled. It *links any country's cooperation with the IMF in reducing its debt with the general privatization policies of such global trade entities as the WTO.* The following decade-old statement should also still be of serious interest both to Canadian farmers and independent business people. "Canada has continued to show its strong support for free trade by passing the legislation needed to implement the Uruguay Round Agreement and signing the interim financial services accord reached last July. *Tariffs have also been reduced on a wide range of manufacturing inputs, and further consolidation and simplification of the tariff structure are intended. In the agricultural area, the elimination of the Western Grain Transportation Act subsidy is welcome.*" The Uruguay Round was a WTO treaty that has become known for its widespread effects in creating more power for private corporations while disenfranchising governments, small businesses, and farmers.

Although Jean Chretien, Paul Martin, and the other members of the new Liberal government had been elected on a platform directly opposed to cutting back or privatizing social services, particularly health care, Paul Martin's maiden budget, for which he is still infamous, ended up delivering, in every detail, precisely what the IMF had suggested. For that, he and his government took the brunt of the public's anger and shock. But the public was never informed of the external reasons for this shocking change in position. This period also saw a remarkable shift in federal responsibilities, which were downloaded to the provinces by the simple expedient of cutting transfer payments. This policy has had noticeable impacts on the services that the smaller and less wealthy provincial governments are able to deliver to the public and has greatly injured loyalty to the federal government. Provinces like Quebec, Ontario, and Alberta, which were also suffering from internal deficits on top of their share of Canada's national debt, were most heavily affected and two of them remain very resentful of the federal system. But as we've seen, all provinces lost primary, secondary, and tertiary health services because of the large closure of hospital beds and the related loss of access to both general and specialized medical care.

As we can see from the government's own charts and figures, the hectic demands for immediate closure of health institutions and beds during the fiscal year of 1994–95 virtually paralyzed the country's hospital sector. Québecers were told that these cuts were the result of the natural and gradual evolution of hospital care, while the federal and Albertan governments said they were a response to desperately needed social service belt-tightening. Now that the previously secret IMF documents are available, these rapid and drastic cuts in health services start to make sense, especially if the haste with which they were implemented was part of the requirements of a structural adjustment program. That is, it all makes sense if governments were being faced with an external and inflexible international financial deadline. And we now know that, in fact, such pressure was being applied at precisely this period.

Of course, international finance was just one more limiting factor that hit hospitals in the early and middle nineties, and we may never know with complete certainty how much importance to grant such things as the IMF Programme to Canada. The "suggestions," actions, and agreements our governments exchange with financial and trade authorities do not have to be revealed to Canadian citizens, although in 2004, at a Liberal Party fundraising dinner in Montreal, then-Prime Minister Paul Martin admitted the whole thing to an audience of a thousand supporters, saying, "I traveled to all the financial centres of the world, and they told me if I didn't decrease health care spending, they would cut Canada's bond rating."[98] Despite the open communications believed to characterize modern society, these politically critical decisions are nearly all negotiated and implemented in secrecy. Agreements like the one for 1994–95, quoted above, are made between the IMF and its debtor nations, as well as between our governments and the trade and other financial bodies, *every single year.* Dozens more of them have been received since then and the public knows nothing about them. We can assume that they are having effects on both internal and external policies, however. And, although trade representatives to the European Union (EU) are elected and therefore mandated to defend both social programs and national protections with noticeably greater vigour, under NAFTA, the people who negotiate trade for Canada, the U.S., and the other signatories in the Western Hemisphere such as Mexico and Chile, are appointed – not directly elected. Voters have no way of knowing their positions on the various issues involved in the negotiations. To make this picture even more alarming, Canada's Access to Information laws have very recently been weakened rather than strengthened, so it's become increasingly difficult, even years later, to find out exactly what we've agreed to do.

SPINNING TOMMY IN HIS GRAVE

> There's not any doubt at all that the present Medicare program in
> Canada is in serious danger of being sabotaged.
>
> Tommy Douglas, 1984[99]

International pressures are not the only issue that influences provincial commitments to health care. Local political shenanigans and economic demands are also responsible for changes to health care policy. That means that Canadians need to pay attention to international trade influences and federal maneuvers, certainly, but also remember that access to hospital care differs widely from province to province and even from city to city. All complex political and social systems have local, national, and international causes and repercussions, which becomes crystal clear whenever a given social situation develops problems.

Alberta's response to this crisis can stand as an example. Kevin Taft, who started his career in Alberta's provincial bureaucracy as a researcher and consultant and who today is a Liberal MNA, writes in his and Gillian Steward's book, *Clear Answers*, that he was hired by the province of Alberta in the early 1980s to study the issue of user fees in health care. "With my freshly minted Masters degree and an earnest desire to do a 'professional' job, I set off to read up on all sides of the issue," he writes. "The logic of user fees seemed clear enough, and I expected to find studies showing that they worked as planned." Instead, he writes, *"Every study I found showed much the opposite: user fees do not reduce total costs, nor do they lower overall demand on the health-care system."*[100]

Taft found that user fees, which are primarily intended to discourage patients who don't really need care from over-burdening the system, instead discourage the last people who should hesitate to see a doctor – the elderly and the poor. Remember Physician Induced Demand, that is, the tendency for institutions to either over- or under-play the need for treatment depending on their own financial interest, and the tendency to use any system, private or public, to its economic capacity? Taft discovered that "Any capacity freed up by reduction in demand is quickly filled with services initiated by physicians, such as minor surgeries, and by people for whom user fees are no barrier – the middle and upper classes." Taft goes further. "While many public issues present genuine puzzles and dilemmas (think of, say, locating garbage dumps, responding to youth crime, or balancing environmental issues), there was a striking clarity and consistency in studies of health economics: study after study – decade after decade and in country after country – has found that *health care is a market failure.*"[101]

How could such a sweeping statement, especially in the face of increasingly popular and widespread modern health care initiatives such as "P–3" (public/private partnership) hospitals and clinics, be true? The concept that private infusions of cash from society's more well-heeled members, along with investment from private enterprises, logically sounds as if it would help. It certainly seems to work in countries such as France and Germany, which have long enjoyed mixed public/private systems. The margins within which this mix can operate successfully, however, turn out to be far more narrow than most North American theorists have imagined, as we'll see ahead. Taft is not the first analyst to point out that the main bone of contention concerning how to fund health care is not whether scientific and economic data support mixed or single-player plans. The numbers on that competition are in and for decades now have demonstrated that, despite their many frustrating qualities, almost every public system is less expensive in virtually every instance than almost any type of private one, and also delivers better overall health care.

Researchers ploughing through the mounds of data that illustrate this fact come to realize that if there still is any debate about how to fund health care, it is not based on scientific or statistical evidence. As with the Climate Change "debate," deciding whether to use private, for-profit or largely public, non-profit institutions is a philosophical and political, rather than a fact-based, decision. That means that any country engaged in the issue first has to decide on its philosophical attitude towards health care. Are such things as inoculations and operations to be considered needed services, provided by each society to its members as a basic right of citizenship? Or should health care be treated as a commodity like any other, a good to be purchased, with its management left to the forces of a competitive market? Should some types of care, for example, operations, be a right, but other types of care, such as prescription drugs, not considered a right? Many, many books have been written on this subject, from both sides, so the conflicting arguments will be presented as quickly and fairly as possible.

MORE PROS AND CONS

The fundamental flaw of the Medicare system is that patients bear no direct costs for the medical services they receive ... the doctor-patient relationship has been corrupted by the "free" nature of the system.

David Gratzer, *Code Blue*[102]

Political slogans about "reducing big government" and "supporting a free market" should not be allowed to obscure the fact that Medicare spends substantially more of each health-care dollar on health services than private insurers do.

Christine Cassel, *Medicare Matters*[103]

Many doctors and health economists today would agree with *Code Blue*, a book written by David Gratzer in 1999. It contends that leaving the basic economic, seller-buyer relationship out of health care, the way that Tommy Douglas' legacy, the Canadian single-payer, universal Medicare system does, is a serious mistake. It means that a service that costs society an enormous amount of money has come to be considered "free." "Patients bear no direct costs for the medical services they receive ... the problem lies in the fact that the doctor-patient relationship has been corrupted by the 'free' nature of the system."[104] Because the "competitive market" beloved by trade and financial organizations and nearly all Western governments has provided "an abundance of inexpensive, high-quality and widely available food, shelter and clothing," it's assumed that the same market "would do the same for Canada's health-care system, if only the constraints of Medicare were lifted."[105]

Gratzer argues, "Consumers tend to avoid waste and inefficiency because they usually result in higher prices. Instead, consumers seek good products at attractive prices offered by efficient suppliers. Producers search for less costly ways of delivering wanted goods – they reduce inefficiencies and develop innovative approaches." This "pursuit of self-interest" by both producers and consumers will theoretically result in a far more streamlined, cost-efficient health delivery system than one run by "bureaucratic institutions" where "normal market incentives have been replaced by bureaucratic rule making." Comparing health services to food, Gratzer notes that an incredible variety of food is available at any time, produced in a cost-effective way, and that, "all Canadians have access to basic foods. True, not everyone can afford caviar and lox, but no one starves."[106]

Many analysts have postulated that a very strong philosophical belief in the concepts of free market operation and especially in each individual's freedom to choose between varied consumer goods explains why a country as rich as the United States has never established a universal health care system. That's one side of the equation, but it ignores another part of the political social contract that's very well understood, even in the United States. Christine Cassel, president of the Board of Internal Medicine in the U.S., points out in her most recent book, *Medicare Matters*, that the ideas on which the United States was founded spring from the Enlightenment philosophies of the 18th century, which "support the maximum liberty for each consistent with the maximum liberty for all." This means that individual freedoms, like the right to have a noisy party, must nevertheless not be permitted to infringe upon the freedoms of others, such as the right of the neighbours to get some sleep. "And the social contract means that we contribute our resources, by means of local, state and federal taxes, only to pay for services and protections for the public good, services that government can provide more effectively than the private sector can."[107]

Examples of these services are "fire and police ... public highways, sewage treatment and a basic public-health infrastructure. It would be ridiculous to expect every private citizen to pay only for that piece of road he or she uses to travel to work every day." By the same token, "Health care is most appropriately regarded as belonging in this category. No one knows what their future health-care needs will be, but all citizens are affected equally when these needs are not met ... Most of us, thankfully, will never need the fire department or police; but, if we did, we would not want to have to pay them before they agreed to put out a fire, rescue us, or prevent a crime from occurring." Cassel goes on to say that universal health insurance systems, like the American Medicare and Medicaid and the single-payer programs used in most of the rest of the developed world, "spread the risk across the entire population so that all of us pay a small amount," even though a relatively small number will be using those resources at any given time. Universal health plans work just like the taxes we pay for police and fire protection; few of us will need the service, but everyone pays into the pot.

However, worldwide, and especially in the United States, there is a "lack of confidence in the ability of government" to efficiently manage such programs. There is also a widespread belief that it is "more cost-effective to have health care provided entirely by private entities and selected and paid for directly by the consumer." This tendency makes the social contract a servant, not of the greater public good, but of the market. Cassel says the two concepts won't mesh; she points out that, "In health care, a successful free market requires that consumers – whether individual patients or businesses purchasing insurance for their employees – be capable of determining and choosing the lowest cost and the highest quality. *Yet our ability to do so is limited by the complexity of health-care issues and the circumstances under which we seek care.*"[108]

As discussed earlier, during the period just preceding Canadian Medicare, patients being admitted to many hospitals were expected to decide the level of room they were to have and also to self-identify their financial limits for care – all this while being admitted to hospital during a health crisis. Just in terms of their eventual ability to pay, even the hospitals realized that medical consumers weren't in a very good position to make wise choices. Cassel asks, "How many of us really shop around for the best bargain when we need to have cancer surgery or a Caesarean section? ... relying solely on the marketplace forces people who are sick and vulnerable to fend for themselves in a theatre of very imperfect information. It drives insurance companies to avoid covering people who need health care the most. It means that medical expenses may dramatically affect the ability of a family to support their children's education."[109] This is what happened in Canada prior to Medicare and what happens in the United States today under a market system. Cassel says the only way to get out of this quandary is not to have more philosophical debates but to go out and study what works, get the facts and figures, and go with the system, however flawed, that has proven to be efficient and have results.

The idea of merging the two systems, trying to get the best of both worlds by partially privatizing public systems, like Canada's or Britain's, has led to many schemes, including Medical Savings Accounts (MSAs) where compulsory insurance programs bank a certain amount of money from each citizen and their employers that will be available to pay major expenses of a serious illness. This method, recently being pushed in the U.S. as "consumer-driven health care" and tried in Singapore, is supposed to motivate people to "shop around for the best prices on health care and to avoid unnecessary treatments because they can keep the surplus in their account at the end of the year."[110] In Britain, hospitals and other health-care institutions are now locked in another kind of competitive battle. They are vying with each other for the *right* to serve patients and deliver certain forms of care, all in the name of keeping costs low. The hospitals offering the best services at the lowest prices win the contract, for example, to do pediatric care. But putting a public system into a competitive, private jacket has generated a great deal of controversy in Britain, as we will see.

In Canada, doctors and hospitals in public systems are increasingly able to "contract out" certain services to private entrepreneurs. Private X-ray, knee surgery, and cataract clinics are now widespread and have proven so popular in Alberta, B.C., and Quebec that there are already good statistics showing whether or not they are economically or therapeutically attractive. Finally, as Steward and Taft point out, "In the United States, where the effects of market forces on health care are most strongly felt, huge hospital corporations vie for patients, pharmaceutical companies own many medical clinics, for-profit insurance companies have enormous influence on the demand for and supply of health care, and for-profit Health Maintenance Organizations (HMOs) manage huge, diverse private systems." Steward and Taft sum up the situation by saying, "There is no shortage of experience in mixing [public] health care and [private] market forces."[111] The question now is not to determine which of all possible systems *sounds* most reasonable, but to *measure* which one actually delivers the best health care at the cheapest cost. As Cassel says, we have no other choice than to look at the evidence.

Throughout this book, there have been repeated references to reliable and widespread studies showing that, to everyone's surprise and disappointment, mixing the public good with profit-making businesses does not seem to save any money. Research studies and other formal investigations undertaken by esteemed universities including McMasters and Harvard, amassed by government and international agencies such as Statistics Canada and the World Health Organization, and published in the most prestigious medical journals, such as the CMAJ, the *New England Journal of Medicine*, and *The Lancet*, all reveal the same thing. What they say is apparently so philosophically disappointing that additional studies are undertaken almost immediately by governments and other bodies anxious to find some other way to fund and manage public health care. This philosophical disbelief is no doubt why we have such a richness of statistical and economic studies on these subjects, dating from the early 1980s right up to the present. Along with the surprise that closing hospital beds doesn't save money, the sad fact seems to be that the distressing waste and staggering expense evident in a single-payer health system like our own is as nothing compared to the social and economic costs of a for-profit system, or even a mixed one. Apparently, hospital care is faulty, scattered, and frighteningly, unendingly expensive, no matter how you fund it, which is not to say that Canada's methods of dealing with this fact can't stand considerable improvements, as we'll see in chapter 7.

For example, in 1999, in an important editorial on the costs of investor-owned, for-profit hospitals, the *New England Journal of Medicine* outlined a situation that has not changed in the years since: "for decades studies have shown that for-profit hospitals are 3 to 11 per cent more expensive than not-for-profit hospitals." In fact, the article goes on to say, "*no peer-reviewed study has found that for-profit hospitals are less expensive.*"[112] In a detailed study published in the same issue, costs were higher yet for profit-making hospitals, from between 13 to 16 percent above those of non-profit hospitals. Moreover, health care spending was increasing faster in areas served by for-profit hospitals than in areas served by not-for-profit hospitals. In other words, the cost gap between for-profit and not-for-profit care is growing. The study took in all 50 U.S. states, age and race differences, and places of residence.[113]

Today, all across Canada, patients are being encouraged to jump waiting lines for elective surgery to correct conditions such as cataract and hip or knee joint failure and go to the newly established private clinics mentioned above, which are proliferating, especially in Alberta and Quebec. Although costing the patient thousands of dollars out of pocket, promoters of private clinics reason that not only will the patients' pain and worry be alleviated more quickly, but their actions will take pressure off the rest of the line-up, letting poorer patients move closer to their own surgery dates. And of course, because the private clinics operate in a free, competitive market, costs per procedure will be lower and efficiency will be greater than in a public system, which, quite truthfully, really is often stifled by bureaucracy and admittedly has no profit incentive.

Alberta has had private clinics for cataract surgery for many years now. In 1999 in Calgary, where the greatest number of eye surgeons live, a full 100 percent of cataract operations were being done privately. This is not to say the surgeons weren't being paid by Medicare: they charged the province their normal fees, but their patients also paid extra costs, so it was a true mixed system. Waiting times were 16 to 24 weeks and the most common charge, beyond what was covered by Medicare, was $400 per eye for an upgraded lens. In Edmonton, there were fewer eye surgeons, but 80 percent of them were working in the public system. There the waiting times averaged between five to seven weeks, that is, operations were done 65 percent faster, and the extra charge for the same upgraded lens was $250, almost half-price. In Lethbridge, where there was no competition at all from private clinics and 100 percent of the cataract surgery was done in public hospitals, the waiting time was even shorter, four to seven weeks, and there was no extra charge for the upgraded lens, "which was purchased by the regional health authority for well under $100." In short, the private clinics got a 300 percent mark-up on the lens alone and the customer received much slower service.[114] These figures fly in the face of everything we believe about free market systems, but there they are. They, and thousands of other studies like them, are the reason for the ongoing, increasingly exasperated editorials and articles coming out of the big medical journals and international associations about the merits of public and private health care funding.

In *The Journal of the American Medical Association*, researcher David Himmelstein goes further than exasperation. His article announced that a study within the United States that compared fully half of the country's for-profit HMOs with not-for-profit HMOs showed that market-based medicine could cost people their lives. "If all 23.7 million American women between the ages 50 and 69 were enrolled in investor-owned, rather than not-for-profit plans, an estimated 5,925 additional [annual] breast cancer deaths would be expected." The authors of this article make their anger very clear. "The decade-old experiment with market medicine is a failure. The drive for profit is compromising the quality of care, the number of uninsured persons is increasing, those with insurance are increasingly dissatisfied, bureaucracy is proliferating, and costs are again rapidly escalating."[115]

Two of the public/private combinations described above, the MSAs tried in the U.S. and especially Singapore, as well as Britain's scheme to introduce competition between hospitals, are also dismal failures. One decade after introducing Medical Savings Accounts in order to control costs and improve efficiency, the government of Singapore concluded, "The health care system is an example of market failure." This must have been difficult to admit. Wealthy Singapore is one of the most enthusiastic bastions of free enterprise and capitalism on earth. Until 1985, they had a tax-funded health care system based on the British, single-payer model. That year, the government introduced MSAs and discovered that when the goal of an institution is profits rather than care, profits are what you get. Hospitals competed not by streamlining costs but by offering the most expensive equipment. "Ten years after the reform, Singapore is saddled with widespread duplication of expensive medical equipment and high-technology services," including seven in-vitro fertilization clinics for a population of only 3.3 million. Fees and incomes of the physicians who chose to enter private practice "rose at a phenomenal rate, which caused experienced physicians to migrate from the public to the private sector. The [remaining] public sector had to raise compensation for its physicians and other health care workers to retain qualified health professionals."[116]

Despite such experiences, MSAs, also called Health Savings Accounts or HSAs, were President George W. Bush's 2006 answer to health care needs in the U.S. The Republicans liked the rhetoric about "personal empowerment," also referred to as "consumer-driven health care." But M- or HSAs not only increase costs, they also have the potential to exacerbate the phenomenon called "adverse selection." People who don't expect health problems choose bare-bones insurance, whereas those with a family history of something like asthma or cancer end up in the now smaller pool of traditional insurance. "Without a variance in risk profiles," writes health care analyst Cindy Zeldin in a January 2006 article, "insurance costs for those in the traditional insurance pools can skyrocket." HSAs are good tax shelters for the rich, but Zeldin says such plans mean that other Americans are going to be even more likely to start paying their health bills with their credit cards and add to the number of personal bankruptcies in the U.S. caused by illness.[117]

In Britain, analysts say the "internal market" schemes introduced by the Thatcher government in the late 1980s did help "loosen some of the overly-centralized administration of the National Health Service" and seem to have improved "the responsiveness of hospitals to doctors and patients." However, this was also "accompanied by the fastest increase in spending on the NHS since the 1960s." The reforms did not "substantially reduce the numbers waiting for at least a year for elective procedures, and they have required substantial additional funds to cover the larger transaction costs of a price-based health market."[118] In fact, in a March 2006 article in *The Economist*, the NHS, despite tax funding that has doubled in the past seven years, is now described as "grappling with record deficits." The chief executive of the now corporate-organized NHS, Sir Nigel Crisp, responded by taking early retirement, and the government is dealing with the problem by doing more of the same: intensifying the competition for efficiency between hospitals. A new payment change, originally set up for elective procedures, will now extend to ERs and outpatients. It will encourage hospitals "to shed services when they cannot provide them competitively." Managers are looking forward to this change but it's reasonable to wonder what people in the locality of the hospitals that have decided to close beds or ERs or other services are going to do about their health problems.[119]

The primary goal even of publicly owned health services like the NHS seems to have become economic efficiency. The subject of health is seldom mentioned with as much interest in articles reporting their success or failure, and no wonder. Concern about the social good is peripheral to the interests of any for-profit or partly for-profit institution. Canada's system is still largely public, even though more than 30 percent is now private. But as much as we jigger, realign, and malign it, it is still held up as an economic beacon by people in many other countries, especially in the U.S.[120] The success of the Canadian method of taking care of the public health is reflected in the mortality statistics quoted earlier and its cost per capita is low compared to other countries. Ironically, this is one reason it's being eyed hungrily by the private corporations that make their money from the business of health.

Critics of the move towards privatization are alarmed about increasing pressures to privatize those plans that are still largely public. They also bring up the subject of international trade treaties and financial entities. As Erika Shaker of the Canadian Centre for Policy Alternatives puts it, "Canada's trade treaty commitments could make health care commercialization a one-way street, not [an] easily reversible [experiment], as is often assumed."[121] Shaker and Maude Barlow, who has also specialized in investigating these treaties and international financial arrangements in terms of their legal power over Canadian internal policies, point out that although health care was exempted from NAFTA, which is why most big U.S. for-profit health corporations haven't yet entered Canada, "*the exemption ... applies only to a fully publicly-funded system delivered on a non-commercial basis.* Once privatized, the system must give 'national treatment' rights to American private hospital chains and HMOs, which must not be treated differently than Canadian for-profit companies."[122]

Barlow reminds Canadians that even though most reformers say they don't want an American system, but a "kinder, gentler" public/private combination on the lines of those in Germany or Sweden, "the fact is that Canada has not signed a free trade agreement with those countries." Barlow goes on to say, "There are also 140 private health insurance companies [now working in Canada] ... at least 37 of them American." NAFTA rules make it clear that the U.S. health corporations granted the right to set up shop in Canada "also *have the same right to public funding as Canadian companies.*"[123] It is one of the facts of the modern economy that the private health insurance industry has become one of the most powerful in the world. This industry spent $169 million in lobbying in the 1999–2000 U.S. election alone; only the pharmaceutical industry has more economic and political clout, which means that put together, the health care business is the richest on earth, outstripping oil or any other industry. And today, they have four lobbyists on Capital Hill for every congressman and woman.

It's clear that most of the rhetoric implying that a private system would be better for Canada comes from an industry that – like any other for-profit business – always needs to expand. "They are the direct beneficiaries when currently listed health services are removed from Medicare coverage," Barlow points out. It is a matter of concern how public facilities and insurance plans will be maintained once the private ones are able to make equal demands on government budgets. But even more worrisome are those trade treaties. "Best estimates suggest that these foreign firms receive as much as $2.5 billion in private health premiums from Canadians ... [almost a third of the market]. Any attempt by any [level of] government to wrest back Canadian control of this business, or to bring it to the public sector, would trigger billions of dollars of trade challenges under NAFTA's Chapter 11 provisions."[124] Back in 2001, it was estimated that the Canadian health care market is potentially worth at least $95 billion to private providers.[125] So there's a lot at stake for an industry that's already done a great deal to cripple public initiatives in the U.S., discussed ahead.

TEMPTING THE ELEPHANT

> Canada is already farther down the path to ... private-sector involvement
> ... than most European countries ... Canada is integrating our economy
> with the US, not with Germany, Sweden or France ... and it is US health
> care corporations, not European ones, who are pushing for access to the
> Canadian health care system.
>   Diana Gibson, Research Director, the Parkland Institute[126]

Privatization isn't creeping into Canada's public health care system simply because governments are convinced that it will be more "efficient" for doctors to opt out of public health care and establish pay-as-you-go clinics, or for governments to build hospitals with private partners. Dr Gordon Guyatt, who teaches Clinical Epidemiology and Biostatistics at McMaster University, writes that most Canadians believe that "P–3" facilities, a term that means Public/Private Partnerships, such as P–3 hospitals, mean that private dollars will infuse outside money into the public health system. Two new hospitals in Ontario, the William Osler Health Center and the Royal Ottawa Hospital, as well as the projected McGill super-hospital in Montreal, have announced that private companies will help design, build, finance, and/or operate these institutions and also assume investment risks. "That makes it sound as if private dollars are [at least partly] paying for the hospitals," Guyatt writes, citing a letter to the *National Post* by Ontario Health Minister Tony Clement, who claimed that one new, "publicly owned hospital" would be built and maintained "without taxpayers' money."

Guyatt has done the math to figure out why, in the countries such as Britain and Australia where P–3 hospitals have been adopted, they have turned out to actually cost more. "First, the cost of borrowing is higher for the private sector ... typically 0.5 percent to 2.0 percent higher" than government rates. Secondly, *the private companies have to make a profit*, usually of at least 5 to 10 percent. Thirdly, there are special costs involved in such deals. "The Royal Ottawa Hospital ... required $8 million to put together a P3 deal." Where does all the

extra money come from? Not from the private companies, as one is led
to believe, but from tax coffers. "All of these costs are ultimately
charged to the publicly-funded hospitals ... and any additional donations you make to your hospital end up, in part, as profits for the investors."[127] That means even the community funds donated by
individuals, which hospitals like the Queen E used to depend on to buy
special equipment or get them through lean times, will, in P–3 hospitals, have a significant bite taken out of them so that private company
investors can get their profits.

Allyson Pollock of the London School of Public Policy analyzed the
decade-long British experiment with P3 hospitals for a series of articles
published in the *British Medical Journal*. She explained that the accounting strategy used to camouflage these increased costs places a dollar
value on the risk transferred from the public to the private sector. For
some P3 hospitals, this estimate adds up to 50 percent of total capital
costs. This large amount translates to profit because when problems
arise in P3 hospitals, the private companies do not typically take that
capital and use it to fix the problems. Instead, the public system is
almost invariably forced to step in.[128] It's difficult for the public to
understand these financial deals, Guyatt claims, because "with public
financing, auditors have full access to a hospital's financial and performance records." But private or mixed facilities "routinely use commercial confidentiality to keep financial information and performance
data away from auditors."

Dr Guyatt cites several examples in Britain and two in Australia,
where "the Victoria government had to buy back LaTrobe hospital
from a private company because its losses 'meant that [the company]
no longer guaranteed the hospital's standard of care.'" In another
case, vital equipment, supposedly paid for, was missing, and in yet
another, the Recovery Room was too far from the OR and had to be
rebuilt. In all cases, the public, not the private, partner had to make up
the costs to get the hospital in question operational. "These examples,"
Guyatt writes, "show that risk [often] is not transferred to the private
sector." Public money eventually ends up paying capital costs such as
building and borrowing interest. "When private provision of necessary
public services fails, public money bails out the private sector."[129]

If there's so little in it for governments, why then do they agree to
these deals? Guyatt explains that Ontario Liberal leader Dalton
McGuinty reneged on an election promise to scrap P3 deals in
Ontario. He did so largely because he had also promised not to raise

taxes and balance the budget. "Under current procedures," Guyatt explains, "if the government borrows money to build the hospitals, the entire capital expenditure counts in the current budget. That means [the] deficit increases and the government is left with a political black eye." If the government leases or mortgages to a private company, however, "the expenditure is charged to the hospital and doesn't appear on the government's books, allowing them to claim prudent management ... The deal will make the current year's accounting look better, but ends up costing more in the long run. Never mind that the public ends up paying much more for their hospitals," Guyatt says. "Leave the unpleasant options of raising taxes, incurring a deficit, or cutting services – including hospital services – to future political leaders." There are solutions, such as simply changing accounting practices so that the cost of the hospital could be spread out over its useful life instead of over the first few years. But meanwhile, Guyatt predicts, "How will our hospitals respond to the increased costs they will have to bear if they are part of P3 schemes? If they follow the British model, they will cut beds, doctors, and nurses, which means more hospital waits, and poorer care."[130]

This chapter has been about the death – or threats of death – to the hospital care and health systems that Canadians have spent generations building and supporting. There seem to be pathological monsters threatening the future of public health systems in every direction, from emerging diseases and spiraling costs to trade treaties, and there is at least one more ahead – the scariest of all – the dragon known colloquially as Big Pharma. But it's always darkest before the dawn. The last chapter in this book is about the rebirth and regeneration of a kind of hospital that can carry people into the future. Analysts who have studied these systems worldwide are well aware that there is no need to fund more studies on whether public or private systems are the most efficient – there are literally thousands of these studies, all saying exactly the same thing. Instead, it's crucial to face up to the fact that the private market doesn't seem to work for health care, take a big breath, and then figure out some other way to control costs. Once more, we have to look at the basic hospital/health care cost equation. Administrators have spent 150 years fiddling with the methods of payment – public, private, taxes, donations, charity, for-profit, and every imaginable combination, ad infinitum. However, except to cut services and access within the system, they have never tried very hard to do anything to control medical costs in terms of analyzing the desirability of new drugs and technologies or challenging the bigger-and-more-complex-is-better paradigm of the past century and a half of modern Western society. Changing entire paradigms is always hard for anybody. That's not to say it's impossible.

6

Social Pathologies

GOING TO THE DRUG MALL

Depression is a serious medical condition with a variety of symptoms. Emotional symptoms can include sadness, loss of interest in things you once enjoyed, feelings of guilt or worthlessness, restlessness, and trouble concentrating or making decisions.

official Eli Lilly site for the anti-depressant Cymbalta[1]

Attention deficit hyperactivity disorder (ADHD) ... consists of a persistent pattern of abnormally high levels of activity, impulsivity, and/or inattention that is more frequently displayed and more severe than is typically observed in individuals with comparable levels of development ... Treatment of ADHD with stimulants such as Ritalin ... help to improve the abnormal behaviors of ADHD, as well as the self-esteem, cognition, and social and family function of the patient ... It is estimated that 3–7 percent of school age children have ADHD.

U.S. government website on Ritalin[2]

Earlier chapters in this book have pointed out that our health care systems are faced with funding what seems to be a never-ending demand for treatments that require expensive technological interventions and pharmaceutical products. Hospital administrations and various levels of government bureaucracies have responded to these rising costs by continuously tinkering with one side of the health care equation: sources of funding. As the recent history of Queen Elizabeth and so many other Canadian hospitals illustrates, persisting in this method of control means that funders everywhere must try to reduce patient load by closing hospital beds – essentially denying care – as well as by limiting the number of doctors and nurses working in the system. On the opposite side of the equation, the providers of the medical goods, pharmaceuticals, equipment, and the health insurance companies have naturally countered any trends to limit their markets by attempting to medicalize more conditions. They also work hard to create new products targeted to serve old needs.

Those entrusted with making decisions about health care, whether in a Manitoba hospital or a Kansas HMO, can only continue trying to put some kind of cap on drug and equipment costs and limit the number of health professionals available to patients. This explains why it's so hard to get a GP, an MRI, or hip replacement in Canada – or anything approaching full insurance coverage in the U.S. Oddly enough, however, apart from trying to control the number of people working in the system, as well as those who have access to that system, there has never been a high-level effort in North America to control demand for medical services, either by funding the kind of unbiased research that would educate professionals as to which treatments are actually worth the money or by trying to legislate against intrusive marketing for drugs, therapies, or equipment. Investigating treatments more carefully with a view to controlling wasteful demand would be one of the most effective things governments and hospitals could do to control costs without damaging care, but that has rarely been attempted in a serious or consistent manner. Hospital administrators, government bodies, and universities could try a lot harder to use research science less as an endless marketing tool and more to help limit the demand for technologies and drugs that can be demonstrated to be unnecessary.

As we all know, even commonplace ailments are being technologized and medicalized these days. Although there is still a crying need for better drug treatments for diseases like TB, malaria, and the other diseases such as cholera that decimate the poor around the world, pharmaceutical manufacturers spend most of their research dollars on drugs for common complaints experienced by middle-class populations – for the simple reason that these products are far more profitable. Physical and mental sensations that have never before been seen as pathologies – things such as shyness, restless legs, riotous behaviour by little boys, and occasional sleeplessness or sexual dysfunction – are now being touted as medical conditions that require expensive drug therapy and even hospital treatment. Human beings are always ready to drop the mundane for the new and exotic, so this trend has been supported by consumers and, to a significant extent, the medical profession. It is only relatively recently that advertising legislation and tradition have been amended to allow profit-making entities with a vested interest in creating more diseases to participate in the diagnosis of ailments. These interests are even permitted to suggest treatments. Today's typical television drug ad that almost as an afterthought ends: "Ask your Doctor" is really just telling consumers where they can get the new product that promises to solve their problem. The result is that the consumption of medical care is no longer clearly differentiated from any other industry-driven consumer good. People are encouraged to demand branded, high-end products – the medical equivalent of plug-in air fresheners and computerized flashlights – instead of plain, dependable, and reasonably priced tools such as hot milk before bed or more exercise. This trend has the potential to destroy any attempt to keep medical treatments reasonably priced and available to all. As public health advocate Laurie Garrett puts it, "by 1999, the real question facing policy makers was no longer whether insurance companies, governments and individuals could afford the costs of hospitalizations, but whether they would be able to afford to *buy the drugs* intended to prevent those hospitalizations."[3]

Since the earliest days of tertiary-care institutions, the lure of modern technologies, like the latest CT, MRI, or fibre-optic scanners, has proven irresistible. Even the struggling Homeopathic purchased its first X-ray machine in the 1920s – two decades before anyone really knew how to use it. Shiny machines are bad enough, but hospitals and health care systems have also displayed remarkable credulity when offered a new batch of pharmaceutical potions. The history of their often-precipitate over-usage of new drugs – thalidomide, breast implants, NSAIDs (non-steroidal anti-inflammatory drugs) – is reminiscent of many of the gruesome stories that litter the history of anesthesia and can best be addressed by a more critical approach to pharmaceuticals in med school. That's not the way medical education is going, however.

The outside providers of medical products – both drugs and machines – often began as public institutions and tiny, altruistic, science-based mom-and-pop businesses like Merck, which used to work so closely with Harold Griffith, or the family-owned and operated firm Johnson & Johnson. Today these same companies have become ruthless, global business giants. Novartis, Bristol-Myers Squibb, GlaxoSmithKline, Eli

Lilly, Pfizer, and Merck & Co, to name but a few, control annual profits that dwarf many nations' GDPs. For example, Johnson & Johnson is now the world's second-largest drug giant and reports an annual net income of more than *8.5 billion dollars*.[4]

The tools these rich and powerful companies have at their disposal to aid their continuing expansion have become frightening and, in terms of influencing important social and political decisions all around the world, socially pathological. They include an astonishing degree of political, regulatory, and academic influence on top of sophisticated marketing techniques. As illustrated further on, many companies are also guilty of falsification of data, corruption, and bribery. When discussing the purposes and goals of these firms, it is important to differentiate between brand marketing and business reality. The activities of large medical and pharmaceutical corporations are intended to serve an economic goal that makes good business sense for their shareholders, but need not have any actual medical value. The enormous industry that has grown up over the last 60 or 70 years to service hospital systems is not legally bound to honour concepts like government or private budgetary limits, protecting the public health, or saving lives. Like any publicly traded business, the structure of these firms mandates that they concentrate on selling more and more products to make increasing profits for their shareholders. That is their goal; the medical usefulness of their products is only important insofar as it serves to support that intention to continue to make and increase profits.

Since in theory they know this, publicly funded health care systems have displayed more resistance to the suppliers' sales talks than privately funded ones. But even they can be suckers for the latest products. As well, they're often pressured by professionals and the public into buying a new machine or drug protocol as soon as it comes within their means, regardless of whether it has been demonstrated to serve a real purpose in their institutions. In private systems, this tendency is stronger. It has been demonstrated over and over again that private clinics will ignore the normal, widespread medical needs of the populace in order to provide fancy services, like in-vitro fertilization, for a few rich clients.[5] In fact, to an ever-increasing extent, the providers of medical goods have used their growing powers to revert back towards the snake oil salesmen and hucksters of the earliest days of medicine. The only rein on an economically lethal combination of hospitals, doctors, and patients who are lusting for the new and companies whose only motivation is greed has historically been provided by government regulatory bodies and professional and academic institutions. The latter two bodies, by conducting careful scientific research, are supposed to be able to control both desire and greed by ascertaining and pronouncing on both the safety and usefulness of every new drug, procedure, and device. In theory, such assessments enable purchasers to make safe and economically wise decisions.'

Unfortunately, political and economic pressures, traceable to the wealth of medical technology providers, have transformed the functions of these regulatory bodies. Today, both governments and academic institutions see themselves as one of the "engines of the economy." The worst thing they can do from either a political or funding point of view is to hamper the growth of profitable companies developing new technologies with which to "be competitive on the global market" – especially if those companies are providing their institutions with lots of grants or their political parties with contributions. Regulators have also fallen for glamour, glitter, and the immediate rewards of expansive actions and are frequently staffed by a "revolving door" of people who work for the very industries that are being regulated. Although scientific research has helped eliminate many useless treatments and technologies, it has also pushed some of the commercialized treatments that are instrumental in crippling hospital systems today.

ARE CONFLICTS OF INTEREST HAZARDOUS TO OUR HEALTH?

The ... medical school faculties who had once dedicated themselves to raising the scientific and ethical standards of their profession by clearly separating medicine from the marketplace [are] now pushing to tear down the walls dividing academia and business.

Jennifer Washburn[6]

As we saw in earlier chapters, the medical profession struggled valiantly throughout the second half of the 19th century and the beginning of the 20th to establish its members as individuals who were far more altruistic and trustworthy than public servants, teachers, academic experts, government employees, or even scientists. They were right up there with men of the cloth, in fact. Professional bodies such as the AMA and the CMA spent those years sweating over ethics codes. The first, adopted in 1847, affirmed that physicians should not own patents, surgical instruments, or medicines – a restriction that has definitely gone by the wayside and was never very stringently enforced. Subsequent codes instructed members to avoid unnecessary patient visits and forbade fee splitting, financial kickbacks, owning pharmacies, dispensing medical products, or running advertisements.

Members voted to accept these codes at annual conventions. Enforcement usually avoided outright disbarment or any other clear penalties, "leaving it entirely to the discretion of individual physicians whether to abide by them or not," as Jennifer Washburn, author of a recent book investigating academic ethics, explains in a section entitled: "Universities, Medicine and the Market: A Short History." Washburn goes on to say that these rather weak ethics codes had a huge hole that has led to today's worst medical scandals. "Unlike lawyers, public servants, and other professionals who serve as fiduciaries for their clients, the medical establishment never implemented any normative conflict-of-interest standards – an omission that has haunted the profession [ever since]."[7]

As we have seen in the microcosm of the Queen Elizabeth, the halcyon years of the 1940s through the 1970s saw vast increases in efficacy, public trust, and the prestige of any sort of medical institution. But when costs finally ballooned out of control in the 1980s and 90s, governments in all countries slashed budgets, especially to the small community hospitals that had been the lifeblood of the profession in terms of training, research, and medical innovations. Washburn sums up the situation: "Having grown accustomed to an extraordinary degree of autonomy, physicians now found themselves operating in a far more commercial environment, with diminished control over both their professional lives and their medical decisions."[8] This tendency was particularly true in the U.S. following the famous HMO revolution. Doctors all across North America, like those at the Queen E., fought single-payer health care and government control of hospitals tooth and claw. As we have noted subsequent events have shown that they misconstrued who would end up holding the professional power they wished to retain.

It bears repeating that doctors operating in countries such as Canada or France have massive clout as united professional partners in national and state systems. Even though they may feel thwarted at times, they actually retain more control over their professional and treatment decisions, as well as over patient relations and even, to some degree, their benefits and salaries, than do their counterparts working in fully private systems. In the U.S., most doctors, especially in hospitals, are nothing more than employees of one or another of the extremely powerful health corporations. Because there are many such corporations, each doctor is relatively isolated in her or his unique situation and never enjoys the power of physicians represented by a union that negotiates with only one entity – the government. And unlike a government, a business corporation organized to be profitable is not required to take arguments involving professional quality or the state of public health very seriously.

Even in Canada, however, economic and privatization pressures on the health system have resulted in many physicians responding to a medical landscape of less money and less control by, as Washburn puts it, "becoming more entrepreneurial themselves." Today it is common, even in countries with national health programs, to find doctors "investing in an array of health care businesses, including diagnostic laboratories, dialysis units, free-standing surgical centers [especially for orthopedics], nursing homes, and hospital chains." – To say nothing of drug companies.[9]

As early as 1980, Arnold Relman, the editor-in-chief of the *New England Journal of Medicine*, warned of a new "*medical-industrial complex*" that has come to wield remarkable power over the public health, even in countries like Canada that have single-payer systems. Washburn says that Relman was worried about the same things that concerned doctors like Harold Griffith and inspired them to found professional organizations in the first place – namely, that "physicians' direct financial stake in health care businesses would destroy the public's trust in the medical profession and the doctor's ability to serve patients as an 'honest, disinterested trustee.'" Relman was pointing out that, as we have seen throughout this book, "health care services [are] not like other market commodities." For one thing, patients lack the education to confidently assess medical matters. This "informational inequality" makes patients highly dependent on the doctor for unbiased medical advice. As well, other market actions such as "shopping around" for cheaper or safer hospitals or surgical procedures are rarely an option for a sick person.[10]

Today, many doctors, even in Canada, are working as the paid partners of this medical-industrial complex. When medical professionals try to go against the prevailing economic interests, they can lose their grants, reputations, professional autonomy, and their jobs, especially within academia. There are too many examples of this growing tendency for an exhaustive list and more are accruing every year. One of the best known stories in Canada, however, is how David Healy, a respected Welsh psychiatrist, was hired in the year 2000 as the director of the Mood Disorders Program at the University of Toronto. He was then fired almost immediately, right after he delivered a lecture on the history of psychopharmacology in which he voiced concerns about the mounting cases of suicides associated with the use of antidepressants. Although the university did not admit why Healy was suddenly not, as they put it, "a good fit," the same firing email mentioned "your recent appearance ... in the context of an academic lecture." The University of Toronto had just received a $1.5 million gift from Eli Lilly, the manufacturer of Prozac. And in fact, as a whole *was receiving the majority of its funding from corporate sources.* Apparently so much money was at stake that the University found it worth its while to settle a $9.4 million lawsuit filed by Healy for violating his academic freedom.[11]

The University of Toronto, as any Canadian knows, is one of the most important and prestigious academic institutions in the country. It's arguably the most respected in terms of medical research. But another medical professor there, Nancy Oliveri, was another victim of corporate censorship. In 1995, Oliveri was working on a medication called deferiprone, which is used in the treatment of thalassemia, a genetic blood disorder that afflicts millions of people worldwide. At first she had favourable results in her study but, as the clinical trials progressed, "she found disturbing evidence that the agent was frequently ineffective and possibly even harmful." Oliveri felt she should notify the patients who had volunteered for the trial, a normal ethical response for a professional physician. But when she tried to, her sponsor, the generic drug giant Apotex, insisted her interpretation of the data was incorrect. She then approached the Research Ethics Board, a hospital committee that monitors clinical trials; it agreed with her assessment and prepared to send out consent forms to notify the participants. At this point, Apotex terminated Oliveri's research contract and shut down her trials. When they learned she planed to publish the story in the *New England Journal of Medicine,* they threatened to sue her. Despite all this, trials of this possibly dangerous drug were not really terminated. Oliveri's coinvestigator, Gideon Koren, was given even more research funding to complete them. He published favourable assessments of Apotex' deferiprone without disclosing who had given him the money to do so.[12]

It would be nice to hear that the University of Toronto and the Hospital for Sick Children supported Oliveri, who worked for both institutions. In fact, they refused to provide any legal assistance and she was fired from one of her most prestigious positions at the hospital. Oliveri had signed a contract barring disclosure of any of her findings without "the prior written consent of Apotex." This is apparently an increasingly common agreement in the academic field that is intended to effectively prevent any public revelation of negative effects. The National Cancer Institute of Canada and John Hoey, then editor in chief of the *Canadian Medical Association Journal*, were both shocked. "That an internationally renowned children's hospital would have no normal mechanism to scrutinize contracts ... is astounding."[13] John Hoey, the world-respected editor of the once-prestigious *Canadian Medical Association Journal*, the CMAJ, has also had his contract terminated by the periodical's owners, the Canadian Medical Association, for exercising journalistic integrity in exposing a variety of medical system failings. Before he was fired for this and other criticisms in 2005, however, he had uncovered financial discussions between the University and Apotex. They were "part," as the CEO of Apotex later put it, "of a[n] ambitious and generous philanthropic discussion" that could have totaled $55 million in grants for the University of Toronto.[14]

Hoey wrote that despite increasing professional outcries, the Hospital for Sick Children fired Oliveri as director of the Program in Haemoglobinopathy and issued a gag order that prohibited not only her but the entire hospital staff from discussing the case. So many faculty associations and health experts expressed outrage that Robert Pritchard, president of the university, reinstated Oliveri a few weeks later. However, nine months down the road, it was revealed that Prichard had left to become, as the *Toronto Star* put it, "a drug lobbyist." On behalf of Apotex, he had pressed top government officials – including then-Prime Minister Jean Chrètien – to change Canada's drug patent regulations in the drug companies' favour. Pritchard explained that he was afraid new regulations would affect the company's promised $20 million donation to the university's new molecular biology centre.[15] Obviously, situations like these are the talk of the medical community and they send very clear and chilling warnings to any doctor, researcher, or medical journalist who wants to maintain objectivity. They can follow Hoey, Oliveri, and Healy's lead and lose their jobs and their grants or they can comply with funders' demands, as Pritchard and Gideon Koren seem to have done, and risk nothing worse than some public disapproval, assuming anyone ever notices.

Such cases are not abstract problems for doctors alone. Even back in the 19th century, the pioneers of medical professionalism realized that this kind of commercialization of medicine would result first in a public body count, and second in the steady weakening of the social contract between sick people and their health providers. That is why they worked so hard to try to convince the public that doctors are above the normal temptations and influences of business or political life. Physicians are still rated as having more honour and altruism than any other professional group except firemen. In fact, given the utter dependence of sick people on that honour, if patients don't trust their doctors almost implicitly, the system could hardly work at all. But today there are increasing numbers of horror stories of gatekeeper doctors in HMOs sacrificing patients' lives to save a little money, and worse yet, medical researchers who subject people to worthless or dangerous treatments – also in exchange for money.

It's said that Nancy Oliveri's experience was part of the inspiration for the blockbuster book and movie by John Le Carre, *The Constant Gardener.*[16] In many other countries, most notably the U.S., doctors and researchers are also succumbing to the virus of greed. In the middle 1990s, for example, Rezulin, a diabetes drug made by Warner-Lambert, was suspected of causing liver failure deaths. The FDA, the U.S. government drug watchdog, whose pronouncements are generally echoed by Health Canada, entrusted a panel of doctors and university scientists to look into these charges, despite the fact that they knew that *every single one of the panel members had financial ties to the company making the drug.* In 1997, there had been an estimated 28 deaths and Rezulin had already been banned in Britain, but the U.S. panel gave the drug their professional blessing. It was three more years and an estimated 363 more deaths before the FDA reluctantly joined the ban.[17] Such conflict of interest controversies are affecting ever-larger organizations and more of the basic research that informs a great deal of medical treatment. This trend is disturbing on every level. Each of the 391 people who died from Rezulin had a life and a family and, prior to the falsification of data that encouraged Rezulin treatment, relatively long futures ahead of them. Simply put, ethical failures in the medical research community kill people.

The two drug families most recently associated with increasingly long trails of bodies are the anti-depressants termed SSRIs, "selective serotonin reuptake inhibitors" such as Zoloft, Paxil, and Prozac, and the NSAIDs, "non-steroidal anti-inflammatory drugs" such as Celebrex, Vioxx, Naproxen, and Motrin. As we've seen in evening news stories about both of these commercial medical compounds, it seems that government agencies finally enact their half-hearted bans only after a remarkable cohort of families have undergone needless tragedies and also only after the medical researchers, doctors, and companies involved have been permitted years of denials and stalling tactics.

To put the afore-mentioned case of dismissing Healy from teaching at the University of Toronto into a broader context, it is now known that Paxil, Prozac, and other anti-depressants of the same type were originally developed for adults but began to be aggressively marketed to children and adolescents following an influential study published in *Child and Adolescent Psychiatry* in 2002. The study's chief author, Martin B. Keller, the respected chair of the psychiatry department of Brown University, virtually raved about Paxil's "safety and efficacy ... in the treatment of adolescent depression." This testimonial led to much wider use of the drug, especially for boys under twelve "with conduct disorders." More than eleven million prescriptions had been handed out by the end of that year. But subsequent investigators in the FDA found no data in the study trials that actually supported the claim in Keller's article. In fact, "seven of the children who took Paxil had to be hospitalized" due to adverse effects Keller described as "not serious." Subsequently, a closer look at other studies available to the FDA, as well as an increasing number of suspicious deaths and parental complaints, revealed that these drugs "increased thoughts of suicide," especially in young patients, by at least two to three times. To make matters worse, "in all but three of those studies, young patients suffering from depression experienced no greater improvement taking an SSRI, like Prozac and Zoloft, than they did with a placebo, or sugar pill."[18]

In other words, a drug was being prescribed to millions of helpless children that, at best, had no effect and, at worst, resulted in a self-destructive or dead child. Because suicides are a tricky thing to link directly to a medication, the companies involved were able to resist investigation. Even so, by 2004, New York attorney general Eliot Spitzer filed suit against GlaxoSmithKline (GSK), the makers of Paxil, for fraud in misrepresenting or burying this data. Even at this point, "nearly all the published literature, authored by many of the leading lights of academic psychiatry, had arrived at the opposite conclusion: SSRIs were safe and effective in treating depression in youngsters."[19]

The public expects an uninvestigated and unregulated profit-making entity such as GlaxoSmithKline to try to hide financially damaging data to some extent. What seriously alarms researchers and the public is the proof that hospitals, universities, doctors, and medical researchers are often doing the same thing. In too many cases, the medical community, at its highest levels, is colluding with moneyed interests. As far back as 1998, the influential Dr. Keller had been found to have received "more than half a million dollars from drug companies," most of it from the same firms whose products he had favourably reviewed in his many journal articles and speeches at medical conferences. This did not prevent the medical community from trusting him.

Jennifer Washburn, author of *University, Inc.*, says, "It is indeed impossible to prove a direct causal relationship between Keller's funding sources and the distortions found in his research." But it isn't that hard to think of four words that unequivocally apply to the whole situation. They are: "professional conflict of interest." In fact, as early as 1999, the *Boston Globe* reported that the National Institute of Mental Health decided to review its conflict-of-interest rules after seeing how many financial ties important researchers had to companies whose products they were entrusted with assessing.[20] The NIMH's concern doesn't seem to have had much effect. Four years later, in 2003, Dr. Keller was still consulting for seventeen major drug firms while enjoying a $25 million grant from Wyeth-Ayerst, and he was still writing influential papers assessing drugs made by these companies.[21] It is obvious that if the regulators and the medical profession itself want to retain public confidence, the old AMA/CMA rule of "voluntary guidelines" for professional standards have to include some real punishments, such as expulsion, probation, or disbarment. Very large fines wouldn't hurt, either.

It's also clear that while it's certainly true that some medical professionals are being corrupted by the drug industry, most of them are simply too busy to investigate company claims. They simply go along with the general trend. And, just as often, they're probably tricked. NSAIDs and "cox–2 inhibitors" originally came on the market as relief for arthritis sufferers who require regular doses of painkillers such as aspirin to cope with their conditions but whose stomachs cannot take the compounds' side-effects. Drugs such as aspirin, ibuprofen, or Motrin can cause pain, ulcers, and even fatal perforations. The new cox–2 family was supposed to bypass all these problems and was widely hailed as a break-through and even more widely prescribed. From a public hospital's point of view, it has been a very expensive experiment; increasing numbers of people have had to come into tertiary care for internal bleeding, strokes, and heart attacks. In an era of evidence-based medicine, one has to question how this drug, which causes precisely the side-effect it claims to avoid, came to be prescribed so frequently.

Dr Michael Wolfe, a gastroenterologist at Boston University, is one of the few medical professionals to have gone public about this class of drugs. He testified that he was duped by Pharmacia, the maker of Celebrex, into believing that their new drug was associated with lower rates of stomach and intestinal complications. Wolfe was given a study by the company that was supposed to have tracked 8,000 patients for six months. The numbers were quite persuasive, so he wrote a favourable review that was one of several that helped drive up sales of what would become a blockbuster drug. However, a year later, when serving on the FDA's arthritis advisory committee, he was shocked to discover that Pharmacia's study had run not just for six months, as he had been told, but for a whole year. When the later data was included, Celebrex's advantages over previous drugs such as ibuprofen disappeared, because patients developed complications with Celebrex the longer they used it. Its inefficacy at doing what it claimed to do, that is, avoid stomach distress, was only the tip of the iceberg. Within a few more years, evidence was amassing that Celebrex and Vioxx were implicated in the sudden deaths of literally hundreds of thousands of people due to heart attacks and strokes.[22] To date, only one of these drugs, Vioxx, is off the market. Celebrex has started a media blitz to point out that it is still available, as are some very close relatives, Motrin and the humble ibuprophen.

What does all this mean to the state of hospital care we experience? Anyone who has gone to a doctor or who has been hospitalized for, say, arthritis problems over the last eight years or so was given care that in all likelihood included a prescription for an NSAID. If the problem was depression, the patient received advice and very likely a prescription for an SSRI. In a system like Canada's, the ensuing medical crises, such as suicide attempts for the latter and bleeding ulcers, heart attacks, and strokes for the former, are paid for by taxpayers when the patients present themselves in hospital ERs. Unbiased, scientific assessment of drugs is therefore of major concern to any public health system and to any hospital's bottom line – quite apart from the suffering and tragedy it can bring to the patient. Add this to the fact that because of our current systems, which concentrate on specialist rather than generalist care, the rhumatologist who gave the patient the NSAID prescription for arthritis is unlikely to consult with the gastro-enterologist who managed the person's care in the hospital or the cardiologist who saw her die. The rheumatologist will probably never even find out about the adverse reaction. And so fatal mistakes will continue to proliferate.

THE ADVANCEMENT OF MEDICINE

The *Times* uncovered numerous cases in which doctors relaxed eligibility criteria for patient enrollment in trials, fabricated data, and handed off their professional responsibilities to untrained nurses and staff. In once case, bodily fluids that met certain lab values were stored [and] ... substituted for the urine or blood for patients who did not qualify for studies.

Jennifer Washburn[23]

"Let me congratulate you and your writer ... Perhaps I can get you to write all my papers for me!"

letter from Richard Atkinson, obesity expert at the University of Wisconsin, whose name appeared on a company-authored article supporting the now-banned diet drug Redux.[24]

However hospital or research costs are paid, doctors and patients base their decisions to use a particular drug or therapy on government recommendations, which in turn are based on articles published in the professional journals, which in turn are based on clinical trials like the ones mentioned above. And we are learning that clinical trials, on which the whole system depends, are frequently manipulated by people with a financial stake in the outcome. John Abrahamson of the Harvard Medical School charges that there's been a virtual takeover of medical knowledge by the pharmaceutical industry, even at the highest levels – the professional journals and government guidelines. A recent CBC radio series on *Ideas* recounts that he began to distrust the quality of information required to guide him in his work as a doctor and decided to research the situation. He discovered that, like the clinical trials themselves, "Seventy percent of the clinical trials that are published in even our best, most respected journals are funded by the drug companies." That number is now pegged at at least 80 percent.[25]

Abrahamson says we expect the editors of these journals "to be able to discern whether articles are accurately representing the data from the study and drawing appropriate conclusions." But in fact, they can't. "Not only do the editors and the peer reviewers of these major journals not get all the data to look at to see if it's been accurately represented; but many times the authors of those articles don't even get to see all of the data from *their own studies*. The drug companies actually parcel out the data so that sometimes only one and sometimes *no* authors have had free access to all the data." This is the practice that fooled Michael Wolfe, mentioned above, who subsequently had the rare bravery to go public and admit how he was tricked. Dr. Abrahamson adds, "I think that many of the articles serve the same social function as infomercials. Their purpose is to sell product, not to improve our health."[26] The money the industry is now having to pay in lawsuits creates a slight disincentive, but it's not much compared to disbursements like the $41 million the drug industry spent to get candidates open to their needs elected in the 2002 U.S. election. Spending their profits this way helps companies control legislation so they won't be held responsible in the first place, and riders such as the one on the Homeland Security Bill described just ahead have become commonplace.

The sad fact is that the pharmaceutical industry doesn't just have friends in high places – it is often entrusted with policing itself. After the recent George W. Bush Medicare bill that forbade the government from even attempting to negotiate prices with the big pharmacological companies was passed, the accredited "principal author" of the bill, Republican Congressman William Tauzin, immediately resigned his seat to become CEO of PhRMA, the Pharmaceutical Research and Manufacturers of America, the industry's political action committee. "In his new home, Tauzin is paid roughly $2 million a year in salary, perks and benefits," says Eric Lotke of the Institute for America's Future in a recent article that gives many other examples of the political/industry "revolving door" that operates in both directions. "The nation's capitol is awash in drug money," he charges.[27]

One can only imagine how eager such groups would be to fund efforts to privatize hospital and medical care in Canada and to influence how a large public system uses its products. The recent complete refiguring of the Canada Health Act uses language that makes it clear that the federal government now considers the drug industry to be its "client," rather than the citizens, who are now referred to as "consumers" of the Health Canada/drug industry product.[28] To illustrate how far Health Canada has strayed from its original, protective purpose, there's the recent evidence of how it treats its own scientists. As we saw earlier, just because medical researchers have figured out how to keep people healthy doesn't mean they have the political power or backing to do so. That's the job of public health departments, whose status in Canada has become increasingly vague and compromised. Failures on the part of public health systems fill hospitals and vastly increase the costs of health care.

When Quebec ignored its own public health guidelines about water and milk in the 1920s, cases of typhoid and typhus flooded the hospitals. In fact, they did so also because of industry resistance to government interference – in this case, a big Montreal dairy that killed thousands of people before its filthy holding tanks were finally unmasked by a municipal government that had been reluctant to antagonize it.[29] The same rules apply today; when the public finally demands it, public health systems will attack an individual industry. Yet the regulations that could help prevent many other emerging and returning diseases are considerably weakened by increasingly fuzzy professional standards, as well as the contamination of all levels of medical research by industry money.

For example, three Health Canada scientists warned in 1998 of the dangers of the genetically engineered growth hormone rGBH, that increases milk production in dairy cows. They also exposed an attempt by a life sciences company closely allied with pharmaceuticals, Monsanto, to bribe that drug's way into Canada. Their criticisms led to a Senate inquiry and a decision not to approve the drug. Canadians, like the Europeans who also banned this drug because of animal cruelty and its connection with human illnesses, felt smug. Then, during the anthrax scare after 9–11, Shiv Chopra, one of the four original whistleblowers on rGBH, criticized then-Health Minister Allan Rock for spending millions to stockpile antibiotics, "saying the fear of bioterrorism was overblown," which it turned out to be. In 2003, Chopra and his colleague Margaret Haydon again went to the public to warn that, "measures to prevent mad cow disease were inadequate." Canadians are well aware of the disastrous effects on the beef industry when the federal government ignored this last warning. Instead of promotions for being right in three high-profile cases, Health Canada initiated disciplinary proceedings against the scientists, "who in turn filed grievances in a complicated tangle of cases, most of which they have won." So Health Canada fired them.[30]

Ever vigilant to society's well-being, Shiv Chopra has said that although he applauds his union's support in getting his job back, "the grievance appeal process will only deal with the technical and legal aspects of the department's action." He says that the substance of the issue, the part of greatest concern to health and hospital care costs, will be left out: the ability of the powerful food and pharmaceutical lobbies to pressure Ottawa to bypass scientific concerns about the introduction of suspected cancer-causing hormones and the excessive use of antibiotics in animals." The sub-therapeutic use of antibiotics, not to cure meat animals of infections but to create an artificial appetite so they will continue to eat in overcrowded conditions, has been singled out by the Canadian Medical Association as the primary reason why antibiotics are declining in effectiveness. In an ominous return to 19th-century conditions, we all now face new fears of dying in hospital from antibiotic-resistant infections like *C. difficile* and MRSA. The normally very conservative CMA has called for a full moratorium on industrial farming, especially of hogs, for this reason. They are seeing more and more common infections that cannot be treated with our current drug arsenal as well as "super-bugs" like *C. difficile*, vancomydin-resistant *enterococcus* or VRE, methicillin-resistant *Staphylococcus aureus* or MRSA, *Pseudomonas, candidiasis*, or *Legionella*, better known as Legionnaire's Disease, all of which add to the expensive worries that afflict modern hospitals.

CAVEATS

Medicine has no choice but to deal with Big Pharma ... nobody wants it to go away. But clearly [it] must be better regulated."

Arthur Caplan[31]

When Arthur Caplan, chair of the Department of Medical Ethics of the University of Pennsylvania School of Medicine, reviewed three recent books that vehemently attack the industry colloquially known as "Big Pharma," he argued that, despite its greed and power, the pharmaceutical industry is not "inherently evil." Even if, he added, "its products may sometimes be sold at bloated prices and ... some of those products may even turn out to be dangerous or ineffective." Many of the drugs manufactured by the big pharmaceutical are beneficial, even necessary to people's survival. We would all probably agree with Caplan that, "Medicine has no choice" except to deal with these companies.[32] It's also important to emphasize that most drugs and procedures used in Canada are both safe and effective. The large majority of sick people will come out of hospital or physician care in better shape than when they went in. To hark back to what Harold Griffith once said, it really is nothing short of miraculous that so many people, machines, and treatments are waiting, twenty-four hours a day, in all of our hospitals, to try to save our lives and alleviate our pain. But it's also important to recognize that the increasing economic bias of both the FDA and Health Canada can actually sicken or kill a significant percentage of the citizens that look to both bodies for protection. We all need to get more concerned about the fact that both of these government agencies approved a drug like Vioxx, which is now implicated in causing 100,000 mostly fatal heart attacks or strokes in the U.S. and another 10,000 in Canada, and that both were extremely slow in banning it.

Evidence shows that the FDA and Health Canada were actually "aware of the increased risk of cardiovascular adverse events long before the drug was withdrawn from the market. There is also evidence that the manufacturer (Merck) tried to play down the risk in its promotional material for doctors." This drug was recently being prescribed to arthritis sufferers with the same confidence that all forms of statins (cholesterol-reducing drugs) are today. Vioxx is a slightly stronger version of all the other NSAIDs still on the market but so far, the other brand names' connections with increased morbidity have not been investigated. The *Canadian Medical Association Journal* chastised both regulators for "putting their resources into assessing drug *benefits*, not harms ... [T]he built-in bias toward approving drugs without adequate assurance of their safety is a fundamental and (often literally) fatal flaw ... The current FDA/Health Canada emphasis on partnerships with industry and rapid drug approval conflicts with the public's expectation that these agencies exist to protect them."[33]

Today, the Canadian government is not moving to solve such problems. Instead, there is a move to actually scrap the Canada Food and Drug Act and replace it with something dubbed "Smart Regulation." This is a part of SPP or the "Security and Prosperity Partnership" trade agreement brought in under the George W. Bush, Paul Martin, and Stephen Harper governments. In the interests of "trade and security," these legislative changes are intended to "harmonize" Canadian health services, environmental protections, and foreign policy, even in terms of who is allowed to enter the country. Its health pilot program, the aptly named "Therapeutics Access Strategy," is described as "market-oriented and industry-friendly" by the Canadian Health Coalition, a non-profit research group trying to analyze trends and offer policy advice on health matters. With so many lives at stake, so much money being poured into health care systems, and so much pressure to privatize, Canadians must pay more attention to conflicts of interest in government and regulators as well as in doctors, hospitals, educators, and the medical sector in general.[34]

TREATING THE PATHOLOGY

Meaningful reform might include ending the industry's patent
extension tricks, licensing drugs developed with public monies on a
nonexclusive basis to permit price-reducing competition ... and
considering rollbacks to the 20-year patent term and the adoption of
price controls.

Russell Mokhiber and Robert Weissman[35]

The first thing we need to realize about drugs and equipment is that once any medical drug is developed, no matter how complex or life-saving, it is cheap to manufacture. The expense lies in the research, which is why patents giving pharmaceutical companies exclusive right of sale are awarded. The industry says this is the only way they have of making back their research and development investment, which they describe as being, on average, $800 million per drug. This is obviously an amount so crippling that no company would ever develop a new drug again if their patents were to be infringed. Although this does make sense in a general way, at least to those outside the industry, insiders have been taking issue with this system and objecting to the amount of money the companies claim the whole process requires. Many hospitals and public health systems in the world demand their doctors use generic medicines – those that are off-patent – when possible. But the pharmaceutical companies fight even that small brake on costs.

Dr Marcia Angell, in a recent *New York Times* article says, "Only a handful of truly important drugs have been brought to market in recent years, and they were mostly based on taxpayer-funded research at academic institutions, small biotechnology companies, or the National Institutes of Health."[36] Angell, former editor of the *New England Journal of Medicine* and author of one of many new books skewering the pharmaceutical industry, *The Truth About the Drug Companies*, suggests we take the case of Taxol, "the bestselling cancer drug in history," which is used to treat cancers of the ovary, breast, and lung.

The initial idea for using the bark of the Pacific yew tree as a cancer therapy came from the ancient practices of Native American groups on the West coast. They did not benefit in any way from the commercialization of their medicine. The taxpayer-funded National Cancer Institute (NCI) worked on the components of the yew tree for more than thirty years, at a cost to American taxpayers of $183 million, although they didn't benefit much either. In 1991, Angell says, the drug giant Bristol-Myers Squibb signed a "cooperative research and development agreement" with the NCI, made possible by new legislation called the Federal Technology Transfer Act that was voted in under Ronald Reagan. Bristol-Myers Squibb's part of the deal was to provide NCI with 17 kilograms of paclitaxel, the active compound in the tree, which it got from a chemical company. "In 1992, after Taxol was approved by the FDA for treatment of cancer of the ovary, entirely on the basis of the publicly supported research, Bristol-Myers Squibb was given five years of exclusive marketing rights." Then publicly funded scientists at Florida State University devised a method to synthesize Taxol, "which they promptly licensed to Bristol-Myers Squibb in return for royalties. No company ingenuity [or monetary investment] there," Angell remarks. [37]

Worldwide, the sale of Taxol has generated between one and two billion dollars each year since 1994 for Bristol-Myers Squibb as well as tens of millions in annual royalties to Florida State. Those are the profits. As for the cost of this medicine, *each woman suffering from breast or ovarian cancer (or her insurance company) has to come up with between $10,000 to $20,000 per year for the treatment.*" [Bristol-Myers Squibb] ... has undoubtedly spent substantial sums since then to test the drug for other cancers. But that takes no ingenuity, either." The U.S. government, which funded the research that made the drug possible, has also spent "hundreds of millions of dollars [to buy] Taxol through the Medicare program." "The story of Taxol," Angell concludes, "is a prime example of a taxpayer-supported research discovering a valuable and lucrative drug that was virtually given as a gift to a large drug company for marketing, commercial exploitation, and further development. The public pays again when it buys Taxol at the exorbitant price Bristol-Myers Squibb [charges for a drug] it neither discovered nor developed."[38]

The U.S.-based Pfizer is rated as the largest drug company in the world. Hank McKinnell, the current CEO of Pfizer, has written a book in which he admits that the patent protections demanded by such companies on the basis of their research and development expenses are completely fallacious: "high ... drug prices have nothing to do with past R&D expenses."[39] Later he also states, "It's a fallacy to suggest that our industry, or any industry, prices a product to recapture the R&D budget spent in development." Yet that's the basis on which patents are granted and is also the excuse given for costs of more than $15,000 to $30,000 per year, per patient, for cancer-inhibiting drugs or antivirals such as AVIS (anti-viral compounds). Those same drugs can be manufactured and sold at a profit by a generic company for a fraction of the cost, say around $200 a year.[40]

Z Magazine, a left-of-centre source with a bit of an ax to grind, has provided a list of the board of directors of another American pharmacological giant, Eli Lilly. Lilly's current and recent board members include the former president of the United States, George Bush senior. Mitch Daniels, George W. Bush's director of Management and Budget, used to be vice president of Lilly, and Sidney Taurel, the current CEO of this company, was named to be on Bush Jr's Homeland Security Advisory Council in June of 2002. In November of that year, *New York Times* columnist Bob Herbert discovered a provision, "buried in this massive bill," the new 2002 Homeland Security Act, "that – incredibly – will protect Eli Lilly and a few other big pharmaceutical outfits from lawsuits by parents who believe their children were harmed by thimerosal," the mercury-based preservative used in many children's vaccines that is increasingly associated with neurological problems, including the epidemic of autism and syndromes like ADHD.

This rider was so markedly unrelated to military security that "even some Republican senators became embarrassed" and in 2003, "moderate Republicans and Democrats agreed to repeal this particular provision in the Homeland Security Act." Just to complete the picture, Ken Lay, the infamous CEO of Enron, was also a member of the Eli Lilly Board.[41] This single company's most profitable product, Zyprexa, an antipsychotic drug now in disrepute for causing diabetes in some patients, grossed $4.28 billion U.S. in 2003. Lilly's second most successful product line – the components of which all happen to be diabetes treatment drugs, including Actos, Humulin, and Humalog, collectively grossed another $2.51 billion the same year. These are just some of the products and part of the influence of a single pharmaceutical company. Worldwide, this industry is estimated to gross no less than $400 billion every year and is more profitable than any other industry, including oil, arms, and banks. Such figures make it clear why the drug corporations have become a collective political force all over the planet and are perfectly capable of influencing legislation and regulations, manipulating academic research, and clouding such serious sci-

entific issues as medical drug efficacy. It also explains the proliferation
of what are termed "me-too" drugs, that is, new and sometimes more
dangerous or less effective versions of a current drug whose patent has
run out. Such introductions make it even harder for patients in many
countries to access generic versions of even quite old medical drugs.[42]

MARCUS WELBY BECOMES ALAN GREENSPAN

> because of the vital importance of health, consumers are disinclined to
> argue about its price.
>
> Christine Cassel[43]

As in most hospitals of the 1920s and 30s, in Harold Griffith's early
days at the Homeopathic/Queen Elizabeth, he and his friends, working out of hospitals and universities, together with fledgling chemical
and drug concerns, rigged up their own medicines and treatment
delivery systems in basements or the family garage. In the middle, halcyon years, the newly active drug companies were welcomed to present
their products in hospitals, as they did at the Homeopathic's stimulating teaching lunches. By the late 1970s, when Harold retired, the pharmaceutical companies themselves were paying for nearly all these
educational lunches, helping doctors attend important conferences,
and whisking them off to Hawaii and Europe for increasingly luxurious
research and networking trips. This industry began by giving doctors
grants to investigate their products with the unspoken understanding
that the recipients would at least try to find if the product was useful.
Inexorably, by the 1990s, business interests were paying physicians to
"oversee" research papers on new drugs that in many cases they did not
even have to bother to read and enlisting them as assumed collabora-
tors in every new drug offering.

Fortunately, some doctors realize that they have been used as the
delivery arm of a vast sales machine that they have no means of investigating or regulating. As Arthur Caplan puts it, instead of regarding the
drug industry as a scientific godsend, there is an increasing amount of
"moral opprobrium" directed at this influence today, from within as
well as without the medical profession. Many medical professionals are
aware of the industry's "legions of lobbyists, the politicians awash in its
campaign contributions, and the doctors it has bought, free meal by
free meal, junket by junket, free sample by free sample, and trinket by
trinket." Today, increasingly informed doctors, including Montrealers

John Hughes and Michael Sonea, have banned pharma reps from their offices. But many more have become cogs in the big chemical industry wheel, too overwhelmed with work to look into the details of every government or industry recommendation. It's a sad but understandable fact that most physicians find themselves rushing through their patient overload by simply dispensing the latest, greatest drug to a public more prone to consult their television set or computer than their busy doctor.

Canada's health system has a lot to lose in this equation. Drug companies are known to be using their economic and political clout to encourage private or mixed-funded health care systems rather than single-payer ones like Canada's. They have a good reason to do so. Arthur Caplan points out that, "data in [all the] books [attacking the industry]" show that "in the United States, patented, brand-name drugs sell on average for 80 percent more than in Canada and 100 percent more than in France or Italy."[44] This is simply because a national health system is such an enormous buyer that they are in a position to get better prices, even from the most powerful drug companies, than are isolated private hospitals, insurance groups, or HMOs.

The larger medical insurance companies and some local governments in the U.S. are beginning "to push back against drug costs," also bargaining for discounts. But the industry is one step ahead. "It fought the state of Maine all the way to the Supreme Court, which in 2003 upheld Maine's right to bargain with drug companies for lower prices." George W. Bush's Medicare Prescription Drug Benefit Act that came into effect in 2006 has a staggering constraint. Arthur Caplan says this is a "windfall for Big Pharma ... [because] it *forbids the government from negotiating prices.*" Canada could easily find itself in this position if the move towards privatization and segmentation of the health system continues, not to mention its attempts to "harmonize" its regulatory bodies with the U.S. for "trade and security reasons."[45]

Such machinations have effects on patients and on medical costs and have a great influence on the future of public health in general. Dr. Ashley Wazana of McGill University wrote a seminal article in the *Journal of the American Medical Association* back in 2000 showing that such sweeping corruption and collusion starts with innocent and altruistic students at the most mundane levels of education. Industries understand that people simply don't want to bite the hand that feeds them. In "Physicians and the Pharmaceutical Industry: Is a Gift Ever Just a Gift?" he conducted his own scientific, statistical study, noting that most medical schools "generally endorse" remarkable closeness between doctors in training and their pharmaceutical sponsors and marketing representatives. The young physicians' interactions with drug corporation salespeople "begin in medical school and continue at a rate of about *four times a month*." Anyone related to a doctor knows their extended family is lucky to see them that often. Despite subjective insistence by the doctors that their behavior was "not influenced by gifts," tabulation between interfaces with the companies and the doctors' reactions tells a different story.

"Meetings with pharmaceutical representatives were associated with requests by physicians for adding the drugs to the hospital formulary and changes in prescribing practice. Drug company-sponsored Continuing Medical Education (CME) preferentially highlighted the sponsor's drugs compared with other CME programs. Attending sponsored CME events and accepting funding for travel or lodging for educational symposia were associated with increased prescription rates of the sponsor's medication. Attending presentations given by pharmaceutical representative speakers was also associated with [this] non-rational prescribing." Wazana concluded that, "The present extent of physician-industry interactions appears to affect prescribing and professional behavior and should be further addressed at the level of policy and education."[46]

This kind of calculated erosion of professional judgment by the manipulation of normal human reactions has extended into the next level of oversight: regulatory bodies like the FDA and Health Canada. Citizens assume that these agencies make sure that dangerous, overpriced, or ineffective drugs and technologies don't become part of our tax-supported health systems. In fact, "The FDA and its Canadian and European counterparts can demand only that pharmaceutical companies provide data to show that drugs are efficacious." The producers obviously have a vested interest to demonstrate safety and efficacy and downplay dangers and side-effects, and their studies are routinely pressed into that service. Most citizens are innocent of the almost universal fact that few government regulatory agencies ever test drugs and chemicals themselves.

The pharmaceutical companies are not even required to prove their products are effective, that is, "that they will work not only in closely monitored clinical trials but also in the real world under a variety of conditions." This explains how drugs such as Vioxx, DES, and Thalidomide end up killing or crippling thousands of people. "Nor," says

Arthur Caplan, summarizing a sad situation, "is there any systematic, independent source of evidence about the comparative value of drugs and medical technologies ... Head-to-head trials comparing a drug with a rival company's similar product or generic version are almost non-existent."[47]

When such studies are conducted, they have tended to show that the "new, improved," i.e., more expensive re-patented version, is no better than the old drugs that the reps are downplaying to their physician customers. And, when large numbers of people complain, belated studies have revealed that the drug companies always knew or at least suspected that Vioxx, breast implants, growth hormones, or even Prozac for teenagers were dangerous because of warning signs in their own data that were downplayed or actively suppressed.

The Bush government moved to lower standards and limit liability for drug companies in the United States, and the Martin Liberals, followed quickly by the Harper Conservatives, have worked whenever possible to bring Canada's national health and environmental standards down to match the Americans'. When it comes to one of the most popular of whiz-bang medical technologies, for example, genetic engineering, whether applied to "novel" food, gene therapy, bio-pharmaceuticals, reproductive technology, zeno- (animal organ) transplantation, cloning, or life patenting, the Canadian Health Coalition states, "No evidence of safety will be required and current legal duties to protect health (in the Food & Drugs Act) will be gutted. The objective is to create a 'competitive advantage' for these industries by means of weaker safety standards."[48]

There has been one Oscar-nominated movie, *The Constant Gardener*, several documentaries, including *Sicko* and *Big Bucks, Big Pharma*, as well as a flock of books crowding the nonfiction charts that deal with the subject of pharmaceutical company malfeasance. They have provocative titles, such as: *Big Pharma: How Modern Medicine Is Damaging Your Health*; *On the Take: How Medicine's Complicity with Big Business Can Endanger Your Health*; *Big Bucks, Big Pharma: Marketing Diseases, Pushing Drugs*. Another is called *The Big Fix: How the Pharmaceutical Industry Rips Off American Consumers*, and also, *Powerful Medicines: The Benefits, Risks and Costs of Prescription Drugs; Big Pharma*; and, of course, *The Truth about the Drug Companies: How They Deceive Us and What To Do about It*. The authors are, respectively, Jackie Law, Jerome P. Kassirer, ed. Ronit Ridburg, Katherine Greider, Jerry Avorn, John Prieve, and Marcia Angell. Most of these books were written by insiders from the medical profession. Jerome P. Kassirer, who wrote *On the Take*, teaches medicine at Tufts University, and Jerry Avorn of *Powerful Medicines* is a Harvard physician and pharmaepidemiologist. Marcia Angell teaches at the Harvard Medical School and is a former editor of the prestigious *New England Journal of Medicine*. There are also scores of websites and blogs that center around this subject.

This means that even though the advantages of wealth, power, and influence that the cost-side of the health equation has achieved over the consumer side are daunting, there is now increasingly widespread awareness of the seriousness of this influence. Between the 1930s and 1950s, this unfair balance of power was held in check by a variety of means, including a much smaller supply of "miracle drugs" and technological treatments and a lower consumer demand and expectations. One purpose of all the new books, articles, movies, and programs critical of the drug industry is an attempt to counter some of the demand that direct advertising has created with a dose of reality.

THE BEST-SELLING DRUGS OF ALL TIME

When medicine has a business aspect to it and becomes an industry, then what do you do? You try to magnify consumption, and when you have a $1.8 trillion industry, as it is in the United States, then the medical-industrial complex requires everybody to be dying.

Dr. Bernard Lown, cardiologist, author of *The Lost Art of Healing*[49]

Back when the Homeopathic/Queen Elizabeth was young, a continent-wide epidemic of heart disease began. In the 1920s, heart attacks, which had not previously been seen in so many people, became the major cause of death, especially in the male population. To this day, they continue to be so in all of North America, and they are also the primary cause of death for women. At first, people with "bad hearts" were sent to the seaside – or home to die – with prescriptions for bed rest and no excitement. So even when patients managed to survive a few years, quality of life was severely reduced. Thanks to the advances in surgery made possible by better anesthetics after the 1940s, however, it became increasingly possible to do chest and thoracic surgery and to dream of understanding the progress of this disease. Pretty soon, the whole concept of "hardened" or blocked arteries that could be alleviated by surgical intervention was embraced, and even small community hospitals like the Queen E had lively cardiac treatment departments.

Because surgery is always a risk, cardiologists today are leaning heavily in the direction all medicine must take – prevention. The theory of "hardening of the arteries" progressed in the 1970s and 80s towards the idea that cholesterol, a basic protein in the body that measurably increases in heart attack victims, is allied to a fatty diet. "Control the diet," was the first cry, and people across North America – but significantly, not around the world – began to eshew beef and eggs and to gobble up margarine and oatmeal. The second cry, when diet proved not to be very effective, was to reduce the production of cholesterol by the body, and pharmacologists developed a new family of drugs, the statins, to do so.

Drugs like Lipitor, Crestor, Lescol, Zocor and the like are now used by millions of people worldwide to lower blood cholesterol. They are complex drugs that are capable of physically blocking the body's production of cholesterol. Research on the action of cholesterol has continued, however, and cardiologists are now learning that cholesterol is not really some gluey monster hiding in rich foods that exists only to clog up people's arteries, as we have been led to believe. In fact, the body makes cholesterol whether there is any in the diet or not; removing all dietary cholesterol only cuts the blood cholesterol level by 20 to 25 percent. Even many doctors aren't fully aware that, as neurologist Beatrice Golomb says, "About 50 percent of the dry weight of the brain is actually cholesterol ... evolution has mandated that every cell in our body produces it." So controlling the production of a substance so integral to an organism's structure logically becomes a proposition that must carry risks.

Cholesterol's "absolutely pivotal functions in the body ... include delivery of antioxidant vitamins to tissue. It's important for the development of synapses, the nerve connections that allow neurons to communicate with one another. It's the precursor for all the sex hormones, like testosterone and estrogen ... as well as the sugar-regulating hormones." Dr. Golomb adds, "What's surprising is that when we lower cholesterol things [still] work as well as they do."[50]

We're all familiar with the many ads asking healthy, non-smokers, who are generally young students, to submit to drug tests for a weekend or two in exchange for a few thousand dollars. As Bernard Lown, professor emeritus at the Harvard School of Public Health and founder of his own cardiovascular center in Boston, says, "When drugs enter the market now in the United States [and Canada], they've been tested for a year or two in a small subset of highly selected, healthy people. You exclude those who've had strokes, those who have severe heart disease, those who have diabetes ... and then you give them a pill, and nothing happens. And then you launch it in the community of everybody," including older and sicker people, and for a much longer time. In many cases, the side-effects from new, complex drugs like statins do not manifest in this larger population for five or six years or even longer. It apparently can take quite awhile for a drug that alters the production of vital cell and hormone components to express itself.[51]

Now just to keep things straight, as another cardiologist, Jim Wright, professor in the Department of Pharmacology, Therapeutics, and Medicine at the University of British Columbia, says, "These drugs are clearly useful and should be prescribed to people who have had *proven* coronary heart disease, which means they have had a heart attack or they have angina, plus proven cerebral-vascular disease, which means they've had a stroke ... or proven peripheral vascular disease, which means they have obstruction of the arteries to the legs. And in that setting, the benefits clearly outweigh the harms." However, "in the people who've never had an event, the benefits are extremely small, and *they may not outweigh the harms.*"[52] Dr. Colin Rose, a cardiologist at McGill, agrees. "I can show you lots of patients with a blood cholesterol level of 4 who've had heart attacks. I can show you patients with a cholesterol level of 10 who've never had a heart attack. What you measure in the blood has almost no connection with what's going on in the wall of the artery."[53]

In fact, many studies, including one undertaken by Dr. Dariesh Mozaffarian of the Harvard School of Public Health and published in November of 2005 in the *American Journal of Clinical Nutrition*, have found that high blood cholesterol can actually be good for you, especially if you're an older woman! The Harvard study found that 235 post-menopausal women at high risk of heart disease, as physically measured by coronary angiography, had *less* progression of their disease the *higher* their saturated fat intake got. "We also found," says Dr. Mozaffarian, "that the higher the carbohydrate intake they had, especially refined carbohydrates, like white bread or cookies or sugars, they had greater progression of coronary-artery disease."[54]

Because heart disease is the number-one killer of women in North America, ahead of breast cancer and other illnesses, and surgery is very expensive, it's of keen interest to strapped hospital administrators. These studies show that *lowering* cholesterol in such patients, on top of the worrisome side-effects already mentioned, can actually *increase* the risk of their arriving in hospital with a heart attack or a stroke. Early studies did not include women,and even based on later ones, like the Ascot Study so often referred to by statin proponents, Dr. Wright says, "You would have to treat 83 people for three to five years to prevent one event, and total mortality was not significantly reduced in that trial." Moreover, "If you break it down by gender, and you look at women of all ages, there's actually *no benefit* ... no reduction in heart attacks and strokes in women, so ... for primary prevention, women shouldn't be receiving these drugs." The same is true *for all people over 65*, yet these pills are widely prescribed for all these non-benefiting groups.

The doctors researching these curious statistics think that higher cholesterol is produced in order to shore up arteries that are damaged, much like a scab over a cut, and that cholesterol, certainly the "good" HLD but possibly also the "bad," LDL, may protect against cancers and infections.[55] This disturbing and controversial evidence, however, has not stopped government guidelines for physicians, in both the U.S. and Canada, from steadily advising lower and lower and lower levels of blood cholesterol as a diagnosis of potential illness – regardless of age, gender, or current physical condition. Cholesterol levels alone are being used as a signal to intervene with drug treatment and what may be individually beneficial levels of cholesterol are now defined as pathologic. Today, according to our regulatory boards, tens of millions more people have fallen into the category of being in need of the brand-name statin drugs. All of these drugs are still on patent. Given the financial windfall such guidelines bring to their manufacturers, it is probably not a coincidence that, "*All four members of the Canada choles-terol guideline committee have received research grants, consulting fees, speakers fees, or travel assistance from makers of statins. And eight out of nine members of the most recent guideline panel in the U.S. have financial ties to the drug industry.*"[56]

As David Alter of the Institute for Clinical Evaluative Sciences in Toronto reminds us, pharmaceutical costs are the biggest expense faced by our health care system, including the costs of our hospitals. "The public-funded, universal medicare system [has] a limited pool of resources ... [We've] got to fund a whole, vast array of health services, aside from just cholesterol-lowering medications, and it ... becomes an issue of tradeoffs." Alter happens to think statins are safe but that claiming so many otherwise healthy people should be taking them is problematic because it requires "hundreds of millions of dollars ... to

manage these lower-risk patients" and research shows that very few of
them will actually derive any benefit from the intervention.[57] Paying to
measure the cholesterol and then prescribing drugs for millions of
people is not a negligible public hospital or health care cost, especially
when there really aren't many benefits to anyone except the drug companies.

Beatrice Golomb, a doctor and neurobiologist at the University of
California at San Diego, goes much further. She feels statins are not
only expensive and often useless, but actually dangerous. She has done
some of the most serious studies on the unwanted side-effects of these
drugs. Besides the best-known serious side-effect, muscle pain and
weakness leading to kidney damage, there are cognitive and neurological problems as well, including TGA, or Total Global Amnesia, a temporary but total loss of memory that is very frightening. There are also
other neurological problems and debilitating effects such as pain and
burning in the extremities. Although the manufacturers claim only
about 2 percent of users suffer side effects, other researchers in obser-
vational studies note that *between 15 and 30 percent of statin users are
reporting adverse effects.*[58]

It sounds scary, and it is. But people shouldn't get too angry at their
doctors or the hospitals for prescribing these drugs. They are victims of
the money takeover of medicine, just as patients are. "There's no way
that a practicing doctor can critically evaluate the medical research
that guides his or her medical practice and practice at the same time,"
says Harvard Medical School professor Dr John Abramson. His job
allowed him to take the time to study the 2001 U.S. government guidelines for cholesterol on which most doctors base their recommendations. These guidelines bumped candidates for statin therapy from 13
million to 36 million people in the U.S. alone, and Canada's are similar. Abramson found that if you actually read the studies the guidelines
cite, the conclusions they reach – to prescribe drug therapy to healthy
people with moderate levels of cholesterol – are simply not supported
by scientific data. "There was no evidence from the gold standard of
medical research, randomized controlled trials, showing that statins
benefit these populations." He says we've lost sight of the fact that our
real goal should be preventing heart disease and cardiac events, not
lowering cholesterol. But lowering cholesterol is what statins actually
can do, and this debate "is largely determined by how the drug companies are going to make the most profits."[59]

Sounding eerily like Dr. Harold back in the early days of the Queen E, Abramson says the real challenge is to stick to the commonplace. "We already know how to reduce the risk of heart disease ... exercise routinely, eat a Mediterranean-style diet, don't smoke, drink in moderation, and maintain a healthy body weight The younger people who do this have 83 percent less heart disease; not a bad rate of protection, and even when patients are over sixty-five, these habits will still cut risk by 60 percent. "We know very well how to prevent the majority of heart disease, which, by the way, also improves longevity and decreases the risk of cancer. We know how to do that, but it doesn't generate the kinds of profits that the pharmaceutical industry is reaping from having us all focus our preventive health efforts on lowering cholesterol." Beatrice Golomb emphasizes, "All the major clinical trials were pharmaceutical company-funded, and it is perhaps not unexpected that studies that [they] fund are focused on identifying benefits. And the very small number of individuals who are interested in looking at harms as well as benefits have had a significant difficulty trying to get funding to perform their studies. There really isn't anybody who perceives it in their interest to focus research dollars in that direction."

Abramson says that in our era of television and Internet advertising for Big Pharma, many family practitioners point out that "lifestyle interventions would be a good thing if we could do it, but we can't." As Montreal family practitioner Adam Gavsie says, with so few family or general practice doctors available, there's simply not enough time in either private insurance-funded or publicly funded systems to "talk to the patient, understand their lives and stress levels, and follow up on their reactions to medical advice." Moreover, what has become valued in our medical system "is specialty care and technological intervention." As Abramson says, "When that's our folk medicine, it's very hard to say, 'Wait a minute. I understand that these statins are being pushed, but if you really want to prevent heart disease, I need to help you figure out why you're not able to start exercising and change to a healthy diet, and I will work with you on those issues.' That's what good medical care ought to be, and what's happened with this commercialization of our medical knowledge is that it takes the doctor-patient relationship away from serving the patient's interests and moves it toward serving a medical corporation's interests." And that puts us on a gradient of patient demand and corporate greed that no publicly-funded health or hospital system can survive.[60]

BLAME WHERE BLAME IS DUE

> When should help be sought? We throw resources at people who won't
> take them. And the other extreme: congenitally anxious people looking
> for explanations of every deviant sensation their body perceives.
>
> John Hughes, GP

In our single-payer system, many doctors, especially the GPs and rural physicians who are on the preventive frontlines, complain that too much of their energy – and the system's resources – are taken up by people who either do not need, won't accept, or cannot benefit from medical help. Ex-Queen E GP John Hughes can go on at some length about people who show up every year for their physical. "They want an entire work-up; blood, urine, you name it. And there's nothing wrong with them! But it's free, or at least they don't realize they're paying for it, and they think it's their due." It's true that evidence has refuted the once-sacrosanct medical command that you must visit your doctor once a year. It was popularized by public interest and advertising campaigns from the 1950s through most of the 1970s. Not only did doctors feel they needed more time for diagnoses back then, they were still working on fee-for-service and they needed those regular, paying visitors. Today, with limits on how many patients can be seen in our crowded system, doctors need to get the word out that this is unnecessary. Naturally, they'd rather be spending their limited time with sick people.

But not too sick. Surgeon Ron Lewis worries about patients who really should be concentrating on quality of life or getting their affairs in order, people with "incurable cancers who will come in for dialysis or other very expensive procedures. Why do they bother? What is the point of prolonging their suffering?" Our society has an unprecedented denial of the reality of death, which impels people to seek treatment even when there's no point and the treatment involves much misery. Moreover, doctors are often caught in the same denial. Lewis mentioned his father, dying at eighty-three. "And the doctors were offering to cut off both his legs because of complications. 'What's the point of that?' I asked them, 'he's only going to live a few more weeks!' And in fact he died very soon after. But they wanted to intervene that way, spend all that time and money and increase his suffering." One big problem with a "free" public system is that, "People – patients and doctors – learn to expect that giving or receiving treatment, even useless treatment, is what should be done instead of balancing the risk of operations with their remaining chance at comfort."

We are now encroaching on areas that aren't the responsibility of the doctors, the hospitals, or the system. That responsibility belongs to us, the medical consumers. "Nothing is for nothing, there are always trade-offs," Lewis says. "The less time you have to benefit from an intervention, the less you ought to consider it ... Doctors are under so much pressure to deliver these services," he adds. "And the patients are often unforgiving as well. The other day, my last patient was a lady whose operation had gone perfectly; she really had the desired-for outcome. But she was mad at me because she had to wait an hour. 'How are you?' I said. 'Awful!' she said. 'I was about to leave.' Even though I apologized, I had to drag it out of her how well she was doing. She wasn't grateful; all she could see was her recent wait."

Lewis explains, "Only spectacular care impresses people. Having a normal outcome with no complications isn't enough. At the Queen Elizabeth, over and over, we used to realize how hard it is for the patient, too. They arrive in hospital, their first hour is a jumble, they wander around, they're sent here and there, everyone's too busy to pay attention to them. How many go out after that and say, 'Boy, that was satisfying!' As hospitals become larger and more like assembly lines, even taking the trouble to arrange home-care falls apart. People are just breathless doing the assembly line. And the patient feels, 'well, nothing too bad happened, but do I feel cared for?'"

The more people are treated this way, the less appreciative they are for what they do have and the more they demand the fancier, more spectacular care they hear or read about being offered elsewhere. Dr Judith Levitan says that today, "patients come in with a grocery list of drugs they want and they don't want to take 'no' for an answer. Simple, effective methods of dealing with these problems, like exercise or better sleeping habits, are rejected because of advertising. Worst of all, doctors used to be allowed a failure rate; people understood we couldn't fix every problem, and our success was also based on our professional abilities, our bedside manner. But now that's gone; what everyone wants from us is a fast pill, an intervention, a cure Right Now!"

Those instant cures, like most quick fixes in life, aren't all they're cracked up to be, and the people demanding them need to be more suspicious and watch for real evidence of safety. For example, patients suffering the agony of an impacted kidney stone are demanding that hospitals offer an expensive, state-of-the-art therapy known as ESWL, extracorporeal shock-wave lithotripsy. In fact, Canadian publicly funded hospitals have been criticized by bodies such as The Fraser Institute for not having enough of it available.[61]

With ESWL, shockwaves, guided by x-rays, are aimed at the kidney stone to physically disintegrate it. Larger urban hospitals in Canada have rushed to try to offer such equipment because kidney stones are very painful for the patient and, apart from waiting for the stone to pass or performing regular surgery, there have been few treatment options. The emphasis has been on fund-raising for the equipment. But the one thing few hospitals are taking the time to consider is that lithotripsy is a pretty violent intervention. It depends on the untested theory that shock waves powerful enough to destroy a kidney stone will not affect surrounding tissues. Like cholesterol-lowering statins, lithotripsy was not subjected to proper clinical trials before becoming widely used, largely because it seemed so much less invasive than normal treatments. Serious tests were not considered necessary.

Today, after thousands of interventions, studies are finally being undertaken. They show that, in a significant number of cases, the process can cause serious problems requiring even more expensive hospital treatments. As many as 25 percent of patients had scarring, and those followed over time suffered increasing and chronic kidney problems such as internal bleeding, kidney hypertension, and even irreversible kidney failure. Patients were not warned of these possibilities because, until recently, doctors didn't really know about them. Nearly a fifth of patients sustained some kind of damage, including lower fertility or abnormal sperm, hemorrhage in the scrotum, and blood pressure and heart problems. Most enlightening of all, in 40 percent of the patients, that is, almost half the time, the stones reappeared. And without any treatment at all, that recurrance is about the same. In fact, like so many other technological interventions, pulverizing kidney stones with shock waves never addresses the problem of why the body was producing the stones in the first place. But as long as fancy, expensive equipment is being sold to eager hospitals and clinics and credulous patients want to try the new treatment, we'll remain in the days of snake-oil and potions. Few researchers will get the funding to look into such questions, and bodies like Canada's Fraser Institute and the U.S.' National Center for Policy Analysis will castigate public systems for not jumping into new technologies more quickly, even though there is good statistical evidence showing that doing so does not improve mortality or disease rates.[62] All this takes us into the very alarming territory of heart surgery.

THE ART OF LISTENING

Trying to get from the patient a sense of what's going on is
time-consuming ... But the moment you listen to your patient, it is
enormously efficient.

Cardiologist Bernard Lown[63]

People at risk for heart disease are currently being prescribed a life-long regime of statins and are also often advised to undergo heroically complicated but very common double or triple-bypass open-heart operations or the somewhat less invasive "balloon" therapy angioplasties that require stents to keep the artery open after the procedure. These treatments are very costly to the health care system and as dangerous as any major surgery. We have come to believe that they are what has enabled our hospitals and public health services to get the coronary disease epidemic under control for the least possible cost, and that these treatments are helping victims live longer, happier lives. Unfortunately, as with the statins, this belief is now under attack. It appears that surgical treatments for heart disease, although useful, have a more strictly limited value than we thought. For many people still receiving them, they are probably useless or dangerous.

Dr Bernard Lown, of the prestigious Lown Cardiovascular Center in Boston, invented the direct-current defibrillator, so he is well acquainted with high-tech, heroic methodology. Today, however, he advises the huge majority of the cardiac patients who come to his center because they have been been diagnosed with serious heart disease not to have surgery. He advises against surgical intervention "in all but 8 percent of the cases," he says. His treatment is to listen to the patient and then to work on the sources of internal stress, the real killer in this disease. Diet and exercise are also managed, and because most of the patients have had previous events, some medication with statins is required. Although nearly all his patients have heart disease and many have already had serious heart attacks or strokes, studies following 750 of the Center's patients show that on average, these "sick" people end up *living longer than the average person* in the general population.

Most cardiologists will insist that the operations that Lown counsels his patients to forego are necessary to save their lives and stoutly defend the clinical value of coronary stents, balloon angioplasties, and open-heart surgeries. But like kidney stone and cholesterol therapy, that's because, until recently, no one had a sufficient cohort of people thus treated to crunch the numbers. Doctors had noticed that arteries that had been ballooned open often closed again within a year, which led to the stent, a device that seems to help keep the arteries open. There is no doubt that these interventions relieve symptoms, the breathlessness and weakness of angina, for example, which is extremely important to the patient. But there's increasing debate over whether they save lives. David Alter, a Toronto cardiologist at Sunny-brook and a researcher at the Institute of Clinical Evaluative Sciences says, "Trials that have compared regions that have high rates of these interventions with other regions that have very low rates ... have absolutely no difference in mortality. In fact, if anything, there might be a tendency towards a higher risk of complications in those regions that do more procedures, and that has been a compelling and consistent message from a number of studies both in Canada and internationally."

This is because we haven't really understood what causes heart attacks in the first place, meaning also that technology is providing us with a highly expensive learning curve. McGill cardiologist Colin Rose says that the new technique of intravascular ultrasound has enabled them to see a wall in the artery and they have discovered that "most of the plaque is buried in the wall of the artery and doesn't show up on an angiogram ... [this plaque] is actually more likely to rupture and cause a heart attack" than the plaque they have been going after. "So if somebody has angina or has a positive exercise test – I often see it, they just have a positive exercise test with no symptoms – they'll say, 'There's plaque there. We better balloon and stent it.' *This has now been shown to have absolutely no effect on future heart attacks and does not prolong life* ... You may be helping some symptoms temporarily, but you're not preventing the heart attack."

The same thing is true with the even more invasive and expensive bypass operations. In the Mass II Study cited in the *Journal of the American College of Cardiology* in 2005, "patients with three-vessel disease, a lot of plaque on the angiogram," were separated into three groups. One was treated for angina with drugs, one with bypasses, and one with balloons and stents. "At the end of a year or so, there was no difference in mortality, no difference in heart attacks. The group that had the balloon actually ... had more heart attacks. And in the bypass group, the procedure tended to relieve the symptoms more, but it didn't prolong life, and it didn't prevent a heart attack."[64]

Many people who are actually at low risk for having a heart attack are undergoing by-pass surgeries and angioplasties. Doctors have even named the knee-jerk tendency to intervene when they should know better the "oculo-stenotic reflex." When they actually see the plaque blockage, they can't resist opening it up, "even if there's no evidence," as David Alter admits, "to suggest that opening that blockage up is going to do any good ... Once we go down the technology route, this aggressive route, we can't [seem to] hold back." Not only are the doctors suckers for technology, the patients hear of such methods being used abroad or in the United States and demand similar opportunities for a "cure."

Worst of all, patients who have invested themselves in high-tech interventions like angioplasty don't want to hear it may have all been for nothing. "Once they're on it," Colin Rose says, they resist diet and exercise protocols. "It's much harder to get them to think that the technology is not going to cure them." Canada as a health provider doesn't want to appear technologically backward, so our hospitals set "volumes" of such procedures, based on comparisons with the rest of the world. We want to be seen as "following the trends elsewhere," as Alter says. It's a real bind; those who criticize public health systems jump on any tendency to have fewer of these heroic interventions as a sign of poor care. In fact, that's one of the ways private-care boosters like the Fraser Institute and the NCPA (National Centre for Policy Analysis) try to convince Canadians their hospital care, despite far better mortality rates, is poorer than the kind available in the United States.

Consequently, scientific assumptions, professional reputations, think-tanks, and patient demand all push hospital care in the techno-fix direction. And of course, there's also the market. Alter says, "There are ... disease-management, exercise, cardiac rehabilitation programs that have been proven to save lives and improve quality of life to the point that they appear to overshadow the benefits of technology, of angioplasty [and the rest]." He adds, "We have very little funding in the public pool for that ... Prevention is neither remunerated at the physician level, nor has it been adopted by industry in any fashion, so there's no marketing driving force." No one makes real money doing it, so it has no real lobbyists on the political stage.

The big problem, according to primary care physicians like John Hughes and Adam Gavsie, as well as specialists like Alter and Rose, is that simple preventative care "takes a lot of time. I have to sit there, listen to [the patient's] complaints, anxieties, and so on, and talk to them for half an hour." Rose says his patients really don't want to hear him say that, "these procedures and drugs are not going to prolong your life to any significant extent. You've got to change your habits. That's the only way to do it." Bernard Lown has not allowed such problems to deter him, however; perhaps his very ill patients are more motivated. In any case, he not only gives each patient the ideal forty-five minutes GPs are supposed to spend; he gives each one an hour. "By the time the hour is up, I know a lot about them ... I don't send them to many tests, because the problem is rapidly resolved." He says it's unusual when that doesn't happen. "I have to scrape my brain to find when in the last six months I had a patient [where] I didn't realize what was going on with them."

THE WAITING IS THE HARDEST PART

A four-year-old Newfoundland boy who has already lost one kidney to cancer is facing a staggering 2½ year wait for a scan on the province's only magnetic-resonance-imaging machine.

lead sentence, Lisa Priest, *The Globe and Mail* [65]

It's a rare week when stories like the one quoted above aren't featured in one of Canada's major newspapers, usually on the front page, accompanied by pictures of patients like this one, described as "a rambunctious, blue-eyed blond." The same journalist featured a similar story a year later about a middle-aged man with cancer who decided to go to the United States "for lifesaving medical treatment." The patient, Greg Ruetz, after having received private American treatment, then sued the Ontario Health Services to recoup his costs. "Susan Warner swallows addictive painkillers every day to ease the crippling pain she endures waiting for knee-replacement surgery," begins another article in the *Calgary Herald*.[66] Few Canadians are able to read such stories without feeling sympathy and indignation or without worrying about finding themselves in a similar situation. So ubiquitous have media descriptions of the misery caused by lack of access to health services become that the Harper Conservative government introduced binding promises to "reduce wait times" as one of its very first actions after being elected in 2005.

It is true that wait times for chemotherapy treatment and especially elective surgeries have been a serious problem in every province, and patients needing pain-relieving elective procedures like hip and knee replacements have been forced to wait many anxious weeks. This has especially been the case since the mass closures in the mid-1990s. There is no doubt that there are serious access problems to hospital beds in some places in Canada, especially with some procedures and for some patients, and that ERs are chronically over-used almost everywhere. Such problems still vary wildly, however, even within provinces. What is unclear is exactly how long Canadians are actually waiting for treatment in comparison with other countries, how often these waits lead to catastrophic outcomes for the patients, and most pertinently, whether there is some kind of indissoluble tie between long wait times and public payment systems, as the people most vociferous about long waits generally imply.

Most of the criticism in the media has placed the blame for long wait times not on local inefficiencies or temporary backlogs, which research has shown are generally the actual culprits, but on the entire single- payer system itself. The media has colluded in the idea that wait times are due to methods of payment and, in this case, government bureaucracy. So, after four decades of only publicly funded care, today there is a boom in Canadian public demand for public/private partnerships to build, maintain, and manage hospitals. People are also demanding access to private CT scans, MRIs, other forms of testing, and surgical clinics that offer the most popular "elective" surgeries. These clinics are actually illegal in terms of the Canada Health Act, but the government so far has turned a blind eye to such infringements of its core legislation.[67]

Having these quasi-illegal clinics in place means that Canadians are now in a position to make comparisons, even within the country, between private and public payment systems, and many preliminary studies are now available. These studies reveal that wait times for tests can be very much shorter in private facilities but that outcome cannot be assumed. The biggest surprise is that many surgical wait times have been shown to be significantly *shorter*, as well as cheaper, in *public* clinics, as Alberta's experience with private clinics, mentioned in chapter 5, has already shown. This is not to say there isn't a "wait time problem" for hospital beds in Canada, or that that problem isn't related to poor government management practices. But it's the tip of the iceberg in illustrating that there is more to wait times than meets the eye.

Media stories about unacceptable wait times for hospital treatments are popular in Canada, but they're even more widespread in the United States. Generally, they serve as a means of scaring those who are arguing for installing a universal health care system in that country. The figures given in American stories are almost universally shocking and damning, but if the source for these figures is traced, the overwhelming majority of the stories refer to just one: the Fraser Institute. Most Canadians know that the Fraser Institute is a right-leaning B.C. think-tank interested in, as its home page proclaims, "promoting free market solutions to social and economic problems." The Fraser Institute has been tracking Canadian health care wait times as well as access to advanced medical technology for years. Its regular reports have become the source for nearly all the wait time figures the general public has been given to judge the system, whether published in *The Calgary Herald*, the *Montreal Gazette*, *The Globe and Mail*, or discussed by other Canadian media outlets, including CBC and CTV. These reports are just as popular with CNN, *The New York Times*, the *Christian Science Monitor*, *The Economist*, and many British papers. The Fraser Institute is also the chief source cited on dozens of websites run by think-tanks, policy analysts and NGOs that support and promulgate free market solutions to health care, including the U.S. National Center for Policy Analysis, Liberty Page.com, and the UK-based CIVITAS (The Institute for the Study of Civil Society).[68]

The Fraser Institute's website states that all its studies are based on figures derived from official Statistics Canada data. However, when analyses of the governments' figures are done by academic and medical researchers, they have shown most of the Institute's most widely quoted figures are either flawed or misleading. In fact, a paper produced by the American Medical Student Association in 2006 concludes, "it is not at all clear that the 'waiting list crisis' that is so often talked about by the media and opponents of single payer [health plans] *actually exists*."[69]

This study explains, "It is a myth that Canadians with serious, life-threatening illnesses are enrolled on a waiting list before they can receive life-saving therapies." What actually happens is that different individuals in different localities are subjected to waiting to see various specialists, waiting for the appropriate tests, and then finally waiting for treatment, as they are in any system. How their "wait time" is measured, whether from the moment they feel sick until they receive appropriate treatment, or any step in-between, varies enormously with each city, province, hospital and even each doctor, to say nothing of who is doing the measuring. One of the most common methods of determining wait times used by the Fraser Institute is to ask the primary care physician what he or she subjectively *estimates* the wait times for a given procedure *will be* – with no subsequent follow-up to see what the patient actually experiences.

The same is true outside of Canada. A major Health Canada study reports that, "Commonly, 20–30% of those on wait lists are found in the international literature to be inappropriately placed, because they have already received the procedure, have died, never knew they were on a list, were placed on the list in the first place for reasons unrelated to medical necessity, or were no longer awaiting the procedure for some other reason." That means a listed wait-time of fifteen weeks should probably be cut to only ten. As P. McDonald et al. explain in their Health Canada paper, "there is an almost total absence of consistently applied criteria (within procedures, let alone across) for determining when patients should be added to wait lists, and how they should be prioritized." Few medical wait lists in general, they conclude, "are sufficiently defined and standardized to provide inter-temporally consistent and geographically comparable databases."[70]

To sum up this singular measurement, upon which we now base budgets and elect politicians, "With rare exceptions, waiting lists in Canada, as in most countries, are non-standardized, capriciously organized, poorly monitored and (according to most informed observers) in grave need of retooling. As such, *most of those currently in use are at best misleading sources of data on access to care, and at worst instruments of misinformation, propaganda, and general mischief.*"[71] All of which may explain why wait-time figures have become so popular with political and economic interests. Because of the lack of standardization, they can be easily manipulated in service of the bias of the researcher. For instance, wait times for *life-threatening* procedures like vascular surgery can be quite short – 2.7 weeks are the Stats Can figures for British Columbia – while wait times for expensive *elective* orthopedic surgeries are much longer in B.C.: 9.3 weeks. Even if the individual rates were based on the same criteria (actual as opposed to estimated wait times), both of these unrelated specialties are often thrown together in official Fraser Institute estimates and media stories to alarmingly elevate "overall surgical wait time" for the province.

There are also different wait times for different procedures, depending on the hospital, the locality, and the density of the population. Although the median wait time for a CT scan in Manitoba in 2005 was ten weeks, some hospitals were delivering in only three weeks, while others took as long as eighteen weeks. Researcher Kao-PinChua com-

pares the wait times listed in Statistics Canada's Health Services Access
Survey of 2003, which queried patients, with those reported by the Fraser Institute in their survey a few months later, which used physicians'
estimates. Stats Can reported patients said that a median wait time to
see a specialist for a new condition was 4.0 weeks; Fraser's sources more
than doubled that, to 8.4 weeks. Stats Can listed non- emergency diagnostic tests, including CTs, MRIs and angiographies, at 3.0 weeks; the
Fraser Institute said 5.2 for CTs and 12.6 for MRIs. That would average
to 8.9 weeks, almost three times longer than patients reported they
actually experienced. PinChua says, "These differences may be
explained by different definitions of waiting times, differences in perceptions between patients and physicians, and source bias."[73]

Of course, truly standardized Canadian wait times need to be combed
for errors and compared to those experienced in other countries if we
are to determine if they are the result of mismanagement, neglect,
insufficient expenditure on beds or machines, or if they reflect relatively normal administrative delays. When effort is expended to do so,
it becomes clear that most citizens in any public system do, in fact, have
to wait longer, particularly for elective treatments, than those who are
prepared to pay whatever is necessary to have faster service. Kao-
PinChua concedes that, "On average, U.S. citizens experience some of
the shortest wait-times for non-emergency surgeries among industrialized countries, although those times vary considerably by procedure."
But he also reminds readers that, "the short waiting times apply mainly
to those who have insurance; for those who do not, the waiting line is
arguably infinite."[73] We need only remember all the Canadians who
lost their lives due to postponing care prior to medicare that are
reflected in our mortality statistics. These shorter wait times also need
to be somehow calibrated with the fact that "the lack of universal
health care in the U.S. means less demand for the system," and they
would significantly lengthen if all citizens did have access to tests and
hospital treatment.

To put the issue back in the individual terms used by the media and
the wait time critics, that means that a hard-working but poor Canadian
cleaning lady with a bad hip might be unlucky enough to be in an
usually crowded surgical area where she would have to wait one of
Canada's worst averages of 18 months months for her new joint. Prostheses aren't cheap. If she lived in the U.S. and, like the majority of
Americans and Canadians before Medicare, had no medical insurance, she would have to find money from relatives, some kind of

fundraiser such as one so often sees in small American towns, or resign herself to being crippled and unemployable for the rest of her life.

Such comparisons illustrate that no system is perfect and we have to be careful that, in seeking to gain one thing, we don't lose another. For example, while approximately 10 to 50 percent more Canadians than Americans in a cross-national survey reported problems waiting for specialists and GPs to see them, three times as many people in the U.S. reported difficulties in getting specialist referrals and almost *six times as many Americans as Canadians reported cost as a significant obstacle* to getting care at all.[74] Finally and most importantly, have the shorter wait times that are admittedly available to those able to access U.S.-style medical care resulted in better survival, mortality, or recovery statistics than in Canada or in other single-payer systems? The short answer to that, as we saw in chapter 5, is "no."

SPP, TILMA, AND NOT-SO-SMART TRADE RULES

Unless Canadians rise up to defend it, our public health care system will not survive this double onslaught from the for-profit sector and deep integration [trade regimes].

>   Council of Canadians "Profit is Not the Cure" campaign[75]

Added to the normal challenges of providing timely care, even large, not-for-profit hospital systems like our own do not have sufficient power to resist the extremely high drug and equipment costs that the powerful and influential pharmaceutical and technology corporations are now able to command. It is fairly apparent that commercial interests are actively trying to undermine public systems in order to create a more fragmented and vulnerable market for their products. As also explored in chapter 5, these private interests are helped by the general world view and policies of the large international finance agencies like the World Bank and the IMF, to whom our governments habitually go for loans. These entities in turn encourage cooperation with international trade regimes like the WTO and NAFTA that favour privatization of government services as a prerequistite to their help. As already established, these financial bodies and trade regimes played a big role in the remarkably rapid downsizing of our health care system in the mid-1990s that has led to many of the crises it is suffering today.

At present, aggressive efforts are being made by North American trade regimes to gain control over any nationally funded service, including health. On their website, the well-known Canadian non-profit Council of Canadians is urging people to oppose "Deep Integration," which is a general term for the current attempts undertaken by signatories to NAFTA to "harmonize" U.S. and Canadian regulations governing environment and food safety, health care, transport, and many other government-controlled services, which include the federal postal system. "Deep Integration" is being fostered especially through "SPP," the Security and Prosperity Partnership of North America, signed in March of 2005 by Prime Minister Paul Martin, U.S. President George Bush, and Mexican President Vincente Fox. Its intention is to find ways to merge "commerce, trade, immigration, food safety, and many other policies," including health.

In many cases, this means the separate health and environmental standards Canadians have enjoyed until now will go down to join lower levels in the U.S. and Mexico. Already, the pesticide residue levels our regulatory bodies will tolerate on our fruits and vegetables have been "harmonized" with much higher U.S. ones. One of the more alarming arms of this initiative is called TILMA (Trade, Investment and Labour Mobility Agreement), already signed onto by Alberta and British Columbia. It sounds at first glance like a commonsense agreement to facilitate commerce between provinces, but under TILMA, *corporations and individuals are allowed to sue any provincial government for anything they feel "restricts or impairs" their profits.* "Even measures designed to protect the environment and public health are vulnerable to attack from corporate lawsuits with compensation penalties as high as $5 million."[76]

Most Canadians believe that health care, culture, and other key national concerns are exempt from such outside trade controls. So far, that exemption has in fact kept the large for-profit health and hospital corporations at bay. However, as mentioned above, it applies only to a *fully* publicly funded system. "Once privatized, the system must treat U.S. companies as if they were Canadian. *This would make U.S. private hospital chains, HMOs, and private insurance companies eligible for government funding,* draining resources from the public system."[77] It could be argued that if governments were the most desirable guarantors of the public interest in the first place, they would guard their own services more carefully and not be so open to financial manipulation by outside interests and foreign powers. That's true to a marked extent, and the electorate in Canada needs to hold all our levels of governments much more accountable for their loan behaviours and the details of the trade treaties they sign, the way European, Mexican, and Indian electorates do. However, turning everything over to the industrial, financial, and trade interests that have undermined public systems in the first place, with no future means of control or public oversight, hardly seems like the proper solution to a government's previous errors.

More Canadians need to understand the direction of the recent Supreme Court decision allowing Quebec to permit the purchase of private insurance for specific treatments. This decision would seem to be a clear violation of the Canada Health Care Act. The Act is very specific about the illegality of private clinics of any kind. Such a decision fragments support and creates serious confusion regarding the public system. Because there is already a crucial shortage of medical professionals, opening surgical, MRI, and other forms of clinics will drain more doctors, nurses, and technicians away from the public sector. So far, that has always been the case where private clinics have been allowed, around the world. This means that we are living in a period in which many forces are combining to return Canadian health care to the two-tier system that it started out with, the one that Canadians managed to change in 1970. That system, although popular with the medical profession, was, as we have seen in the story of the Queen Elizabeth, even more difficult to fund – besides being extremely unpopular with patients. It also gave Canada general mortality and health statistics on a par with those of the U.S. – that is, at the bottom of the industrialized world.

The financial pressures coming from commercial interests, banks, lenders, and sometimes the governments themselves are so crushing that it is becoming clear that currently, the only thing holding up a rapid privatization process of Canadian health care is Canadians themselves. Minority governments like Stephen Harper's and Quebec Premier Jean Charest's do not dare to openly privatize the one remaining focus of Canadian identity and pride, the universal health care system. However, there have been no real debates about the effects of these court decisions in open legislative sessions in Canada, and municipalities and other local governments are not being consulted about the loss of powers that they will suffer once TILMA and other aspects of the SPP are fully operational.

This entire discussion is alarming and depressing because, once again, it expresses helplessness in terms of being able to control the burgeoning costs of health care in the face of modern trends. But that's because we have persisted in looking at one side of the equation: financing those costs. Before we move on to the rather radical solu-

tions ahead, however, we need to look at one more well-researched
effort to fund the pathological money monster of modern health care:
northern Europe's PPP's, or public/private partnerships.

CAN FIFTY MILLION FRENCHMEN BE WRONG?

The World Health Organization ranked the French health care system
as the best in the world, although the high level of premature death and
major health inequalities are serious problems which illustrates there
remains great room for improvement.

High Committee on Public Health, France[78]

In the new context of discussing the partial dismantling of the universal health care system in Canada in general and Quebec in particular,
France has been held up in the mass media as a prime example of a
successful system that combines public and private funding, one which
Canada would do well to emulate. Gilles Brucker, the general director
of France's entire public health system, the Institut de Veille Sanitaire,
is a small, handsome man with an unusually direct manner of speaking,
especially for a top government official. Brucker is a big fan of Canadian Medicare, our own health care and hospital system. He says that in
the 1980s, everyone "made pilgrimages to Quebec" because of the
high level of public health theory and legislation in the province at the
time. He has since learned that much of that international reputation
was due to provincial public health policies that are indeed written
down but rarely, if ever, properly funded and implemented. However,
both Quebec's and Canada's record of relative lack of discrimination
because of income level is the one ideal he knows has generally held
true.

Brucker explains that despite the fact that there is a mixed system in
France, most people are covered through government-regulated private employment insurance or special government programs for the
poor. As always with a mixed system, however, there are a significant
number of people left out. For example, there is a remarkable ten-year
difference in life expectancy between the north and south of France,
which holds true in many parts of Europe, but in France's case has
been attributed to the concentration of higher quality hospitals and
clinics and professional staff in the north. Like the United States,
France has only recently begun to document social differences and disease or death rates, but in general, health officials there are in awe of

the Canadian system, mostly because of the *equality of care.* Particularly worrisome to them in their own system, for example, is the "marked socially based inequality in cancer mortality."[79]

Brucker is now in his fifties and came up through the ranks of public health workers, spending much of his career in NGOs fighting for poor people's rights to health. Today, he admits, with a touch of weariness, his responsibilities are "vast – nothing less than the state of health of the entire population of France." He has to worry about the thousands of HIV-positive African immigrants that France admits every year, about SARS and Avian Flu, about car accidents, Legionnaire's Disease, cancer, cirrhosis, and heart disease. Throughout the 1980s, he was in charge of getting all of Paris' hospital-borne infections under control by designing hygiene protocols. He was appointed to his present position only two weeks before the heat wave of 2003 killed thousands of elderly people in northern French cities, so he's had to work out brand-new policies to register and evacuate people at risk. In the recent past, he organized a national coordination committee for the control of hospital infections throughout the French regions. "Back in 1988, 70 percent of our endoscopes were contaminated with bacteria and causing serious infections. We undertook a huge prevention and teaching program and five years later, we had them down to 5 percent!" He savours that rare moment of success and then adds ruefully, "Nothing is ever fixed forever. As soon as the pressure lets up, people will go back to not washing their hands or sterilizing the equipment again."

The combined private and public programs that France uses to protect its population shoulder 70 percent of people's hospital or health expenses, but as Brucker says, "If you're poor, 30 percent is not nothing!" In statements reminiscent of pre-Medicare Canada, he says, "The Mutual Insurance companies who cover the rich are reimbursed by the government. Organizations like the CMU (Couverture Maladie Universelle) cover the unemployed poor. But to qualify for the latter, you have to make almost nothing – in fact, a little less than what's considered the poverty level. So the 'working poor' – the hard-working, struggling families who run a little shop in an immigrant neighbourhood – they're the ones who fall through the cracks." Echoing what the doctors at the Queen E used to say in the 1950s, Brucker adds, "People come to the emergencies, we care for them; no one is turned away for money reasons. But people suffering from TB or AIDS or other chronic or long-term diseases can only turn to the emergencies when they're in crisis. That's not real care."

The problems in France are very similar to the problems here. Brucker recognizes the serious pressures coming from a public that in France, as here, has come to expect more and more from health care. "Society is becoming increasingly intolerant of risk. People seem to be saying, 'I want everything and right now, but with *no* risks.'" Brucker feels the forces of globalization that have enormously aided the power of the big pharmacological companies and have also helped spread new diseases are a formidable challenge for any public health official. "Globalization has a lot to do with the risks we have today in society. People want the economic development they think is associated with world trade and modern systems of production, like industrial agriculture; they don't want the diseases, though."

Brucker, like Bernard Lown, above, and Paul Farmer, cited below, points out that, "feeding herbivores meat causes mad cow disease, which impacts expenses in the health care system. And that decision comes through trade and economics. There are serious health risks associated with all forms of industrial production, especially food. But before we had local risks only; today, they're planetary." Brucker says all you have to do is follow the trail of SARS from the first doctor who treated it in China, got on a jet, stopped at the Hotel Metropole in Singapore, and then landed in Toronto. "We can no longer treat infectious diseases as if they were national problems. We simply no longer have any borders." The idea that foreigners infected with AIDS are denied entry to the United States makes him particularly angry. He lists potentially deadly disease-causing products like infected meats, genetically engineered viruses and bacteria, and also industrially raised chickens carrying Avian Flu, that are all allowed free passage under our current Free Trade system. "But sick, needy people, that's when globalization stops free exchange!" He adds, with some emotion, "We can't let entire countries die of AIDS. That will come back on us. Each person's health is an international issue."

"Economic development entails health risks. So how much power and importance are you going to grant to the public health?" Brucker asks. "Will you rate health as a little more important? A little less? Today's powerful trade organizations, such as the European Union, are based on economic, not health logic. However, at least the EU has demanded that every signatory nation have a viable public health policy in place." This is not true of North American trade alliances like NAFTA and the FTAA. And that's a global concern because what is done for the public health in Canada or Argentina or Bosnia, Brucker feels, is no longer a matter of indifference to a country like France.

"This is a very small planet. The SARS epidemic, which might have been so much worse, came out of south China and went around the world incredibly fast. This means we all have to work on a better sharing of health policies. Better balances, better prevention. Otherwise, we're helping a natural form of bio-terrorism to spread." In 2005, the Center for Transmissible Disease Surveillance, a Swedish-based, globally focused health organization, was founded. France is also forming partnerships with less functional health services in the Caribbean, Madagascar, Tahiti, and Africa. It all goes back to the egalitarian nature of real health care. "Unfortunately," Brucker says, "rich people don't worry about poor people dying of disease unless that starts to affect them." The nature of modern infectious diseases takes us back to the lessons learned in the late 19th century, and Brucker is not alone in worrying about them.

These facts only lead to one conclusion: public health, with its integral conception of ultimate social equality, is the key to health in general. We noted earlier in this book the fact that much of the misery from cholera, typhoid, and other infections in 19th-century Canada came from the overcrowding of new immigrants into burgeoning urban areas. Today, we realize that tracking the effects of human activities on public health is even more complex. As Paul Farmer, who teaches Medical Anthropology at the Harvard Medical School asks, "Are World Bank policies related to the spread of HIV, as has recently been claimed? What is the relationship between international shipping practices and the spread of cholera from Asia to South America?"

Paul Farmer's research agrees with Gilles Brucker's views: when we design hospital and health care systems, we now have to consider globalized trade regimes, travel, overpopulation, economic inequality, cultural traditions, and especially ecologically disruptive activities like war, chemical and biotechnology use, deforestation, and expanding agriculture, to say nothing of global warming. But in terms of legislation and prevention, we are still acting as if a living microbe will only spread within the human-created concept of national boundaries. "These are concepts that have to be reconsidered, synthesized, adjusted for, or broadened," Farmer says. He asks some hard questions: "What are the mechanisms by which changes in agriculture have led to outbreaks of disease ... and how might these mechanisms be related to international trade agreements, such as the General Agreement on Tariffs and Trade (GATT) and NAFTA? How might institutional racism be related to urban crime and the outbreaks of multidrug-resistant TB in New York prisons [or on Canadian native reserves]? Does the privatization of health services buttress social inequalities, increasing risk for certain infections?"

If we are to avoid the pandemics that could fill our hospitals to the breaking point and destroy our hard-won health systems, we need to stop looking at the incidence and virulence of each new or reemerging disease as a purely scientific problem that exists in isolation from the social world. It is even now being proven that the greatly-feared Avian Flu is *not* being spread by the wild birds and backyard flocks so often in the media, but that the infection has moved along trade routes and primarily comes out of the vastly overcrowded, monoculture conditions of large, industrial poultry farming.[80] Moreover, unlike the fuss surrounding the case of someone with antibiotic-resistant TB who got on a plane in 2007, there is a large amount of similarly drug-resistant tuberculosis on Canadian native reserves and especially in prisons and inner cities, as several public health researchers have privately admitted. Because of their economic, industrial and therefore political implications, however, public health phenomena like drug-resistant TB or AIDS and asthma or cancer clusters have become extremely sensitive information, information that most countries hesitate to share with their own citizens, let alone with other countries.

"Almost all diseases held to be emerging," Farmer explains, "from the increasing number of drug-resistant [hospital-borne] diseases to the great pandemics of HIV infection and cholera, stand as modern rebukes to the parochialism of this and other public health constructs." Farmer agrees with Gilles Brucker that the global emphasis on long-distance, "free" trade, with new rules that actually mandate the cross-border travel of living things and all their viral and bacterial hitchhikers, from cattle and plants to human-engineered bacteria and viruses, mean that political borders no longer have any real meaning in terms of stemming the flow of disease. Globalized trade also means that national borders have become "semipermeable membranes, often open to diseases but [because of patent regimes and legislative influence,] *closed to the free movement of cures.*" If these practices continue, they will vastly affect how big or small hospitals have to be, how they will need to be set up, and how much funding they will require – if we can even begin to expect them to continue to stand as our first line of defense against epidemics.

SIZE REALLY REALLY DOES MATTER

Plus que c'est gros, moins que ca marche. (The bigger it is, the less it works.)
Dr. Anne Gervais, pathologist and infectious disease specialist[81]

Countries such as France and Canada have a lot more in common than just worrying about the same diseases. Ironically, as we have seen in this chapter, the identical economic forces that have increased disease threats by creating Mad Cow disease and aided the spread of SARS are putting pressure on all health systems to either reduce services or privatize and cut down the overall numbers of hospital beds by consolidating them in huge, centralized, and "super" hospitals. The French public, like the Canadian, and even, statistically, the Americans – strongly support their public health systems (or the sections that are public, like U.S. Medicare) at levels between 70 and 90 percent of those polled. But all three countries will have to fight very hard to keep these services. Gilles Brucker is worried about economic pressures in France to close hospital beds and open community clinics on the lines of the Quebec CLSCs that is just now hitting France and is reminiscent of the mid-1990s closure period that killed the Queen E. "This kind of community and home care can be very helpful," he says hopefully, and then, sounding just like Mario Larivière, asks, "but there are limits to what it can do. What is the right size for a hospital? If we close as many beds as we're being pressured to, what will we do in an emergency?"

Every year in France, Brucker notes, there is an "epidemic of bronchitis in babies ... They're brought to the local hospitals; they need oxygen and other emergency care. We don't have enough beds, so they end up being treated miles away from home. Obviously, this is very hard on the parents." The French system, like ours in the early 1990s, is also being pressured to limit the number of doctors, although it's not so much the numbers that are a problem there as the distribution, as in Quebec. "No one has figured out how many doctors we need. In France, they can set up wherever they like ... so the rural areas suffer." There are far fewer doctors, clinics, and ERs outside of Paris than in the city, which may explain the much higher mortality rates the further you get from the capital. In fact, as mentioned, it's so bad that, like a native person in the Canadian North, a southern Frenchman can expect to lose a decade of life, although in the latter case, no one is sure if that statistic is based on the low numbers of doctors or considerations such as climate, diet, or culture.

France is under the same pressures to privatize, consolidate, and make their system "profitable" as is Canada, the U.S., Britain, Australia, and most of the rest of the world. Of course, these are economic pressures; social pressures tend to work in the opposite direction. Natalie Simonnot is the assistant director general of Medecins du monde, a group similar to Doctors Without Borders (Medicines sans frontiers), but with a more local focus. Although France's public/private system is held out as an example for Canada to follow, most of the people suggesting that approach are really hoping to integrate a U.S.-style system of private HMOs and hospitals with our public ones. Simonnot says that France's public/private marriage has managed to be as inclusive as it is because it really is "a falsely private system." The central government has had total control over the private insurance companies, which must go through it to be reimbursed. Their fees are overseen and their profits to a great degree controlled, something it's hard to imagine happening in North America. The country also mass-negotiates for prices with the big pharmaceutical companies, so drugs are 20 percent less expensive than in Canada, on average, and *100 percent cheaper* than in the U.S.

"The keystone to our system," she says, "has always *been that the private sector has to obey the rules set down by the public.*" Private doctors have had government-imposed fee tariffs, as have private hospitals. It all ultimately comes through taxes. "If I go to a private doctor," says Simonnot, "I pay him. But then I get reimbursed by my insurance and also by the government, through social security, for almost the total cost. My primary care physician has to refer me to any specialist, and both are paid by the government. They are very complicated, our taxes!" But in 2004, all that changed with new reforms to the health code, and Simonnot was outraged. "Now the public sector no longer directs and controls the private doctors, it's the private sector having control over the public!" The law was very new when Simonnot was interviewed, and she was one of the few people to have read it in its entirety and to have grasped its significance. By way of example, she said there's a security service for health products, like blood and medications. Now that has to be administered to show a profit. "People don't realize what this means. It means that the sick and disabled have been turned into a market commodity! This is a catastrophe."

Simonnot says that making money off the sick will collapse as there begin to be too many of them. "There is no policy of prevention whatsoever ... and only the acute-care physicians are cared for in this system." She says there are some local, left-wing co-ops here and there throughout the country, "working doctors, maternal health clinics ... but they're starved for money. And two things are descending on us, very fast: advances in technology and pharmacology, which are causing medical costs to sky-rocket, and on top of that, the population is aging. You'd think the Health minister would formulate a plan to deal with that, but [no]." Dr Ann Gervais, an energetic, pixie-like infectious disease specialist who works in the north of Paris, treating mostly poor people, agrees. Many people complain about France's policy of caring for very sick illegal immigrants. She says, "That's not what's costing the money! It's the meds, the huge increases in pharmaceutical prices. I mean, just one quick example, there's Astra, a drug company that came up with a good arthritis medication thirty years ago. They're still demanding and getting these huge prices, even though their investment was obviously paid off at least two decades ago. These aren't really social questions for the medical system; they're political."

Gervais' explanation for the French situation sounds like a re-run of what all the old Queen E doctors have been saying about Quebec's. "Let's say you come in for an appendectomy under this new regime. You're supposed to be in and out in three days, so this new system defines a theoretical cost for a 'normal' stay. It's rigid; it doesn't take things like complications or other illnesses into account. At the same time, there are chic, professionally 'cool' ailments that are also expensive, like liver transplants. They love those in private hospital circles, because the bed-stay is relatively short, but the payment they get from insurance is big. That's profitable for them. But simple, common illnesses like gall bladders and broken bones and so forth – the ones that cause people to lose their independence and really need care – for that you can wait six months for treatment. Not much money for those procedures ends up in a private hospital's account, and there's a lot of time in bed, so it's not profitable for them to take care of basic health needs."

Just as in Canada, as Ann Gervais says, "There's the whole status thing going on. The chic, expensive, super-hospitals, the 'centres d'excellence' and so on, are supposed to spearhead all the research. And then there are hospitals like this one: smaller, public, where they put the old people, the uninteresting illnesses. They get less and less money even to research the very common illnesses." "And yet," she adds, again in unconscious imitation of doctors from the Queen E, "here at Bichat, despite our problems, there is a very high level of technical excellence, very good research. For example – it was written up in the *New England Journal of Medicine* six months ago – Philippe Menascher, one of our surgeons, developed a way to take muscle cells from the leg to graft into the cardiac muscle, which means you don't have to have a heart transplant, you can fix the problem from within your own body! Obviously, you can't do this in every case, there are many conditions that have to be met and you need a really big hospital. You can't do it in your kitchen. But innovations still come out of public, community, overcrowded hospitals like this one, because we're on the front lines!"

So far, the care of the needy is still adequate, she says. "Ours is a system very rich in paperwork," Gervais laughs. "We usually manage, but it can be very hard for some people." She gave a very personal example of how it all works. "My sister has Grave's Disease, a very serious malignancy of the thyroid. She got her first test here, then went to the city for her insurance company to pay for the next step. Les services sociaux booked her at the Hôpital Necker a whole two months later! That's way too long to wait for Grave's intervention, but it's typical of what happens if you have to use the public services. I pleaded and pulled strings and finally got her endoscopy and ultrasound [relatively quickly]. This proves how the system fails people. If you have a pancreatic pathology – that's scary stuff – it's a minimum of two days in the private system but three weeks in the public."

The reasons are recognizable to anyone familiar with Canadian health care. Gervais says, "One common problem might be technological. Let's say the endoscopy machine is broken. First, the public hospitals have fewer of whatever kind of machines. Second, although the private hospitals pay extra insurance on their machines so they're repaired immediately when they break down, the government didn't want to sign that kind of contract when they bought theirs so they have to wait X number of weeks whenever one is broken. These little, tiny economies, all the time in the public service, have big effects on the patients." Cardiac surgeon at the old Queen Elizabeth, Ron Lewis, tells the same story about his practice. "One of the worst things about these constant shortages," he says, "is how they affect everyday care. When you're doing an aortic surgery, you protect your graft by using a clamp with little shoes to make it less traumatic to the tissue. They cost ten to fifteen dollars each. People spend their time trying to save a few shoes. No shoes left, you just use the clamp alone. But of course it does damage, so the patient may end up in the hospital longer and cost the system way more money. The problem is that it takes so long to expose the reality of the link between something like that and the number of people having a rough time in the Recovery Room. It's like cigarette smoking and cancer. You can ignore it at the time, but then the patient comes back with an occluded graft and you have to operate all over again! You know there's only one good clamp and yet you get in trouble using them! You just get worn down by everyone criticizing you for these daily expenses and start to say, 'Oh, just give me the shoeless clamp.'" Like Ron Lewis' story about the aortic clamp, Gervais said the same ridiculous *petits economies* are going on in France's public hospitals with horrifically expensive liver transplants. "It happens when there are obstructions in the liver – a rare pathology, Budd-Chiri syndrome. If you use a cheap stint, the blood flows too fast. We're only issued five good ones a year. When they run out, you use the cheap one and the patient ends up in surgery again with complications that cost a fortune. It's ridiculous."

Gervais, like Ron Lewis and many other veterans of hospital closures in Canada, blames much of the inertia in public hospitals on the fact that it's the public, community hospitals that are usually the ones that are being forced to consolidate, always becoming bigger and bigger. That brings with it the destruction of highly efficient small teams and years of learning which protocols really work best. Then, along come more crowded conditions and "problems like long-term patients, which can cause morale problems in the staff. Trust me," she says, "size matters! Many public hospitals are large, or are being forced to consolidate. *Plus que c'est gros, moins que ca marche!*" Gervais used to work in a smaller community hospital before it was merged with a much bigger one. "I knew everyone," she says, singing a familiar song. "So if I needed something and they hadn't delivered, they'd be embarrassed to see me in the cafeteria. I could say, 'Hey, what's happening, yes or no?' and get an answer. But in the big outfits, I don't even know who to ask!" When it comes to the challenges looming in the 21ST century, which include pandemics and massive public health problems allied to global warming and possible pollution or food contamination events, it becomes more and more clear that depending on one central hospital, instead of many small, decentralized ones, is a very serious mistake.

Gervais also used to work for the president of the *Assemblee Nationale*. She said while she was involved in national health policy decisions, she saw that many politicians "have good will, but they're overwhelmed with all their responsibilities. They also have to defend their ridings all the time. They get these papers from all the super-technicians and they don't have any contact with the reality of health care on the ground ... So things creep into health legislation that can completely change the spirit of the law, and they don't even realize it! These changes get put in by the lifers, the bureaucrats, and the elected officials can't defend themselves. And you know who would have to demand the firing of bureaucrats? The bureaucrats themselves. So that's not going to happen!"

Our current obsession with doing everything the same way all around the world means that even in Europe, "Everyone is more and more committed to this policy of economies of scale. So they're closing or consolidating all our small, community hospitals. Somehow that's supposed to save money, *mais c'est pas evident* ... If they would instead invest in follow-up care, it would prevent so many people getting sick again, and instead of spending money on that later, then they could really save money!" As it is, like our own hospitals in the days of mostly private care, French public care centers often beg for charity from citizens' groups, associations, and former patients just to keep going.

As these problems become revealed, it's even more important to remember that in terms of health care, we are among the luckiest countries in the world. Even if the Canadian system does have plenty of things wrong with it, it is more just, equitable and workable than most. Statistics don't lie; at 4.7 for us and 6.0 for France, even our infant mortality rate is considerably better than that of a country that can justly claim to have the best health system in Europe. Most Canadians instinctively realize that fact and regularly threaten their elected officials with annihilation if they propose to alter the Health Care Act. But recent events – the Supreme Court decision allowing Quebec to offer private care for some patients; the media obsession with complaining about wait times without clearly knowing what they are; the election of a Conservative government, well known to favour more privatization; and the slow erosion, via bureaucratic changes, provincial bills, and increasingly aggressive trade treaties, of both funding and health care integrity – are all breaking down the Canadian system as quickly as citizens try to build it up.

Medical and hospital professionals all around the world are being faced with a similar diminishing of the capacities of their health care systems by economic pressures. Many countries, including Ireland, England, Australia, France, Germany, Denmark, Sweden, Holland, India, and Mexico, are starting to get together at international meetings to try to figure out what is actually practical and workable about what they still have and how they can protect it and work onwards from there. It is at these international meetings that some very surprising solutions and role-models are being discovered – not to mention a whole new way to address that pathological old monster, the funding versus costs equation.

7

Long Live the Queen

MERCY, FORTITUDE AND COMMON SENSE

I do thank God for the new knowledge of disease, new drugs and new methods which are now at our command. I only wish that in making use of the good new things we would not forget too much of the qualities of mercy, of fortitude and of common sense which characterized our doctors and nurses of past generations.

Harold Griffith, 1955[1]

Looking at the early history of a single modern hospital is instructive when we consider our current and pressing health care issues. The choices that some of the pioneers of hospital care once made can help us to assess the options available today. It's surprisingly edifying to read what an experienced doctor like Harold Griffith thought of the middle years of medical history, the decades between the two World Wars. Although it seems to us a Dark Ages, with far too few antibiotics and anesthetics, no steroids, Viagra, Prozac, or cholesterol-lowering drugs – and not even a thought of MRIs and laparoscopy, to say nothing of nanotechnology or gene therapy – Harold Griffith remembered those early days with remarkable cheerfulness. "The old Hospital was a happy place," he reminisced in 1955, "in spite of facilities which even then seemed primitive; for there was good nursing, kindness, and a sympathetic attention to each patient's particular needs. Some diseases, like typhoid, lobar pneumonia, puerperal fever and erysipelas, which we seldom see nowadays, were always prevalent and the cause of much misery; but in spite of this, most of our patients recovered. When I listen to some of the young doctors talking today I think they really believe that all our patients in the old days must have died, because we had no antibiotics, sulphas or hormones with which to save them."[2]

Griffith finished his portrait of the Montreal Homeopathic as he remembered it back in the 1920s and 30s with the comment that begins this chapter. His little list of all-important medical qualities may sound like rather corny platitudes: mercy, fortitude, and common sense – although they do seem to be very Canadian platitudes, especially the idea of using "common sense." Of course, his era of small, community entwined hospitals, staffed with dedicated teams proud of their newly established professions who were able to take the time to really get to know their patients, has today nearly vanished, even in the rural areas where systems like this have persisted. We take this situation for granted, but in the increasingly unanimous opinion of the highest level of experts on the cutting edge of medical care, this loss has definitely not been a good thing.

John Hughes, a general or family practitioner who is much quoted in this book, represents a large number of professionals who think the reason for the change from personalized, family care to specialized, impersonal clinics is relentlessly economic: we just can't afford to pay doctors for the time investment per-patient the old system requires. But such critics don't think we can afford the new kind of hospital systems we're setting up, either. Hughes says, "With these fancy new specialties, we're teaching people to do things that society can't pay for – and that tendency has become a worldwide phenomenon." As we have seen, he is not alone in feeling that the super-hospitals, centres of excellence, and walk-in clinics with interchangeable doctors and technicians are inadequate substitutions for personalized care. Most of the current research clearly demonstrates that such systems will not be able to deliver effective health care or be economically efficient for the whole population.[3]

When policy options are this conflicted, it's wise turn to the scientific method of looking for empirical proofs. Only scientifically amassed statistical evidence – combined with a bit of common sense – can provide the information needed to assess whether assumptions about the best way to deliver health care in terms of time, costs, and medical priorities are true, and if not, what other options there may be. Fortunately, in recent years, governments, universities, NGOs, and international institutions such as the UN and the World Health Organization (WHO) have been amassing exactly this kind of data.

In 2002, McGill's Institute for the Study of Canada held an important conference called "Building Consensus for Health Care Reform in Canada." Experts from all over the world were invited to present papers, submit evidence, and provide input. A variety of politicians and health care advocates, such as Roy Romanow, were in attendance, but most of the presenters were high-level medical and health system researchers from university faculties and government departments across Canada and Western Europe. Ken Fyke, speaking for Saskatchewan's Health Commission on Medicare, listed three key priorities that his province has determined need to be immediately implemented in their provincial health and hospital systems:

1 Focus on quality rather than volume;
2 Restructure both primary health and acute care hospitals;
3 Increase the kind of research that measures, monitors, and evaluates health.

The "primary health" mentioned in point two means first-line contact, that is, the interface between patients and the first person they see when they need help – usually a GP or family physician, sometimes a community nurse or other such team member. Fyke explained that opposing these ideal goals are the problems we have with hospital systems today. They comprise a somewhat longer list, which includes:

1 Overuse of drugs;
2 Great variations in surgical intervention rates;
3 Under-management of chronic disease;
4 Significant inappropriate utilization of professionals;
5 Great variation in health outcomes.[4]

Closing the gaps between Fyke's two lists goes far beyond tinkering with the present system. If the direction our system is going is carefully compared with what actually needs to be implemented to make it sustainable, it's obvious that Fykes is suggesting what amounts to a serious paradigm shift in behaviour and philosophy – not just within health care but throughout the profession and even society at large.

His third and fourth points, "Under-management of chronic disease" and "Significant inappropriate utilization of professionals" both refer to the concentration in hospital medicine on acute or catastrophic care. As we have noted, hospitals spend most of their time, money, and professional skills on life-threatening emergencies such as heart attacks, liver or kidney failures, or invasive tumours. They reserve almost no time or money for dealing with the chronic conditions and behaviours that nearly always precede these catastrophes. "Inappropriate use of professionals" means the tendency to depend on specialist treatments for the acute event instead of the regular, primary care that might have avoided the expensive disasters or could have controlled them longer.

This conference of international experts received this challenging list with nods of agreement instead of surprise because the major focus of the old Queen Elizabeth Hospital, which was the supreme value of the generalist, has come back to the forefront of the health care equation. The importance of primary, that is to say, general practice care, including its undisputed economic efficiency, has recently become strongly supported by unimpeachable data from around the world.

We need to remember that until around 1995 community hospitals, including the Queen Elizabeth, had typically been founded and were still largely run by general practitioners, that is, primary care professionals. Even while GPs like Harold and Jim Griffith were transforming themselves into specialist anesthesiologists and surgeons in the 1940s and 50s, they made certain that real generalists had full access to their patients when they were admitted to hospitals. These generalists sat in on surgeries and other procedures and were also active on hospital boards and in management. In the 1990s, when the specialist hold on hospitals was more advanced even at the Queen E and many other community hospitals, GPs were still routinely contacted about each admission to give *"continuity of care."* Consequently, a woman with a broken leg would have been treated with full awareness of the complications that might arise from her mild diabetes and tendency towards clinical depression. As we saw in chapter 1, a major reason many doctors at the Queen E protested its closing was because they saw losing such a hospital as yet another attack on the "continuity of care system."[5]

As mentioned previously, GPs were banned from urban hospitals across North America in the late 1980s through the mid-1990s as a cost-cutting measure. Because salaries are the largest item of hospital budgets, hospital administrators determined that a person admitted for an acute condition already had the attention of the specialist – the secondary care physician. They eliminated GP involvement because they did not want to pay for the time needed for a patient's primary-care physician to visit the institution and confer with the specialist – or even to be briefly contacted outside the hospital. Today, in nearly all of Canada except for some small, rural hospitals, generalists never see the inside of a tertiary care facility – that is, a hospital. As well, today in Canada, our generalists almost never get a face-to-face meeting with any secondary care specialist, even specialists who are treating people whom the GPs have been trying to keep healthy all their lives.

According to Judith Levitan, GPs are discouraged from calling specialists for help when diagnosing a difficult condition and are rarely granted professional guidance in determining how to prevent the condition from worsening. GPs also report having a hard time getting records about their patients while they were in hospital. Specialists, on the other hand, are rarely informed about a patient's other ailments, histories, allergies, or physiological eccentricities. Therefore, both types of doctor are at a considerable disadvantage when trying to determine whether the problems the patient experiences subsequent to hospital treatment should be attributed to drug, surgical, or other interventions during the hospitalization, or to an evolution of other conditions. In short, without the input of the generalist, the medical system of primary, secondary, and tertiary care has become *fragmented* – only the secondary specialist has contact with tertiary care.

A very important meta-study published in 2004 by HEN, The Health Evidence Network branch of the World Health Organization, makes it clear that fragmenting the system in this fashion is worrisome not just for the patient – it has also been a serious economic and professional mistake. The study is entitled, "What are the advantages and disadvantages of restructuring a health care system to be more focused on primary care services?" In its summary, it states: "*International studies show that the strength of a country's primary care system is associated with improved population health outcomes for all-cause mortality, all-cause premature mortality, and cause-specific premature mortality from major respiratory and cardiovascular diseases.*" This means that all the people in a country live longer when they have regular and easy access to a GP, community nurse, or other primary-care team. Moreover, "Studies from developed countries demonstrate that *an orientation towards a specialist-based system enforces inequity in access.* Health systems in low income countries with a strong primary care orientation tend to be more pro-poor, equitable and accessible." This means that generalist-run health systems are more accessible to all and more just than our current specialist-dominated ones. Finally, "using primary care physicians [instead of specialist services] *reduces costs and increases patient satisfaction with no adverse effects on quality of care or patient outcomes.*" Most of the studies showed such shifts "to be more cost-effective," although the meta-analysis warns that sometimes "costs might not be reduced," simply because using such a system "ends up identifying previously unmet needs, improves access, and tends to expand service utilization."[6] In short, using primary care is either cheaper or costs the same, while making a greater number of people healthier and more satisfied with the system.

More use of and support for primary care physicians within hospitals seems to be the obvious solution to many of our economic and treatment deficits. But even if we wanted to take that path, it would be impossible in Canada at this time. Because of the cost-switch to specialists – to say nothing of the prestige considerations that began to have serious effects on education in the early 1990s – Canada slashed the supply of all its doctors – particularly its generalists. Today, we're paying for another stylish misconception the experts had about how different the future was going to be from the past. John Hughes reiterates that, in what was likely another far-reaching effect of the IMF Report to Canada of 1994, "Paul Martin admitted to shutting down the medical schools in 1995, in order to save money. The governments were under pressure, and couldn't see their way to paying for the new doctors' salaries, so they decided to make sure there weren't any around to pay ... by the fall of 2006, the Quebec College of Physicians and Surgeons was declaring the lack of generalists a crisis, largely to blame for long wait times, ICU, and ER crowding."

It's easy to see why most Canadian families can't find a GP or have trouble getting a timely appointment with their overworked generalist, even if they're lucky enough to have one. There's another reason, too. In order for schools and professional bodies to encourage the training of more generalists, we have to ask the question: Who does the emphasis on specialization serve? The primary beneficiary of large numbers of specialists is the medical profession, because its members can make higher salaries and command more prestige by specializing. The secondary beneficiaries are the manufacturers of drugs and devices for the medical market. Such businesses do not make nearly such high profits from primary care physicians prescribing diets and exercise as they do from specialists suggesting surgeries and drugs. So the overall situation is unlikely to change in Canada any time soon, unless government health departments display the political will to intervene and mandate that more GPs be trained. So far, they are only bending a few rules here and there, such as Quebec's June 2007 decision to amend part of its demands on young doctors, which had all of them fleeing the province on graduation. The province's remarkable disincentives to practice included an extra year of study to qualify for a Quebec license required in no other provinces, and expensive fees to take another exam. These requirements have been waived for now.

Even so, as John Hughes says, "All the demographic studies show that until 2012 at least, even a best-case scenario shows continuing serious doctor shortages all across the country. The World Health Organization is screaming because we're head-hunting physicians in the Third World." In fact, the province of Saskatchewan has more doctors from South Africa than have graduated from its own schools; South Africa has resorted to diplomatic channels, officially asking Canada to desist so they can have some people left to treat their own citizens, especially since southern Africa is in the midst of the worst AIDS epidemic in the world. Libya is also suffering, but its pleas for Canada to stop poaching its trainee doctors have been rejected by the colleges of physicians and surgeons in Alberta, Newfoundland, Labrador, and Saskatchewan, largely because those provinces are so desperate for medical professionals.[7]

Derek Marpole, a Montreal cardiologist, says, "The number of GPs across the country is more and more inadequate, because training them is way down. And CLSCs, which were not entirely a bad idea, are a disaster in terms of serious care. Forty percent of them really can't do medicine because there are never any doctors there. The idea was that specialists would take up the slack of the GPs and family medicine doctors in hospitals, and that the GP and family medicine doctors would be working in the CLSCs. But in rural areas, there are no specialists to do that, so that's where the few GPs end up. Changes like cutting the numbers of GPs being trained, as well as doctors overall, were completely un-thought-out!" Marpole explains that even within Canada, the health of the primary care system varies. "Out west, family practice physicians control the specialists. You don't go to one unless your GP says you should, and the specialist has to send you back to your GP before there can be even follow-up appointments. That's been shown as an efficient and cost-effective method, but it wouldn't work here in Quebec: a third of my patients don't have a GP to start with because there aren't enough to go around! Even people with something like chronic asthma just manage to get referred to specialists when something dire happens. This isn't a cost- or effect-efficient system."

The western Canadian method is termed "gate-keeping" and is popular in many parts of the world. The GP is paid for the time it takes to assess whether a patient needs a specialist or if the condition could be solved with lifestyle changes. Of course, the GP has to be paid for the time investment it will take to get to know enough about her patient that she can judge whether diet, stress, or pathology are the root of the problem. Without even a few harassed and overworked GPs to keep the gates, the specialists' rates are charged to the system, often without benefit to the patient. GP Adam Gavsie says that primary care doctors "don't get much respect any more. They're considered less knowledgeable than specialists when in fact they have to be *more* knowledgeable. When we rely too heavily on specialists, we end up doing what I call 'band-aid medicine' – working on the symptom instead of the root cause." Gavsie goes on to explain, "The patient's stress or pathology breaks out in, say, a bad back, so in our system they go straight to an expensive orthopedist, get drugs, or an operation." But that wasn't really the root cause, he says, so it breaks out again, this time as indigestion, "and they go to a gastroenterologist. By the time they get to the cardiologist, it's too late to heal the original problem, which a good family doctor, who knew that patient and his circumstances, might have been able to head off much earlier by counseling less work or changes in diet and exercise."

In terms of how this situation affects the wait times, overcrowding, and overgrown budgets of community hospitals, it means that the average patient spends weeks or months anxiously waiting for each specialist appointment and for the results of each expensive test done at a local hospital. This costs the health system an enormous amount of money and the hospital staff a lot of work. Meanwhile, the patient's symptoms aren't even being treated; in fact, his or her condition often deteriorates. As many large studies in the U.S. have shown, "absence of a primary care source was found to be *the most important factor* in determining poor health ... *health systems dominated by specialists, such as that of the United States, have higher total health care costs and reduced access to health care by vulnerable populations.* The high cost is attributed to proportionately low numbers of primary care physicians and consequent impairment of the gate-keeping function."[8] Gate-keeping would have kept the patient out of the hospital and drug lines in the first place, and with more of it, U.S. mortality rates might not be among the worst in the industrialized world.

One of the old family of Queen E primary-care physicians, Jack McMartin, a cousin to Linda Griffith, loved house-calls for both their preventative character and their efficiency in helping both patient and doctor anticipate and avoid acute episodes requiring hospital care. "I was shocked when gradually, in the 1950s and 60s, doctors, really good family doctors, all started to refuse to make house calls. I really liked them and hated to see them go," he reminisced at the age of 84. "You can tell a lot by seeing people at home, a great deal more than any number of questions you pose in the office can tell you! Men are the worst; it's hard to get enough answers from a male patient to make a diagnosis. You know, in those days especially, they figured that if they got an ache or a pain, they should just tough it out. Seeing them at home helped me assess conditions that they might not have felt worth mentioning in the office."

McMartin adds, "As soon as you go into somebody's house, you can see their socio-economic situation, their family situation, how likely it is they're under some kind of stress or danger from, say, bad diet, the wrong kind of job, or unsanitary conditions." McMartin, even after 20 years of retirement, is quite aware of the crisis caused by not having enough generalists, as well as the two main reasons for it: money and prestige. He worries about the systemic implications of such a system and thinks that many people with serious problems end up making the rounds of ten specialists, but never find anyone who understands enough about them to make the right diagnosis. "That causes people with chronic diseases to lose faith in mainstream medicine completely. In those days, we knew a little about a lot of things, and that would help us. Now specialists know a lot about a very, very narrow thing and sometimes that doesn't really help the patient."

Jack thinks doctors should all be trained as GPs first, before they specialize, as they all were in the old days. That might sound quaintly old-fashioned, but it's actually a cutting-edge idea in international circles today. Jack explains that "Changing training in this way could alleviate other problems in the system, such as not enough doctors in remote areas. Students could be sent to unstaffed areas right after residency for a year to get that experience while being well paid. Then they could decide whether to continue as a generalist or come back and specialize."

Thirty-two year-old Adam Gavsie agrees, as do the most current studies. Gavsie explains, "It wouldn't really be impossible to go back to that; it's all a matter of how you want to spend the money." He adds, "Anyone who says Canadian doctors aren't well-paid, by the way, is crazy. We get plenty of money. And if we got the same kind of pay, by the hour, as it were, it might be quite feasible for some of us to choose that kind of practice with very old or very sick patients, for example, to spare them the difficulty of coming in. It's really just a question of remuneration and incentive." He mentions Medi-visit in Ontario, a program funded by the government with what he considers, "good remuneration, $90 a visit, and you can usually do two an hour. Several people I know have chosen to do that exclusively. Or you can buttress up a regular or hospital practice with it. But here in Quebec, doctors can get arrested for trying to help their very ill or elderly patients this way!" The lack of primary care physicians, as the meta-studies show, directly results in higher costs for the health system, poorer general health, and higher death and disability rates for the population. But as Adam Gavsie, John Hughes, Judith Levitan, and so many other GPs have noted, there is no real recognition in Canada, either on the part of society, the government funders, or the medical profession itself, of how important generalized care really is. Primary care is, however, the very care described by the Queen Elizabeth's old motto of "patient-centred" medicine and is still the ideal for most small, community hospitals.

As the WHO meta-study states, there are nine established "levels of care" in medicine: "prevention, pre-symptomatic detection of disease, early diagnosis, diagnosis of established disease, management of disease, management of disease complications, rehabilitation, terminal care, and counseling."[9] Only one professional – the primary care physician – practices every single one. But because of its low status and systems of remuneration that pay per patient instead of for time spent, even the few generalists left in Canada are unable to do their jobs properly. Adam Gavsie says, "There are so few GPs now, we rarely get to do the work we're supposed to do. In school we're taught to allot 45 minutes per patient ... imagine! We never get that kind of time. And we're trained to devote a lot of our attention to listening to the patient, figuring out what's really going on. But training and the real world are very different. If you're expected to move a patient every ten, or as some types of doctors do, every three minutes, there's no time to do what you are trained to do. Even the public resists the slower kind of treatment. They're in a hurry too; they want to self-prescribe the latest pill they saw on TV or they want their pain taken 'seriously,' which to them means being referred to a specialist for what they think will be faster and more dramatic results than just cutting down on sweets or sleeping more." In truth, many people still derive a perverse feeling of prestige because they feel being seen by an expensive specialist legitimizes and recognizes the seriousness of their pain and also proves the system is "taking good care of them."

The final section of the WHO meta-study offers both hope and guidance for common-sense approaches to the reality of how primary care actually produces better results for less money. "Despite the evidence for primary care," it says, "resource allocation in most countries still favours hospitals and specialist care ... This explains the paradox of the attractiveness of primary care on empirical grounds and its lack of appeal to national policy-makers and healthcare professionals. [Both] see it as a low-grade activity with little effect on mortality or serious morbidity and [believe its] predominant role is [to provide] triage of access to hospitals." The encouraging part is, "*Given the right incentives in any health system, there is the real opportunity to expand provision of medical services in a primary care setting* ... Policy makers need to be made aware of the concept of primary care and what it has to offer. This will require investment for advocacy and marketing activities to communicate the benefits of primary care to health professionals, policy-makers and the public."[10]

The study points out that in Europe especially, "Much of specialist outpatient care is [now] shifting to primary care via the outreach clinics encouraged by shared-care schemes," but the following comments already apply to Canada. "There is considerable overlapping of roles of general practitioners giving specialized care and specialists providing general practice services ... Even inpatient services traditionally provided in hospitals by the specialist are shifting to primary care through hospital-care-at-home schemes. [In CLSCs, for example,] ... general practitioners are now expected to provide emergency care for conditions that were traditionally provided in hospital accident and emergency departments."[11]

WHO reports tend to be exceedingly moderate in tone, but this one is startlingly strong in its political advocacy. "Primary care has a greater role to play than before, and *resource allocation needs to flow in its favour.*" Of course, it adds the caveat of further studies for determining "limits of substitution" and "configuration of primary care teams and modes of delivery" as well as the obvious fact that although they have been overemphasized and over-funded for the last generation, secondary (specialist) and tertiary care will always be needed. This golden crown of studies sums up the most desirable situation for any government dealing with national health care. "[International] findings support policies that encourage a shift of services away from specialist care to primary, as the substitution does not adversely affect quality but lowers cost."

STRANGE BEDFELLOWS

The central assumption of the World Bank, the largest international health funding organization, is that economic growth is the most fundamental prerequisite for alleviating poverty and improving health.

Spiegel and Yassi, 2004[12]

It's been established that simple, general care is more effective than specialist intervention. But there is a paradox to think about that has to do with current concepts of economics. The highly respected international health journal quoted above exposes this paradox. Most of us share the assumption that economic prosperity and high per-capita expenditure translate to better health. This belief has created the social consensus that has allowed organizations like the World Bank and the many related trade regimes to flourish. However, increasing amounts of hard data suggest that this assumption may be wrong when practically applied. In fact, as the article goes on to say, "*growth that enhances disparity* will most likely generate *more poor health.*"[13] In other words, if full attention isn't paid to distributing wealth in such a way that all the population is cared for, more people *on every level* will get sick. This is the very old public health lesson learned by the medical pioneers of the 19th century who founded our hospitals in the first place. And the functioning example most often cited that embodies this paradox today is an isolated, poor, and very small country that has been reviled and beleaguered for the past forty years.

Cuba, of all places, is being hailed in much of today's international health literature as a possible health care role-model. This is an odd situation: Cuba is, after all, not only a poor and isolated southern country, but a dictatorship; it is rare for such places to be held up as beacons to emulate, particularly in terms of the physical well-being of their populations. Cuba spends 7.4 percent of its gross national product on health care, compared with the U.S. figure of 13.6 percent or France's 10 percent, but its mortality and life expectancy rates are equal to and sometimes better than those of the U.S. and compare favourably with those in Canada. For decades, however, Cuba has been isolated by economic embargoes and excluded from all the economic and trade organizations, such as NAFTA and the WTO, that are supposed to bring the benefits of modern economic development to the widest possible public. The country has not been able to acquire World Bank loans or any sort of guidance from the economic powerhouses of the world and is not a signatory to NAFTA or any of its offspring, like the SPP or TILMA, discussed in chapter 6. It has been abandoned to follow its own course, one outlined by poverty and a large urban population trying to cope with a scarcity of every kind of resource, even food.

Cuba's health system performance has been investigated by many international and academic bodies, however, and although there are many caveats, especially in terms of a unique social situation that does not easily translate to that of other countries, the numbers seem to be surprisingly solid. As Dr. Robert Butler, president of the International Longevity Center in New York and a Pulitzer Prize-winning author on aging puts it, "I know Americans tend to be skeptical, but health and education are the two achievements of the Cuban revolution, and they deserve some credit, despite the government's poor record on human rights."[14] Moreover, although Cubans are in fact restive and unhappy about their civil rights and freedoms, independent polls show great pride and satisfaction with their health system.

As we saw in chapter 5, income and racial inequalities have contributed to giving the United States the highest infant mortality rates in the industrialized world, close to 7.1, which is higher than poverty-stricken Cuba's 6.4 and much higher than Canada's 4.82.[15] As we noted there, such inequities surprisingly affect the general health of even the wealthy, lowering their life expectancy rates to well below those of poor people living in industrialized countries with single-payer health care and also increasing infant death rates above those of several very poor countries, including Cuba and parts of India. These unexpected figures have naturally spawned curiosity and in recent years studies have been proliferating that attempt to pinpoint how such a small, poor country has managed to take care of its population's health so well. Michael Moore's film *Sicko*, in which some 9/11 recovery workers and victims are transported to the island to receive the health care they can't afford in the United States, has made this odd situation even more public and controversial. It also pointed out that when it comes to health, money isn't everything. Lower-class British people have lower rates of every major disease and can expect to live four years longer than even the richest Americans. A study from the *Journal of the American Medical Association* backs up Moore's claim, stating, "individuals in the top of the education and income strata in the United States have comparable rates of diabetes and heart disease as those in the bottom of the income and education strata in England."[16]

Prior to the revolution in 1959, Cuba's health statistics were much like those of any other impoverished tropical country. But in the 1960s, evaluations were conducted by the new revolutionary government; their results ought to sound familiar to any Canadian medical expert. Cuban researchers highlighted the following problems: *emphasis on acute rather than preventative care, the lack of collaboration between professionals in the health system, fragmented care, patient discontent due to inconsistent quality, overuse of ERs, and shortages of GPs.* In short, the Cubans came up with almost exactly the same list of problems enumerated by Saskatchewan's Ken Fykes at the beginning of this chapter.

The new system the Cubans implemented heads in a direction that those charged with planning future hospital care in Canada should at least note; it is one that Harold Griffith would have applauded, because it relies almost entirely on simplicity and commonsense. In its post-1960s system, Cuba now depends heavily on *primary care* physicians and nurses. Each one takes care of about 600 people in the immediate neighbourhood, a per-capita rate of family physicians to patients that is one of the best in the world – it's at least twice as good as in Canada and almost five times better than the 1 per 3,200 in the U.S. These family doctors and nurses are integrated within their communities, like Jack McMartin and the old Queen E used to be, and practitioners typically use every afternoon "for home visits to patients with acute care needs, rehabilitation of chronic conditions, and primary prevention," after spending the morning seeing patients at the clinic.[17]

Of course, experts cite many "non-medical determinants" that partially account for Cuba's good health record. Basic education and housing are subsidized by the state, and the relatively non-industrialized nature of the society provides fairly clean air and water, decent nutrition, and available employment. A significant part of the population seems to be free of much stress as a consequence of social cohesion, fewer income disparities, and the gentle climate. Basic food is available but not plentiful, and transportation is often by foot or bicycle. Most Canadians would probably choose to avoid the latter two circumstances, but they would undoubtedly be good for their general health.

There is also the ideal and the reality. Foreigners, including medical researchers, are generally taken to see the better clinics that are reserved for Cuban party members and tourists. Poorer Cubans most often have to make do with primitive buildings with almost no facilities. Nonetheless, charges that the country's infant mortality rates, for example, are skewed because they include the births but not the deaths of Cuban refugees are rather silly, since other measures are easily accessed. For example, the percentage of children surviving to age 5 has risen steadily over the past few decades, from 95.6 to 99.2, and percentages of low birth weights declined from 11.4 percent to 6.5 percent between 1975 and 1999.[18] And, although visits to Emergency Rooms have risen over the same period, they have declined in comparison to outpatient visits, a situation devoutly to be wished by every national health system.

It should be noted that these improvements were achieved during a period of severe economic deprivation, when the country had lost its Soviet trading partners and the U.S. embargo had intensified. Between the middle 1970s and 2000, the Cuban transportation infrastructure broke down due to the lack of fuel, which means their typically Soviet-style industrialized farming had to be radically revamped, to one that is now almost completely organic. Power outages lasted as long as 16 hours a day and the trade embargo deprived hospitals of everything from machines to aspirins. That children not only survived – but that they survived in greater numbers and in better health than ever before – is an indication of what could happen to our own health care system if similar moves towards daily family care and prevention were implemented.[19]

Nobody is suggesting that western, industrialized countries adopt the governance model of a tropical, Communist dictatorship. What does fascinate researchers is the high level of care provided by this country's very simple and efficient use of resources. Although there are hospitals and specialists for acute problems, Cuba, because it has so little money and equipment, has had to gear its system almost entirely towards primary care simply because that's the proven cheapest way to take care of a population. The country survives on the margins of security, even food security, and because of the absolute necessity for efficiency, Cuban practices seem to have become simultaneously innovative and old-fashioned.

On the old-fashioned side, GPs and nurses keep track of every family in their assigned community on an ongoing basis. Family physicians are expected to diagnose and treat patients in the context of their particular families and communities. This practice leads to reduced hospital care because the way that medical records are organized, by family rather than by individual, makes tendencies towards heart disease, depression, or obesity much easier to spot, before they become acute. This method works much as home visits did for Jack McMartin sixty years ago and recalls the Queen E's psychiatric staff's practice of dropping in on their patients into the 1990s.

Cuba also utilizes a very innovative modern system called "CARE" (Continuous Assessment and Risk Evaluation), to keep track of each person so that risks like hypertension, diabetes, and so on are defined and steps are taken to provide treatment. The follow-up that doctors long for and that is so rare in our own systems is a common feature of Cuba's. Every family doctor has access to her patient while in hospital and is required to provide care when the patient is discharged. Patients are also treated "holistically, as bio-pyschosocial beings," to avoid the very situation the old Queen E and other hospitals like it used to deplore, that is, of perceiving people through their disease instead of as individuals. Serious attempts are made to integrate services such as diagnostics, physiotherapy, tertiary and specialist care, and so on. Specialists are required to confer with family physicians, and access between other doctors, secondary and tertiary care physicians, and medical professors is encouraged, according to official policy.[20]

Its isolation has not prevented Cuban health care from providing on-the-ground examples of many other innovative international medical buzz-words. "COPC" means "Community-Oriented Primary Care" and has been encouraged by medical researchers worldwide. But because U.S. and Canadian physicians have a culture that has increasingly narrowed its view to the "traditional physician-patient dyad," few people think this more comprehensive approach, using doctors as caregivers to whole families and communities, is likely to be achieved in Canada any time soon. As Adam Gavsie mentioned earlier, physicians in our system are not predictably remunerated for serving the community or spending enough time to ferret out family data. In Cuba, however, epidemiologic data, including the number of people with certain diseases, the severity of their conditions, birth outcomes, immunization rates and so on, are either available by computer, or, in rural areas, are physically posted on the walls of the consultation room for everyone to consult. That means that "cancer clusters," for example, or unusually high rates of MS or Parkinson's – situations that plague much of rural Canada but which are almost never publicly tabulated or addressed here – are available for the whole neighbourhood to see and for researchers to consider.

As we have mentioned earlier, the effectiveness of Canadian provincial or federal public health departments has been seriously compromised by a culture of secrecy and fragmentation. Canadian public health researchers could easily have computer programs that would link their work with similar or related studies right across the country. The Internet could even provide the public at large with various kinds of information needed to help prevent unnecessary deaths from exposure to toxins or from compromised lifestyles. Canada's vast access to computers could work the same way as clinic walls that post family and other epidemiological information do in Cuba. Instead, decentralized Canadian researchers jealously guard their turf and information is often unavailable even to people working in the same department, to say nothing of other cities or provinces. Service directors do not remain in place for very long, which creates divisions and fragments knowledge. Very few people know about any one thing, which makes the information far less useful. Our style of public health research also commonly aggregates data over large areas, which often erases the evidence of cancer, asthma, or other disease clusters.

Patient privacy is one excuse for this secrecy, as is the idea that the public "can't handle" frightening situations. This attitude increases the instincts for secrecy in this isolated, academic culture that has increasingly misconstrued the actual mandate of a public health service. But there are other, more self-serving reasons for public health departments to resist transparency. Former researchers and employees in both federal and provincial departments have estimated that tuberculosis rates on Canadian native reserves, for example, are 25 *times* the rate of the Canadian population at large. Moreover, the percentage of the strain that is resistant to antibiotics and therefore highly dangerous is on the increase. This disease is poorly understood by doctors, who often misdiagnose it as chronic bronchitis or some other, non-communicable lung disease. Like the rest of the population, many health care workers think TB is a disease of the past that they will not encounter in their practice. Yet, on our reserves, it is apparently occurring on a par with rates in developing countries. Tuberculosis is a disease of poverty. It thrives in conditions of overcrowding, poor housing, improper water treatment, poor nutrition, and lack of access to health care. Because the federal government is responsible for providing health care services on reserves, it is clearly not attractive to them to highlight their own failures or to implement reforms that would have to be both expensive and sweeping.[21]

The situation in Cuba, at least in this one area of public health, is considerably more transparent, which demonstrates that if better public health transparency is possible in a dictatorship, it ought to be more common in countries like Canada. But perhaps the most radical and interesting of all Cuba's innovations is the inclusion of what we would call folk or "alternative" medicine in the family doctor's repertoire. "Integrative medicine" is another professional buzz-word that is supposed to indicate "the thoughtful incorporation of concepts, values, and practices from alternative, complementary, and conventional medicines." In short, instead of only having the normal "allopathic" arsenal of patented drugs, surgery, and expensive machines when it comes to treatment options, family doctors in Cuba are taught such disciplines as acupuncture, herbal medicine, massage, heat therapy, floral essence therapy, homeopathy, yoga, meditation training, and music and art therapy. Most Cuban family doctors are also trained herbalists and frequently prescribe these remedies, which are referred to as "green medicine," and most neighbourhoods, however urban, have their own organic plots of medicinal herbs for such use.[22] Cuban GPs spend 200 hours on such subjects in their first two years of medical school and their principles are integrated into more advanced physiology, anatomy, and clinical courses. Educational materials on alternative treatments are distributed to all practitioners by the Cuban Ministry of Health, much as we might distribute guidelines for statins, SSRIs, or other drugs.[23]

This may all seem a little too far from the Canadian experience, but in fact, as anyone who has set foot in a North American or European drug store knows, the alternative therapies Cuban GPs are taught constitute an enormous, if fragmented, business all over the world. Total expenditures on such therapies as massage, homeopathy, chiropractic, acupuncture, herbs, and so on, in the U.S. alone, is about $27 billion a year and is increasing by leaps and bounds. Thirty percent of the elderly, 50 percent of the Baby Boomers and a whopping 70 percent of the post Baby Boom cohort are reporting that they use alternative medicine. In Canada, 71 percent of the adult population regularly takes "natural health products," including homeopathic and Chinese medicines as well as supplements and herbs. Most U.S. doctors, 84 percent in fact, feel they should know more about such treatments, if only to address patient concerns. The Society for the Teachers of Family Medicine (STFM) and the Cochrane database include randomized trials on such treatments as well as recommendations for medical school curric-

ula. Even in the U.S., there are several medical schools offering courses
in CAM to complement regular medical skills.[24] The prestigious Sloan-
Kettering Cancer Center, among other treatment clinics, offers alternative therapies such as massage, acupuncture, and mind-body therapies. The medical program at McMaster University has proven to be
one of the most open in this regard in Canada. In general, however,
Canadian doctors who wish to learn more about integrative medicine
are discouraged or even forbidden by their provincial College of Physicians.[25]

HOW TO GET WELL CHEAP

> Primary care, the backbone of the nation's health care system, is at grave
> risk of collapse due to a dysfunctional financing and delivery system.
> January 30, 2006 *Report from the American College of Physicians*[26]

Cuba has been forced by political and economic circumstance to
move ahead of the pack, but even in the privatized, over-specialized
U.S., the same looming public health crisis, involving an aging population and increasingly limited funding, has impelled the American
College of Physicians (ACP), the nation's largest such group, to
demand immediate implementation of policies that are, in essence,
similar to Cuba's.[27] Like all professional organizations, the ACP is
highly conservative. Nonetheless, at the end of 2006, it released an
unprecedented crisis report that is a political call to the total reform
of the U.S. health system in favour of primary care. "The consequences of failing to act," they wrote at the end of 2006, "will be *higher
costs, greater inefficiency, lower quality, more uninsured persons, and growing
patient and physician dissatisfaction.*" This is not a self-interested suppli-
cation in that the College's members are specialists as well as generalists. It is a very important message to the public at large – not unlike
that of the world's scientists warning of climate change. In Canada,
the only step taken so far to address our own primary care crisis has
been to allow more foreign doctors to become recognized, that is, to
facilitate the dangerous poaching from the Third World mentioned
earlier. No overhaul of our provincial health systems currently reflects
the findings of all the international agencies that are behind the ACP's
call for action.

   As Ken Fykes pointed out at the beginning of this chapter, the most
inefficient use of our health care dollars possible is spending them the

way we all do now: we pay for the *quantity* of patients a doctor sees instead of the *quality* of the care she dispenses, and we focus on expensive, acute – rather than cheap, preventative – care. So urgent is this matter that the ACP spends much of its crisis paper outlining ways in which payment and funding could be altered to favour the new system. For example, they suggest paying primary care doctors for email and phone consultations that could reduce expensive visits and increase the patients' ability to get medical advice in a timely manner. That is to say, quickly enough to statistically avoid ER visits and the worsening of chronic conditions that can lead to expensive hospitalization. Moreover, "Medicare [whether the Canadian or American version] reimbursement policies should ... recognize the value of the time that physicians spend outside the face-to-face visit in coordinating the care of patients with multiple chronic diseases, including the work involved in coordinating care with other health professionals and family caregivers." The ACP even suggests implementation strategies that would not penalize doctors who don't choose to be a part of this new system.[28]

In the U.S., as in Canada, perverse remuneration and recruiting policies detailed in this and earlier chapters have left our systems in this crisis position. About 35 percent of U.S. generalists will retire in the next few years, bringing the GP ratio of 1:3200 in that country to more like 1: 4000. Canada's is also far too low, with slightly over 31,000 GPs in total, about one per thousand people. As well, far too many of these doctors are in urban areas and many will be retiring in the next few years.[29] Because generalists in both countries habitually make about half as much as specialists, with a fraction of the prestige and no hospital access, medical school students are unlikely to volunteer to correct the situation. They need proper incentives, and quickly, because the trend is worsening by the year. In 1998, 54 percent of U.S. students were entering general practice; only four years later, in 2003, only 19 percent planned to be GPs. The situation is similar here, and as the ACP warning points out, "Without primary care, the health system will become increasingly fragmented, over-specialized and inefficient – leading to *poorer quality care at higher costs.*"[30]

When we think about the future of our own health care – how much time we'll each have to spend in a hospital, however that care is funded – it's important to emphasize that studies around the world, in all types of funding systems, show that, "Primary care physicians ... have been shown to deliver care similar in quality to that of specialists for conditions such as diabetes and hypertension, while using fewer resources."

Moreover, "hospitalization rates and expenditures are higher in areas with fewer primary care physicians and limited access to primary care."[31] GPs can actually reduce mortalities caused by using inappropriate specialists, a situation common in our current system. "Patients receiving care from specialists for conditions outside their area of expertise have been shown to have higher mortality rates for community-acquired pneumonia, congestive heart failure and upper gastrointestinal hemorrhage."[32] The cost of taking care of such illnesses also happens to be lower when GPs do it.

Because the population is aging in both Canada and the U.S., the remaining generalists that we do have also need *more* time with each patient, rather than less. Older people typically have complex, chronic problems, so more drugs or therapies must be reviewed or implemented and more screening, diagnostic services, and counseling are required for every encounter. Because most of the population is without a generalist in the first place, the ability of all of our hospital ERs, especially community ones, to manage public care has become crippled by pointless expenses and inefficiencies as well as increased demand. There will be no viable public health care very soon in countries like ours, whether a system is publicly or privately financed, if nothing is done about recruiting and remunerating more generalists.

Basic shortages of trained physicians are probably Canada's most serious medical problem right now. As with every shortage, it's worse in rural areas. There are a variety of programs to encourage or force young medical graduates into the hinterlands. Quebec, as usual, emphasizes force. Adam Gavsie, a recent enough graduate that he is still coping with such legislation, admits, "There are still better bursaries in Quebec for medical school students and a more liberal loan structure. In fact, Quebec subsidizes its young doctors' educations, but then it makes it almost impossible for them to practice here! It's weird, how the province acts as the alternately tyrannical and benevolent parent." American students flock to Quebec for the McGill medical school's government-subsidized, bargain-basement tuitions and then are forbidden by the province to stay and care for Québecers when they graduate. For example, Gavsie mentions that in 2005 a highly experienced U.S. radiologist was not permitted to practice in Quebec, despite her many degrees and the desperate need for just that specialty in the province, because Quebec refused to recognize her credentials.

Gavsie says, "That's because in Quebec, they like to believe their standards are so lofty that no one else in the world can meet them. I guess if they were, they might have a point, but according to all the normal ways the UN or WHO measures such things – infant and child mortality, longevity, and especially doctor-to-patient ratios – they're only average, or for the latter, below average. And it's not just foreign doctors who are forbidden to help us with their expertise because of some cultural or linguistic prejudice. I know several Ontario francophone young doctors who can't get accepted to set up here!" To make the prize of Quebec practice even rarer, until the summer of 2007, Quebec was requiring young graduates to pay $1,500 to take a special exam that required a year of preparation. Gavsie say, "After all they've been through to become doctors in the first place, it's pretty hard for these recent graduates to find that time and money, especially as they're simply studying things they already learned years ago. Of course, they're prepared for some costs, like licensing, but they have to pay that, too, on top of the cost for that test. And then they'll be forced to practice anywhere the government wants and have no say in setting up a practice or living where they want to live." This practice is just now being eased, but it's a tiny little band-aid on a huge wound.

"Today," Gavsie explains, "we're still trying to fill hospital schedules on a shift-by-shift basis! I get these postcards, asking me if I can fill Monday, 11 November, or two days later, whatever, with practically no warning time, as far away as Chibougimou, Rimouski, and Rivière du Loup. Eight, nine hours of driving each way. I used to get scared when I'd get them, but that law forcing us to go, which only lasted six months, was repealed. So many people refused or threatened to leave the province, they had to back down. The fines were incredible while the bill was in effect, though; one guy refused and they were fining him, I think, something like $5,000 for every hour he wasn't where they'd demanded he be."

Gavsie understands the accessibility problem and has voluntarily set up his life to regularly take care of First Nations populations in northern Quebec. He doesn't suggest that we allow doctors completely free run, because we would end up with far too many in one place and none in another. But he points out that simply using a few carrots instead of punitive sticks could solve the whole problem. "It's the cultural differences here in Quebec that attract so many doctors in the first place, native as well as foreign. Why not promote that, not enforce draconian rules? They use a culture of fear to get doctors to do what they want when they could make it attractive by offering tax breaks or tuition breaks or interest-free loans in setting up a practice. They could help you re-locate here or there for a few months or years." Many developing countries, such as Mexico, offer free tuition in exchange for a couple years' practice in the rural areas. In Mexico and Cuba, doctors are sent to rural areas or to help other Third World countries as a matter of course; it's an understood part of a free school tuition program open to med-school students who otherwise could not afford to get an MD. As numerous national stories in newspapers and on the CBC have recorded, desperate communities across Canada have organized some freelance sponsorships of young med students in exchange for a promise to practice in their town for five years after graduation. This method, unlike those in Mexico or Cuba, will continue to concentrate doctors in richer parts of the country. The only difference is that some of those rich communities will be rural.

Faced with the situation of no generalists even in urban areas, the U.S. medical profession, represented by the American College of Physicians, is therefore suggesting a complete overhaul of how we manage the public health, just as happened in Cuba in the 1960s. Their suggestions are also remarkably like Cuba's. The ACP wants to certify general practices scattered across the country as "advanced medical homes," a word choice that reflects the urgency of bringing community and family into the practice of medicine. Doctors, the ACP insists, should be rewarded for quality, prevention, and coordination of care, not volume and catastrophic and acute care, as is now the case.

"The advanced medical home model is based on the premise that the best quality of care is provided not in episodic, illness-oriented, complaint-based care, but through patient-centered, physician-guided, cost-efficient, longitudinal care that encompasses and values both the art and the science of medicine." The College of Physicians also recommends "the promotion of *continuous healing relationships ... in a variety of care settings* according to the needs of the patient and the skills of the medical providers."[33] This opens the door to "integrative medicine" techniques. The American College of Physicians report goes on to talk about working "in partnership with patients" to navigate both their illnesses and the medical system. This new system echoes precepts used in Cuba and also espoused by "old-fashioned" doctors like Jack McMartin and Harold Griffith. It also reflects the conclusions of scores of international studies by every type of prestigious research body, from WHO to *The Lancet*.

In general, the whole question of how we can best manage our populations' health and hospital care is analogous to the "debate" on public vs. privately funded health care outlined in chapter 5, or, for that matter, the "debate" on global warming. Scientific studies have overwhelmingly provided irrefutable and very simple and easy to legislate answers to these questions for many years. For a variety of reasons, from professional and philosophic bias to modern economic theory and outright governmental, institutional, and industrial corruption, our health systems have simply chosen to ignore their own studies. Unfortunately, reality is inexorable, and it is nearly time to pay the piper for all our years of inaction and denial. As the ACP puts it, "The consequences [of inaction] will be higher costs and lower quality as patients find themselves in *a confusing, fragmented and over-specialized system* in which no one physician accepts responsibility for their care, and no one physician is accountable ... for the quality of care provided."[34]

COMMONSENSE

Pray for peace and grace and spiritual food, For wisdom and guidance, for all these are good. But don't forget the potatoes.

> The Griffith family's favourite grace

As we discussed in chapter 6, current global economic activities – what have been termed the policies of "Free Trade" – favour the importation of exotic pathogenic agents from around the world, from ebola, bird flu, and SARS to antibiotic-resistant bacteria from industrial farms. This means that the big, consolidated, hospitals that depend on heavy technology and fancy specialists may not the best place for treating increasing numbers of people stricken with infectious diseases. Although it's all to the good that a few hospitals have created wards or wings with state-of-the art ventilation systems that can be sealed off or purified, most are not set up this way. But even when there is plenty of fancy technology, simple human habits and policies spread diseases. The reason that the SARS epidemic made the rounds of so many Toronto hospitals without infecting those in other Canadian cities to any significant degree is an example.

Dodie Gibbons, the Queen E's former Intensive Care nursing specialist, now lives in Toronto. She says, "Because of the Ontario government cut-backs, most nurses have become part-time at each hospital – that's so the government doesn't have to give them full-time benefits. In order to have full-time work, they had to move from hospital to hospital, carrying infections with them. The same thing holds true for ambulance workers." Another nurse mentioned "parking lots, entrance halls, gift shops, cafeterias" as unchecked infection centres. "If there's an epidemic," she continued, "you want a lot of geographically separate – and that includes separately staffed – care facilities, so that if one hospital gets a lot of cases, it can be in effect sealed off and people sent elsewhere." It's the old adage about putting all your eggs in one basket. And medical personnel, as experts such as Gilles Brucker remind us, not only bring illnesses from one hospital to another – they also spread them within a hospital. They are often resistant to proper hand-washing, changes of clothing, and other disinfection procedures. They are extremely stressed from overwork, and all that cleaning up just takes too much time.

Other social habits mitigate against the idea that advanced technology and fancy experts translates to proper care. Quebec hospital General Director Mario Larivière says, "These days, we have professionals – nurses and doctors – who never work in hospitals. They haven't experienced the system, they don't understand the reality of where they're sending their patients, what kind of treatment will actually happen." Larivière adds, "The government bureaucrats who've created this [approach to care] are like [former Montreal Mayor] Jean Drapeau, with his dream for an Olympic Stadium. It's that kind of grandiose vision the politicians have in Quebec. They want to make a reputation, too, and so they're not thinking about the realities of health care." As we have seen with heart disease, even without professional incentives, people tend to get caught up in plausible theories, especially if they have an immediate economic advantage. But when it's a question of an entire society's investment in its own future, actions should be based only scientific studies and hard evidence.

Larivière says the doctors and hospital administrators watching politicians pushing for super-hospitals and "centers of excellence" are already wondering whether our governments will build super-hospitals and then just let them fall apart. "There has to be money spent on day-to-day things! Orderlies, housekeeping, upkeep. Our hospitals' windows leak; at Sacre Coeur, it's ridiculous in winter. Instead of replacing them, they've chosen to invest in fancy machines. For four years I've been trying to raise $18 million – which is peanuts – for my desperately needed expansion, to deal with all the people in our overrun community hospital who have to be treated in corridors. But we still don't have it. And yet the government can find money to invest in some brand-new huge, dream structure." Larivière says bitterly, "They simply don't give a damn about us, the population, or the professionals."

Building large super-hospitals is still portrayed by politicians and the mass media as a cost-cutting strategy, despite all the studies that show it seriously compromises care and also costs *more* money. Typically, consolidation closes beds. One of many examples is the New York City Hospital occupancy crisis of 1987 and 88, which resulted in ambulances being turned away for a "protracted" period, and "delays of days for urgently sick patients waiting for an open bed." Under the circumstances, the hospitals involved did not think it wise to tabulate mortalities, but it's very likely that people died needlessly. The crisis was caused by "the simultaneous 9 percent decline in [bed] capacity ... that was largely due to new regulations linking Medicaid reimbursement to occupancy levels that were regulated to be 85 percent as well as an unanticipated 18 percent growth in admissions, which was largely due to a rise in AIDS and drug abuse."[35]

A paper published by the Center for Studying Health System Change that investigated the impact on patient service of cutting beds noted that, "Using target occupancy levels (still the major methodology) as the primary determinant of bed capacity is inadequate and may lead to excessive delays for beds. Also, attempts to reduce hospital beds by consolidation of different clinical services into single nursing units may be counterproductive."[36] Nonetheless, Montreal's new super-hospital will consolidate four others: the Royal Victoria, the Children's, the Shriner's, and the Montreal Neurological Institute. The new institution may seem exciting, with lots of new machines and impressive, world-class specialists. But it will leave the city of more than three million with *500 fewer beds* than it has now; that's the equivalent of two Queen Elizabeths. The very tight bed capacity is still being calculated based on that highly dangerous idea of 90 percent occupancy.

Hospitals have only recently begun to pay more attention to international health care. Their concern arose because of professional desires not to fall behind civilized standards, but has now increased because of a desire to protect their facilities and patients from global epidemics. International exchanges have resulted in enormous gains in knowledge while at the same time making everyone realize that when it comes to funding hospitals, we're all in a very similar boat. Kieke Okma, a Dutch professor of social history who also attended the "Building Consensus for Health Care Reform" conference cited at the beginning of this chapter, uses the all-important cost-control methods as an example. "In the EU ... we do fairly similar things as Canada and the U.S. We try to squeeze budgets, [and] ... the political measuring rod is ... the average of OECD country spending, [that is], between 8 and 10 percent of GDP."[37] All countries that spend more than that percentage on taking care of their citizens get nervous. They begin to cut budgets to individual institutions, try to get pharmaceutical costs down, institute fee schedules for services, and close beds or limit the numbers of doctors and nurses being trained. But who decided what is appropriate to spend on health care? Doctors, elected officials, social research experts, citizens? Apparently not – our societies depend upon the expertise of economists for such decisions. In short, cost is the primary consideration, not the public health.

Even so, the advantage still lies with single-payer, government-funded hospitals and health care, as both Canada's share of 9.7 percent of GDP and Cuba's of 7.4, compared to the U.S. 13 percent and mixed systems like Germany's 10.7 percent, prove.[38] Private systems will always be at a disadvantage in such negotiations, partly because they cannot bargain with the providers of medical products as well. "I think the Canadian provinces are too small to deal with the very complicated processes of ... negotiating with international industry and the pharmaceuticals," Kieke Okma pointed out. "[this would probably] call for a national scheme." He also noted that although "there are no easy global solutions," the most useful elements of public systems really do stand out. For example, experts all over the world agree with Okma that, "Canadian Medicare has been extraordinarily effective in protecting the incomes of Canadians against the risk of hospital care and medical care." Carolyn Tuohy of the University of Toronto returned the compliment. In terms of public/private systems, the Netherlands has about 40 percent of its population – the wealthier minority – using private insurance. Of course, as Tuohy says, "Private insurers will risk-select [that is, cover only healthy people] unless carefully regulated and the genius of the Netherlands system is the tight, overarching framework of regulations that cover private insurance, as well as social insurance." As in the French two-tier system, control of the private sector by the public is key to health management success. But all the studies also remind us that a fragmented system will end up ultimately costing more, simply because of divided responsibilities, more administrative overhead, and a lot more paperwork.[39]

So, while there are plenty of lessons to learn, it's not possible to completely "import another system," as Okma pointed out. Canada can't decide to become Americanized or just like the French or the Germans or whomever. Okma emphasized that all health systems, like their agents, the hospitals, have evolved over a great deal of time; they are creatures of history and local politics. Except for the U.S. system, which is globally regarded as a failure, the rest have a great deal in common. "You need the common sense and pragmatism," Okma concluded, "to look for things that *really* work and not for things that *should* work." The former include the preference of most experts, based on statistical analysis, for "continuum of care" and "primary care-led health reform," while the latter include private/public funding as currently recommended by such groups as The Fraser Institute.

Richard Freeman, from the University of Edinburgh, agreed with this meat-and-potatoes approach. "You have to be realistic," he said. "Health systems are complicated and contradictory ... And, there's an inevitable tradeoff that must occur between cost [to the taxpayers] and quality [for the users]." If you want good prenatal care for everyone, you can have it because it's fairly cheap per capita. But you probably can't afford liver transplants for all your 75 year-olds. France's system, Freeman pointed out, is popular because it responds well to the user, but it is also very expensive for the government and hence to the taxpayer. "There is no simple answer ... If you're a politician, please don't promise. If you're a patient, please don't expect. If you're a journalist, don't pretend otherwise!" He suggested looking for things that work not just in similar countries but in places like India, Cuba, or Mexico, where systems dependent on general practice intervention and almost no money are reaping infant and general mortality rates so exemplary that they have made even the wealthy UK "rethink some fundamental questions of the reorganization [of primary care]."[40]

The important thing, Freeman said, is to "*Be wary of lessons everybody else seems to learn* ... For example, [U.S.-style] 'managed competition' was enormously disruptive [in the UK]" and in Singapore. Economic panaceas, like two-tier care for Canada, are another experiment that has been proven again and again not to work, either in terms of general health measures or economic efficiency. "Beware of those lessons which seem to be forced upon you," he added, in a nod to what happened to all our hospitals in the mid-1990s. "*Many countries have their health policies shaped by investment policies indirectly forced upon them by the World Bank.*"

Richard Freeman also spoke at length at this important conference about the pressures of "domestic politics ... and in terms of the international political economy ... globalization, competitiveness, and so on." Australia is much further down the road from a single-payer system towards privatization than Canada, although it is not yet dominated by the U.S. model. Since embarking on increased "economic rationalist" (that is, public/private) health care funding, Australia has experienced a number of scandals and a great deal of political fall-out. For example, the American company Health South has a record of massive Medicare fraud in the U.S. and has also fallen into disrepute in Australia, where it owns a large hospital in Melbourne. Privatizing general practice and community hospitals in Australia was tried over the last decade but has gradually been abandoned, largely because these institutions were not sufficiently economically attractive to the giant American health care corporations that had quickly moved into the new vacuum in the formerly more public system. New Zealanders attempted more privatization as well, but have become disenchanted with it; today their government has reversed some of its pro-market policies.[41]

In Quebec, the new super-hospital that may have been one of the incentives for closing the Queen E, is finally being built under a "public/private partnership" that the public is being assured will not bring the risk down upon them. Maybe it will work out. If so, it will be in contrast to the overwhelmingly disappointing track record of such ventures.

For-profit HMOs and hospitals are probably not a good idea for Canada, if only because of the ways in which they have proven to be as dangerous to the customer's health as they are to her wallet down in the U.S. Dr. Linda Peeno, working in a private San Diego hospital, testified to Congress that she was rewarded for restricting care to a patient who died as a result of her decision rather than being investigated and fired. She said, "It brought me an improved reputation in my job and contributed to my advancement."[42] Peeno talked about the "severing" of job and character under a corporate medical system. "I learned how easy it is to do many things diametrically opposed to everything medicine stands for, not only willingly, but often with great belief (supported by my peers and prevailing sociologic/economic/scientific assumptions of the organizational culture) that I was right and my actions were good. It was even easier when I was 'rewarded' for such professional action." Peeno was a medical gatekeeper for a for-profit HMO.[43]

Huge health corporations like Tenet/NME and Healthscope have moved into specialty psychiatric and rehabilitation hospitals in countries other than the U.S. Their record in these areas of care in the U.S. is extremely unpleasant. The U.S. House of Representatives tabled an inquiry entitled "Profits of Misery" in April of 1992 that found that profits in such hospitals were maximized by giving each patient large amounts of unneeded treatment every day. This was billed as therapy, although these programs were not performed by professionals and "could be inexpensively provided in alternative settings." A job specification ad for an NME hospital reads "the objectives of the case manager are: increase the ALOS (Average Length of Stay) of all inpatient admissions; attend weekly staffing of all patients under concurrent review to maximize LOS (length of stay)."[44]

Canadians are often described as equating their universal health care very closely with their identity and their values as human beings. Some maintain that this is irrational and detrimental to careful decision-making. But at the conference mentioned above, Sylvia Creuss, of McGill's Medical School, countered with the argument that, "public policy in the health care field has got to be evaluated not just on what it costs but on its impact on the *values* of health care. This is really what the core of the social contract [between doctors and patients] is." She quoted William Sullivan of the Carnegie Foundation: "neither economic incentives, nor technology, nor administrative control has proved to be an effective surrogate for the commitment to integrity evoked in the idea of the profession." In short, the major thing that doctors have going for them is the confidence of the public in their goodwill and integrity. That is being eroded, and if it is ever lost, the profession, as such, will cease to exist.

Creuss added that if national values are subverted, the resulting public policies will not succeed.[45] Pierre-Gerlier Forest, attending the Future of Health Care Conference of the Commission sur l'avenir des soins de sante au Canada, as Cruess was, emphasized the contract with the public that any relationship between health care administrators and professionals demands. "The notion of utilitarianism," he says, "the idea that you can sacrifice the interests of a minority to the interests of the majority, is not widely shared by the Canadian public. The public is expressing a lot of mistrust in the kind of deliberative exercise we are doing, pitting experts against decision-makers, professionals against politicians." Forest believes that in structuring any kind of health or hospital care system, "the more you will consult the public, the more you will have [the right kind of] safeguards." He adds, "Egotism is not part of the discourse of the Canadian public on health care," drawing attention to the overwhelming national support for an egalitarian public system, paid for by all.[46]

FORTITUDE

In regard to hospitals, people are inclined to say – this one is good, or that one is just ordinary or even mediocre. What makes one institution 'better' than another?

Harold Griffith, Annual Report, 1955[47]

Back in 1955, Harold Griffith found it easy to answer his own question about what really works, in terms that have lost little of their power in the 21st century. "It isn't just size," he wrote, "for the largest hospitals can sometimes be the least efficient. It isn't just money, or glamorous new buildings, or even a famous history. I am sure the answer lies in the very human element, which might be summed up in the words 'a dedicated staff.'" Unable to contain himself, he tried to characterize that staff – his own, of course. "The Queen Elizabeth Hospital, ever since it was founded," wrote Harold, "has been blessed with dedicated men and women – doctors, nurses and board members – who have served to the point of sacrifice, and who have been willing to make the welfare of our patients their first interest in life."

Of course, this is a highly subjective assessment, and there are plenty of people who could take issue with it. However hard people work or however high their standards, mistakes, on both the individual and the systemic level, will be made. The old Homeopathic/Queen E heroically saved some patients and tragically let others down; it opposed Medicare but championed primary care; it embraced new drugs and medicines, sometimes too quickly, constantly expanding funding needs with little thought of self-control, but it also made sure that patients – and staff – were seen as human beings and part of its own community. Hospitals, even the best, are institutions made up of real people, reflecting the limitations and restrictions of the place where they work and the culture at large. They are all, by definition, flawed. That doesn't mean we shouldn't honour them when they manage to be as good as the situation can get.

The challenges being faced today are more intense than in Harold's era, especially with the arrival on the scene of such powerful entities as the big pharmacology companies, private HMOs, and rapacious trade regimes. However, it's important to recognize that even if the economic landscape changes, the challenges of taking care of sick human bodies are unlikely to alter much. Harold Griffith straddled the era that went from worrying about typhoid and cholera to dealing with heart attacks and cancer. If indeed the infectious diseases of the 21st century surprise everyone and don't create pandemics, hospitals will still have to deal with all the chronic problems that flood their hallways now, including the alarming rise of diabetes and hypertension that accompanies obesity. These are threatening to grow to even more epidemic proportions, and the way we set up hospitals is simply not ready for either kind of future – chronic or contagious.

No one yet has a real handle on the effects of social problems such as AIDS and drug abuse. We do know that the huge cohort of baby boomers is beginning to age and will need care. There are also potentially just as large a group of obese young people with incipient coronary disease and Type–2 diabetes. There could also be an Avian flu or other sort of epidemic. Canada could try to organize its hospitals to have one wing for patients infected with the new, emerging diseases and another for heroically complex operations such as heart, lung, and liver transplants. There could be yet more specialists in another wing, madly trying to deal with the blindness and gangrene of diabetes and the many cancers that accompany chemical contamination and our longer lifespan – all on an enormous and unending scale. This kind of increasingly expensive acute care would destroy any hope for a publicly funded hospital system – only rich people would get any care at all. And we've seen what that does to everyone's life expectancy and the survival of the humane values of the society in question.

It is clear that the only way for hospitals, and countries, to cope with the situation directly ahead of us is to get serious about preventative care. Similar to the heart disease epidemic of the 1920s to the 1960s, researchers understand that Type–2 diabetes is attributable to diet and to the quality of the food people eat. In terms of other concerns about diet, the large quantities we're encouraged to gorge on are not the only problem. Food carrying pathogens and contaminants, which trade regimes encourage to cross borders, also contributes. Trade with China brought antifreeze to toothpaste. We also have to worry about long-term effects from genetically engineered foods like soy or corn that have insect-killing bacteria or systemic herbicide resistance encoded into all their cells. With Free Trade, regulatory systems have to keep track of cleanliness standards from Chile to Africa and mad cow disease in ground beef – all in addition to monitoring North Amer-

ican problems such as *E. coli* in mass-produced produce and the daily
dose of unwanted antibiotics we are absorbing with every bite of indus-
trially-produced chicken or ham. Apart from trying to track and control episodes of contamination, our governmental health systems are
being advised to teach us to go back to eating in a way that promotes
our health. We don't need super-sized fries, but we do need very small
amounts of protein and fats, lots of whole grains, fruits, and vegetables,
plenty of water, and almost no sugar – librally mixed with lots and lots
of exercise. That's what makes people healthy, and high-tech lipo-
suctions and heart transplants aside, there doesn't seem to be much we
can do about that fact.

How we save our hospital and health care systems from collapse,
along with our bodies, is embarrassingly simple and commonsensical.
We know what is proven to help people lead healthy, long lives. Our
health systems have to spend more time fostering those habits and less
time investing attention and prestige in fighting the catastrophes that
an unhealthy lifestyle can cause. Moreover, to be healthy, humans not
only need the right diet and exercise, they also need rest. Rest includes
not just adequate sleep but an absence of stress, the old-fashioned
"peace of mind," which means not only fewer pressures but also more
comforts, especially of a community and spiritual nature.

When we think about treating and preventing heart disease, still the
number-one killer, we have to remember that what is going on in our
bodies that hurts our hearts and sometimes causes other problems,
too, is often simply an inability to cope with the stresses of life. Remember the old-time doctor who used to "order" people off to the moun-
tains or the seashore for "a complete rest"? Dr. Bernard Lown, the
cardiologist quoted in chapter 6, still does that kind of thing, regularly.
He says, "We ... have an atmosphere [in the clinic] where dreadful
things are *not* going to happen. If somebody comes in who's 40 pounds
overweight, I don't act like the Angel of Death about to smite them. I
say, 'You're carrying a little too much weight. I'd like to see you again in
6 months. Let's say you lose 8 pounds.' 'Oh, doctor, no problem. I'll
lose 20 pounds.' 'No, no, I don't want you to lose 20 pounds. I want
you to lose 8 pounds. That would make me enormously happy.' So, I
invest myself in that."

That last sentence is a real throwback, not just to doctors like Jack
McMaster, but as far back as the days of A.R. Griffith. Lown is saying
that *the doctor is investing himself in the patient, not the other way around.* He
lets the patient know that he or she has the power to make him happy

by making themselves healthier. When doctors are real clinicians, healthy patients actually do make them happy. Adam Gavsie likes to tell the story of one of his patients, a man with terrible physical symptoms of anxiety, sleeplessness, palpitations, stomach distress, and so on, who had been working nights as a Wal-Mart manager for years. He never saw his young family and was obviously suffering from the unnatural hours, but Wal-Mart would not change his schedule and he could not find another job. Because even the largest retail outlet on earth does have to comply with minimal health standards, Gavsie was able to order a change to day shifts "for the patient's health," and all the ominous symptoms, obviously leading to heart disease or hypertension, quickly disappeared. "I loved that!" says this doctor. "It's one of the few things I can do where I know I will be able to permanently help the people who come to me." This approach is far more common in Europe, where doctors routinely order time off work and changes of scene, and their statistics bear out the effectiveness of this approach. It may have some up-front costs to society: the doctor's extra time and the patient's time off work. But in the long run, it saves health systems, the society, and the patients millions of dollars in bills and suffering simply because nothing dramatic happens. The chronic problem fails to become acute.

One could protest that Lown can afford to provide this kind of luxurious, old-fashioned care because he serves wealthy patients in a private clinic. But the initial investment of paying a doctor to take more time would save a public system an incredible amount of money. Although deaths from heart disease have gone down slightly since the epidemic of the 1950s and 60s, the incidence of the disease has not budged, and the obesity in the young today will certainly see it increase if nothing is done. In fact, the technological advances in recent years have done surprisingly little to reverse these trends. Lown says, "For the first time in history, we know enough about the risk profiles of patients who do develop heart disease not to abolish it entirely but to reduce it by 50, 70 percent or even more. If we do that, look at how many billions and billions of dollars we can direct to focus on healthy communities."

Today Lown has had time to look back over his career and make some startling realizations. The first one is of consummate importance to the survival of adequate and inclusive hospital care. "Medicine's profound crisis," he says, "is only partially related to ballooning costs; the problem is far deeper than economics ... Healing is replaced with treating, caring is supplanted by managing, and the art of listening is taken over by technology." Like Harold Griffith and many of the doctors interviewed for this book, he considers himself very fortunate to have received his training and to have been practicing before the advent of so many high-tech tools and medications. The CBC radio documentary that featured him cites a 1997 study showing that four out of five recent medical graduates couldn't identify the sounds of common heart abnormalities through a stethoscope. Lown thinks they are unable to hear a lot of other things, too.

"Now you don't have to put a stethoscope on the chest. You can get an echocardiogram and look at the heart beating in three dimensions. You can look at valves functioning. You can look at coronary flows. You can look at electro-physiologic aspects of the heart." So doctors don't spend time talking to their patients and listening to their histories. They spend time figuring out what kinds of tests to order and how to interpret the results. He says that when he looked back on his experience with hundreds of patients, he came to a jarring conclusion. "Coronary disease is [in fact] a very benign disease. It's compatible with a normal life expectancy." Within the huge cohort of people who are identified as being "at risk" for heart attacks, or even among those who have had a heart attack, most can simply be taught, as Lown puts it, "how to live." And the prime component of that is not being forced to never taste a steak or climb a mountain, but the "exorcism of dread." Of course, there are exceptions. "There is a subset of patients who are quite malignant in the sense that they will have a brutal disease with a short life expectancy." But today, just as we are doing with the statins, we're treating the vast majority of manageable cases as if they were the rare and dangerous ones.

As most primary care physicians will tell you, a doctor who knows her patients, who "listens, observes, and takes a careful history" can actually rule out heart disease 90 percent of the time. The usual causes of chest pain are arthritis, indigestion, psychological stress, or some other chronic but non life-threatening problem. When the diagnosis actually is heart disease, even then, "in 92 percent" of the cases, Lown says, these patients can be treated medically. That is, they don't have to undergo expensive and dangerous procedures like angioplasty, stenting, or bypass surgery.

Lown asks if we could do tiny little things, like possibly legislating a little less salt in bread, say 10 percent, "which is not detectable by the human palate. It will result in less elderly stroke ... We could create walkways ... so attractive that you want to walk, or cycle paths, or places

where kids could go swimming – a whole array to encourage sport activities." This is done here by public health departments to some degree,
but Canada and North America in general lag far behind most of
northern Europe, where every tiny village in France has a "*piscine
municipale,*" a town swimming pool, and most larger cities have large
car-free centers that tempt one to walk for miles, to say nothing of doctors who regularly prescribe vacations, psychiatric therapy, and time
away from work. "Of course that can be done," Lown says, "at a fraction
of the resources we spend now on intensive care units and [secondary]
and tertiary care!"

WHAT WOULD PARADISE LOOK LIKE?

I feel like shouting 'Hallelujah!' We have a little hospital which we
should praise God for giving to us, and of which we can be proud.
Perhaps we have been too modest, so I am going to take a few minutes
to boast about some attributes, which, when they are gathered together,
make the Queen Elizabeth Hospital absolutely unique. There just isn't
anything quite like it anywhere.

Harold Griffith, Annual Report, 1955[48]

Like many non-fiction books, this one has had to spend a lot of time
talking about what's wrong with everything. It's just as instructive to
consider the good things about Canadian hospitals and the Canadian
single-payer health system, as well as the good things about Canadians,
period. The first thing to appreciate is the way societies have organized
themselves to create hospitals and health care in the first place, to say
nothing of the benefits of universal access that every Canadian enjoys.
Even though it's under attack, in Canada we still have a health care system that is the envy of most of the rest of the world. The reason for that
envy is not just that sophisticated, modern health and hospital care is
available; it's that it is available equally, to every one of us. But there are
a lot of hints we could take from the studies quoted above to keep it
that way and also to make it work the way it was intended to.

As Cuba has already implemented and the American College of physicians has suggested, regular allopathic medical systems could benefit
from working with their alternative and integrative colleagues in developing more effective therapies for chronic diseases. In the mainstream
system, for example, the current treatments for arthritis are dangerous
and costly drug therapies. These drugs are often as debilitating as the

original complaint and sometimes considerably more damaging; it does little good to trade arthritic pain for a perforated stomach or a stroke, for example. Because of a lack of success with drug regimens, many health systems in Europe and South America are working more closely with a few of the most scientifically interesting, traditional therapies, like naturopathy, osteopathy, acupuncture, yoga, Chinese and Ayurvedic medicine, and even various kinds of massage. When a woman gets breast cancer in France, Holland, or Germany, she is almost always helped to find an acupuncturist, masseuse, naturopath, and/or a psychologist, after completing her mainstream treatments. The MDs there know that treating the whole person will help prevent relapses. Besides providing encouragement and information about such therapies, the government at least partially funds the costs.

Sports medicine clinics in Canada and the US are now combining treatments, too. They offer the entire gamut of chronic illness care, starting with a regular medical doctor who diagnoses the ailment and makes sure that no dangerous pathologies exist under the presenting symptoms. Patients can try out acupuncture, herbal treatments of various kinds, osteopathy, exercise regimes, and more, all with their MD nearby to help them judge whether the treatment is helping or hurting. If such clinics were more widely available, public hospitals might be relieved of some of their ER visitors and possibly even have their surgery and hip replacement lines shortened. They would also discover cases in which chronic ailments such as skin allergies, asthma, chronic indigestion, high blood pressure, or lower back pain responded to varied approaches. This would also eliminate some of the expense of treating allergic or multiple-drug reactions that strike patients who are forced to self-medicate without guidance. As years of research into therapies such as acupuncture have shown, by overseeing instead of merely disapproving of foreign or alternative treatments, mainstream researchers can amass more data on what therapies show promise and which seem to be largely be a waste of time.

The quirky but well-sourced British journal, *What Doctors Don't Tell You,* has a point when it states that, "The fact that doctors are now turning to potentially hazardous cancer treatments to combat [chronic conditions like] arthritis shows just how desperate is the need to find anything that may work. As many sufferers ... have discovered, medicine's track record in [chronic ailments like] arthritis has been disappointing, at worst, an abject failure. It has been a long history of hyped-up hopes followed by painful climb-downs, as one new drug [or surgical procedure] after another has been glowingly brought to market, only to be revealed to be no better than its predecessors."[49] The same kind of track record with MS, Parkinson's, stomach problems such as IBS, and many other common chronic miseries is why the sales of herbal supplements are so high and the waiting rooms of the many kinds of alternative therapists are full. In Canada, waiting three months to see an acupuncturist or homeopath is not unusual. Of course, many vitamins and supplements may be only marginally better than chemical snake oils, simply in that they have fewer dangerous side-effects. But evidence has to be applied in every quarter, not just on man-made chemicals that are profitable to industry, and more and more classically trained doctors are longing to get into this field.

One of the strangest medically accepted alternative healing methods is the mental "imaging" of cancer cells being destroyed by chemotherapy or visualizing other symbols of returning health. "Positive imagery" techniques were found to be so clearly effective in clinical trials that today most oncology departments, even in Canada and the U.S., offer brochures teaching people how to imagine light and flowers and other symbols dissolving their cancers away. Alternative therapies like qigong, tai-chi, or yoga can be as cheap as positive imagery and can usually be learned in a relatively short time. The length of time before they become effective can vary widely, though, and they do not always produce the same results, even on the same problem, for different people. Nonetheless, with even minimal public system support, they could significantly help to lower the number of patients who currently move inexorably from chronic to acute status because they are not given the more gentle, long-term, psychological approach that chronic conditions often require. In other words, if doctors can't spend an hour with each patient, like Adam Gavsie yearns to do and Bernard Lown already does, they could think about recruiting lower-level, alternative helpers under better oversight and direction to do it for them.

John Hughes, the former Queen Elizabeth GP, is involved with another promising new trend: medical informatics. In this case, it's the application of systems engineering to health care. The concept was first suggested in the 1960s by Laurence Weed, a professor of family medicine at the University of Vermont, but computers were too slow at the time to deal with Weed's ideas. These days, we have faster machines and more efficient ways to store and retrieve data. In fact, a doctor can now pull up vast amounts of information on his desktop computer, right in the middle of a hectic consultation. Hughes says, "We are beginning to realize that the practice of clinical medicine in particular, and even the entire healthcare delivery system in general, will be revolutionized by what amounts to medical spreadsheets of evidence-based data."

Even poor areas not served by the Internet can partially access this concept, as Cuba does with its postings of epidemiological data in every community clinic. What we're really talking about here is fixing the problem of public health transparency discussed above. What the system seriously needs is not free access to the records of individual patients, which would be protected, but access to the information that languishes within our provincial and federal and even international public health departments. This vital information is currently not available to the general public or to their busy doctors. In the St Remi area outside of Montreal and up into the Chateauguay Valley west of the city, for example, residents and their doctors have known for many years that there are severe cancer clusters and a very high incidence of brain tumours. Public health departments know this too, but don't release the data. If citizens were aware of this, prevention, relocation, and clean-ups – should the cause turn out to be a waste dump or pesticide use – would be greeted with cooperation. Many lives, as well as medical expenses, could be saved if medical informatics gave GPs free access to not just individual and family history but to community and public health archives.

Researchers are fine-tuning this new approach. Enrico Coiera, who is featured in a *British Medical Journal* article in May of 2004, and scientists at the U.S. National Academy of Science, who described their efforts in a 2005 publication, "Building a Better Delivery System: A New Engineering/Healthcare Partnership," are in the forefront of this work. These medical experts believe that the only way to ensure universal health care in the face of ever-increasing medical capabilities, coupled with ever-increasing demand, is, as Hughes puts it, "through the thoughtful application of these technologies." In other words, so much new information is available that no one physician or nurse can retain all of it. Now they won't have to. They'll be able to access what they need, when they need it, even in some rural, bare-bones clinic. Hughes believes that in the very near future, we will have access to timely and dependable medical information on everything both doctors and patients require to make truly informed decisions with far less manipulation by vested interests. "From access to one's personal medical history to the latest and most reliable drug information and alternative medicine research," he says, "doctors and patients will gradually be able to help each other and also help publicly funded health systems ensure that we really are using the best practices."

MERCY

One recovers from pneumonia or typhoid fever [not just] with help from drugs like penicillin, sulphas, insulin, vaccines, and so on ... but because of some internal reaction, whereby the normal balance of body functions is restored. All that drugs do, or surgical treatment does, is to help in restoring that balance – to remove obstacles to nature's efforts to return the body to health ... All healing comes from within.

Harold Griffith, ca. 1960[50]

When a modern doctor like Harold Griffith – after all, he revolutionized the practice of surgery – talks like this at the end of a long career, two things are at play. In one, he is obviously A.R.'s son, a trained homeopath and a very old-fashioned, caring healer. Homeopathy, like virtually all the alternative and traditional theories of treating disease and injury, postulates a state of balance from which the body, for some reason, becomes "un" balanced, and falls into "dis-"ease. Then, these disciplines all theorize, "something" happens, a kind of internal clicking back into place, aided by their herbs, exercises, or homoepathic pellets, and health mysteriously returns. At the same time that he shows his roots in alternative medicine, Harold is also admitting to a belief that all really good doctors, even the most scientifically invested, will admit to sharing. He's making it clear that he's a person sufficiently humble enough to acknowledge – despite his years of medical mastery in which he had learned to take thousands of very sick people to the brink of death and then bring them back alive – that the delicate membrane that separates life from death and health from disease is ultimately beyond his, or any other doctor's, power to fully understand.

Public health and hospital systems have, since the 1970s, worked medical and social miracles in Canada as well as in all the other countries with similar systems. They protect us from the catastrophic loss of income that strikes along with serious illness and make identical treatments for even the most catastrophic diseases available to all citizens. They have created optimum life expectancies and given many people who are stricken with slow but controllable maladies a vastly improved quality of life. All Canadians share in this amazing achievement. But it

cannot be expected to survive the business approach to health that has
taken hold in medicine over the last few decades. The Queen Elizabeth
Hospital of Montreal and its staff were not wrong in thinking they had
a good hospital. They were not alone, of course, but hospitals like the
Queen Elizabeth were successful for so long mostly because the
"commonsense, fortitude, and mercy" that had characterized the
beginnings of medicine managed to survive in them into the present
era.

The lessons we can learn from the life and death of such a hospital
are as commonplace as bread and salt – obvious, necessary, but seldom
sufficiently noted. Dr Bernard Lown, the renegade cardiologist
described earlier, could not sound more like Harold or A.R. Griffith
when he says that vastly improving survival rates for patients stricken by
serious coronary disease by avoiding surgeries and using a minimum of
drugs "takes a certain trust-engendering activity, where the patient
feels so much at ease and unpressured that they can relate to you what
otherwise would not emerge." Getting this to happen, he adds, "is an
art that is being lost, really. It seems the very opposite intuitively ... a
doctor's time [is supposed to be] too valuable. But the minute you *listen* to your patient, it is enormously efficient." He adds, with complete
confidence, "doctors find the greatest satisfaction in doing it."

Today's science-based medical education has come to favour high-
tech solutions to the acute and catastrophic ills that the profession has
emphasized. Today's most ambitious medical specialists and researchers are now looking to nanotechnolgy, zeno-transplantation, gene therapy, and other futuristic trends for cures to almost any imaginable
human ill, even though these cures generally involve patented products and are therefore going to be too expensive for public systems to
afford. These technologies also have very alarming downsides that may
prove to be extremely dangerous to both the public and the environment, because they are highly invasive as well as therapeutically
unproven by evidence-based studies.

Nanotechnology and zeno-transplantation therapies both carry the
spectre of escaped living organisms that can infect healthy ones and
today remain very far from safe on any level, even experimentally. Even
plain old gene therapy, touted with such enthusiasm beginning in
1990 and lavishly funded, has yet to produce a single clear success.
Very few illnesses can actually be treated with it, even in theory; only
rare, one-gene conditions like hemophilia and SCID (severe combined
immunodeficiency, "Boy in the Bubble" syndrome), for example.

Although use of gene therapy on children with these statistically rare disorders initially produced a few hopeful trials, such as recent ones in France on SCID, the therapies were ultimately deemed to have been equivocal or outright failures. As a U.S. National Institutes of Health committee that was looking into the technology a few years ago concluded, "While the expectations and the promise of gene therapy are great, *clinical efficacy has not been ... demonstrated at this time in any gene therapy protocol,* despite anecdotal claims of successful therapy ... Major difficulties at the basic level include shortcomings [involving] all current gene transfer vectors and an inadequate understanding of the biological interaction of these vectors with the host."[51]

Despite their many failures and serious restraints on some research, such therapies still command far more funding and social attention than the simple, practical treatments listed in the past two chapters, which, unlike them, are already proven to work. This frustrating paradox is due to society's susceptibility to good marketing and its general philosophical belief in technology. Faced with continuing down the high-tech, acute-care path, society more than ever needs to review the most basic aspects of what hospitals are and what medical service should be. As Harold Griffith reminded the young doctors gathered for his retirement speech, "*The pre-eminence of the commonplace* is what should be the principal concern for most of us. Ninety percent of our work will continue to be the provision of ... *efficient and safe* [treatment for] hernias, varicose veins, appendicitis and other such common, human problems."[52]

In the early part of the century, the first edition of a staple medical textbook, *Harrison's; Principles of Internal Medicine,* emphasized that there are few, if any, greater opportunities, responsibilities, or obligations that "can fall to the lot of a human being, than to be a physician." Doctors must not only be humble in the face of their chosen tasks, they must also remember that "the patient is no mere collection of symptoms, signs, disordered functions, damaged organs, and disturbed emotions. He is human, fearful, and hopeful, seeking relief, help and reassurance ... The true physician has a Shakespearean breadth of interest in the wise and the foolish, the proud and the humble, the stoic hero and the whining rogue. He *cares for people.*"[53] It is a reflection of the many truly scientific studies quoted above concerning the efficacy of certain hospital treatments and medical therapies that, "The significance of the intimate personal relationship between physician and patient cannot be too strongly emphasized, for in an extraordinarily large number of cases, both the diagnosis and treatment are directly dependent on it." As Harold Griffith put it when he tried to analyze the measure of a hospital's success, "I am sure the answer lies in the very human element, a staff ... dedicated to the patients."

The most scientifically and technologically centred hospitals, health care systems, and medical professionals, and especially the publicly funded systems hoping both to survive growing budgetary constraints and somehow adequately serve their populations, would do well to follow the advice of this old book and of doctors like Griffith. Evidence is amassing that primary, secondary, and even tertiary medical care does not need to cost an arm and a leg. We will be able to have the hospitals we need if each society's health structures pay attention to all the boring, commonplace evidence about what people's illnesses and disabilities actually respond to, not just briefly, but *over time*. Health systems will not be able to serve us the way we want them to if they are centred around rare, expensive, high-tech miracles that are applicable to only a tiny handful of people. They have to concentrate on the commonplace, key elements that are proven to lead to success in responding to a sick, aging, injured, and growing population.

Innumerable studies from the highest levels of specialized literature are urging that today's hospital systems must be more concerned with primary care and less fragmented. Indeed, there is one, single, underlying principle that becomes obvious in 150 years of stories recounting the actions of "good" doctors, nurses, therapies, hospitals, and health care systems – they are centred around the care of the patient. Today's bureaucrats, politicians, planners, and especially medical professionals need to remember only this one thing, which is also the principle that was central to the birth, literally in charity, of the Queen Elizabeth and all our systems of hospital care. This is essential if we truly want a healthy population. Our hospitals and health care systems cannot be centred around money and power, as is currently the case. If this continues, they will quite naturally focus on making money and serving power; because it is only their secondary concern, they will not be as efficient at healing human illness and injury. In short, there really can be no third parties – no for-profit facilities, catastrophically indebted governments, insurance companies, or drug giants – intimately involved in proper healing equations.

Experienced researchers and increasing evidence agree that healing is fundamentally between people who are sick and the people who are trying to help them get well. The money-making producers of medical

products therefore have to be firmly kept in their place, as distant helpers, by legislation designed to serve the general public interest. This is
not an impossible criteria: it used to exist fairly strongly in Canada and
is still largely in place in Holland, France, Germany, and even parts of
Mexico, Cuba, and India. It's time to recognize that the intention of
making money from helpless, distraught people afflicted with disabilities, injuries, and disease cannot be the goal of any serious medical professional. If such intentions persist, there will be neither real hospitals
nor scientifically effective healing in our future. The old textbook was
serious when it reminded doctors, "the secret of the care of the patient
is in *caring* for the patient." That means caring for the patient above
any other consideration, including fame, money, or power. That book
is still revered by many doctors and nurses. They will hopefully be able
to reclaim their roles as healers when society learns to use past wisdom
and modern research and technology. Many countries already have the
legislative base to help them get the vested interests out of the centre,
and back in the controlled margins, of the health equation.

Afterword

Knowledge unattached to ... a sensible balance of human qualities –
such as ethics, memory, common sense and reason – is powerless ...
[and] merely encourages the passive acceptance of what we know to be
wrong.

John Ralston Saul, *The Doubter's Companion*

When I began this book, I thought I was going to have a complete vacation from my former interests, which in recent years had focused on the sustainability of natural systems. In 2002, I co-authored a book with Dr David Suzuki on whether there are ways to sustain the planet's beleaguered biological systems over the long term. To our surprise, we found out there are already established ways that people can live that can enable us all to survive on our overheated, overused little planet for many centuries to come, although they require some serious shifts in cultural and especially economic attitudes. We called the book *Good News for a Change*. I had spent many years of my professional life studying assaults on our biological systems, including soils, climate, forests, habitat, water, and so on, and that book enabled me to finally meet people who, working on the margins of society and often in situations of great poverty or catastrophe, were evolving methods to actually restore dead rivers, contaminated soil, decimated wildlife populations, and clear-cut forests.

When I undertook this book, on the history of a well-known Montreal community hospital, I didn't expect any of that biological work to be germane. I was brand new to the study of health care and completely open. That is, being humble about my ignorance, I had no preconceptions about what actually does make a good hospital or good health care. Like most people, I figured some kind of mixed system probably works best and also, like most people, I hadn't thought very much about all the challenges that have faced doctors, nurses, and hospital administrators over the past century or so, not to mention every day since. I was also ready to find much to criticize about the little hospital I was profiling since I am well aware of the flaws and faults within many of our social systems; I will add that I was careful to do so when the facts warranted.

Like it or not, health care is hedged on every side by economic concerns. And western society's current economic theory establishes management strategies, such as vertical integration, industrial farming, dragnet fishing, biotechnology, and a burgeoning industrial/medical complex, that are intended to generate the maximum amount of profits for a few groups of people in the minimum amount of time. This is seen to be a good thing, in that wealth is "created," many people are employed, and the formerly central interest – producing food, goods, or caring for health – is also taken care of. However, we are now learning that the apparent profitability of enterprises organized in this way can only be sustained for a few years without either new markets or new resource sources. We have learned that they almost universally leave behind decimated natural and social systems that can rarely be restored to their former productive power. The money they engender is also rarely used in ways that benefit all of society.

In seeking to counter these unfortunate side-effects of how we have set up the economic life of the planet, we discovered that there are five basic criteria that can enable us to judge if any management system – no matter whether it is trying to increase forest growth, produce food, bring back an endangered species, or run an organic restaurant – is not only going to be able to do what it intends to do but also if it will be able to keep on doing it over the long term. Like everything that works, the list turns out to be pretty simple. We discovered that sustainable systems have to mimic nature. That is, if they produce wastes, those wastes have to be recycled or reabsorbed by the process, the way they are in nature. They must also pay attention to the rhythms and requirements of the physical planet we live on in terms of natural systems and cycles, and reproduce them as much as possible. We should not set up water-intensive farming in a desert, for example, or take fish during spawning season. Part of this criterion requires that the management system stay as local as possible, and also that it remain small enough to respond to local needs and local differences. This type of management is the exact opposite of centrally controlled enormous business or management entities like Wal-Mart or the WTO that have proliferated in the past few decades. Once systems are centralized, they lose track of the

small differences that naturally occur every few miles in any environment across the planet and, however well-meaning initially, they
become inappropriate and even destructive to local situations.

Local people know the most about and are usually invested in staying
in their particular area. Therefore, they must be involved in the management of any operation that will affect them. Together with using local
management, the daily workings of the local water, fish, or forest or
food-harvesting systems have to be as "democratic" as possible, which
means that they have to be set up to be transparent, accessible, and non-
hierarchical for the people running them. In short, the human component always has to be considered and the management style needs to be
as egalitarian as possible. Employees must feel free to take part in adding
to the success of the endeavour regardless of their position in the organization. Additionally, we discovered that these localized, egalitarian management systems have to contain a large element of *fun*. Organizing
many festivals, parties and celebrations, we discovered, was a shared
component in every sustainable management system we studied. Management systems also need to be both varied and extremely flexible.

This is another reflection of nature: nature always has more than one
way to do things and attains its goals of fostering the health of a local
environment and its many life forms through variety and flexibility,
from the cellular to the ecosystem level. It is a biological law that the
more variety, the healthier the system. That's how physical reality
works. This flexibility is the other side of a basic and very deep humility.
For example, the key component of the Holistic Management theory
that underpins many current ideas about how to sustainably run a farm
or a business was developed by a wildlife biologist, Allan Savory. When
talking about his own recommendations to ranchers and farmers, he
always includes a caveat: "Assume Wrong." He means that when it
comes to dealing with changeable, intricate, and interdependent natural systems, human theory has to recognize the superiority of physical
reality. What works in a lab or in someone's head does not always (if
ever) work on the ground, especially over the long term. And even if it
works well for many years, things change. So this humility has to be part
of any farmer's attitudes when dealing with a cow that does not
respond to a drug, a soil that does not respond to an amendment, a
field that somehow does well despite a drought, or even to a business
that has a great location but is still failing.

We also discovered, really in retrospect, that the practical, workable
solutions we were finding were nearly always coming from what is

termed "the margins of security." That is, it was not the thousands of government agencies, expert think-tanks, university departments, or NGOs devoted to these issues that were figuring out how to restore a grassland, a river, a habitat, or an urban neighbourhood. It was nearly always the poor, local fishermen, residents, or ranchers. When faced with losing their land or their livelihoods, these people were forced to ignore all the expert advice and theory and pay attention only to what produces real returns over the long-term. Later on, the experts, NGOs, and university professors arrived to confirm through careful research these practical discoveries. Their studies also helped us confirm the efficacy of what the more humble innovators had developed.

Finally, oddly enough, we discovered that the most important characteristic of a sustainable management system is an extremely lofty vision of its purpose. The "vision" of nature, we might say, is a very ambitious one: the continued thriving of all its myriad forms of life that give rise to the air, water, and soil that support still more life. On a management level, we found that human groups that gave themselves remarkably ambitious and lofty goals, and kept these goals in mind as much as possible, were able to achieve amazing results for a very long time. That is to say, a vision demanding that its participants maintain the highest level of ethical and human values came remarkably close to attaining its objectives, however impossible they had seemed at the outset. Interestingly enough, organizations with more practical or pragmatic ambitions rarely came close to even their low-level, short-term goals. In this context, we need only think of what a serious visionary like Tommy Douglas set out to attain for Canadians, and what he ended up getting: fully public schools, a forty-hour work week, and universal, single-payer health care.

In *Good News*, we were mostly working with biological systems. However, we found that when any management organization, including governments and private businesses, contains all – or most – of these criteria, it can be productive and sustainable *almost indefinitely*. That seems to be because these are natural laws of physics, and when they are in accord with our practices, our endeavours fit in with the reality of where we happen to live.

It was only after I was well over halfway through researching the book you are holding in your hands and had read all the minutes, Annual Reports, diaries, and letters and had also interviewed the many alumni, not just of the Queen E but of hospitals elsewhere in Canada, that I realized that – of course – a hospital is like any other management system. I was belatedly recognizing what all the reading and interviews had been telling me: that the Queen Elizabeth as an individual institution, along with many of its equally celebrated sisters like the Wellesley, the Calgary General, or indeed the French or Cuban health care systems, exhibited nearly all the criteria for sustainability that David Suzuki and I had observed in natural systems, always allowing, of course, for the type of institution they were and their particular social and historical surroundings and constraints.

Modern hospitals could go a great deal further in coping with their own chemical and biological wastes – bio-medical wastes are among the most dangerous and inappropriate creations on the planet. But the Queen Elizabeth did at least attempt to follow the more obvious natural cycles and systems of the physical world, which is one reason why it fatally ignored government demands for fewer beds and higher occupancy. Generally, it tried to stick to its mandate of taking care of people who needed that care, even if government budgets did not want to recognize the reality of those needs. The many small community hospitals that were closed or lost beds in the mid-1990s were, like the Queen Elizabeth, entirely locally based, very much a part of the small communities they served, and closely responsive to the particular needs of those local neighbourhoods.

Possibly more than any other hospital I studied, the Queen Elizabeth also practiced a rare egalitarianism from its very beginnings: between the sexes, between the different levels of the medical profession, and between every member and level of its staff. That's why former orderlies still hang out with surgeons at reunions and the hospital cleaning lady had no qualms about approaching the director general and forcing him to eat his dinner. Such equality makes people feel valued and happy; it makes their daily work fun. Enjoyment is a very key component of sustainability, and in this context, the Queen E could almost have been said to be sustainable on the strength of its lunches, sports events, and parties alone.

Egalitarianism feeds into the variety that is a key component of the long-term sustainability of any management system. Nurses and GPs as well as specialists had serious input into all the innovations that eventually made the little hospital a national and international medical pioneer. The same embrace of variety and flexibility can be traced in that hospital's general culture. From Albert Nixon's highly creative budgetary allocations and the teamwork between nurses and doctors, to Joe Mammaza and Ron Lewis' being allowed, even as very young doctors, to pursue their most creative ideas, the institution showed the unusual flexibility that only a small, humble, local, and egalitarian organization can. And it was rewarded by nature, or, one might say, by physics, with an outpouring of success on every level.

Evidence has been mounting that hospital systems that work in other countries share these same qualities. The best ones are also tailored to local needs; they have lofty goals, but fundamentally humble and flexible policies, and they respond well to democratic input. The most remarkable achievements in public health very often, just like the biological solutions, come from the "margins of security." Cuba, like the Queen Elizabeth in its earliest days, has been forced by economic circumstances to concentrate on very basic, commonsense methods of primary and preventative care: holistic attention to families and neighbourhoods, to cleanliness, exercise, and diet. As this book has noted, good community hospitals like the Queen Elizabeth were never far from bankruptcy throughout their history. For most of their existence, they hovered at the edge of economic security. Such a position forces people to pay attention to what brings the most efficient tangible results. Many hospitals dedicated to the poor – Bichat in Paris, for example – have nonetheless managed to come up with innovative ideas that have transformed both patient care and hospital management. All of which implies that heavily endowed super-hospitals and clinics are not always the best way for a country to spend its limited amounts of health care money or even for the profession to foster innovations.

Perhaps most importantly, the Homeopathic/Queen E and so many other community hospitals like it were built on the exceedingly ethical and altruistic values expressed by all its founders and supporters, in its case, those of the Griffith family. These values, which considered each participant's work, no matter how lowly, as an opportunity to be of service to others, were more lofty and sustained than most and may finally be the reason why the Queen E's vision of itself within the community never failed. These values may also explain why the people who worked in it still get tears in their eyes when they remember it today. We should all get tears in our eyes when we think of how a full 20 percent of Canada's hospital system was destroyed in 1995, without our input or clear knowledge, and continues to be attacked today by the very same forces that crippled it back then. Hopefully this book has done something to elucidate how that happened. I also hope it helps us recognize the kind of institutions we need to support to keep everyone in society well and in step with the basic physical laws of this planet.

Notes

Many quotations in the text are taken from interviews conducted by the author in Montreal and Ottawa between 2003 and 2006. Because this material is not publically available and the source is clear, there are no notes for such quotations.

Neither "Some Reminiscences" nor "Highlights in the Life of Harold Randall Griffith" have page numbers.

CHAPTER ONE

1 Levy, from "Clippings on Closure," 10.
2 Riga, from "Clippings on Closure," 17.
3 Sutherland, Stewart, and Cuthier, "Marchers Decry Hospital Closing."
4 Ibid.
5 Curran, "Don't Tell Mrs. Taylor That Cutbacks Won't Hurt."
6 Eisler, "An Unprecedented Hospital Closing in Calgary."
7 Ibid.
8 StratCom (Strategic Market Research and Communications), "Health Care in Canada," as cited on the Health Care in Canada website.
9 Canadian Auto Workers Union, from "Campaigns & Issues, Conservative Government Record on Health Care."
10 HEN, "What Are the Lessons Learnt by Countries That Have Had Dramatic Reductions of Their Hospital Bed Capacity?"
11 Taft and Steward, *Clear Answers,* 34–40.
12 Hamilton, "Reprieve for Hospitals Seems Unlikely." See also Hamilton and Lalonde, "Seven Local Hospitals Slated to Close, MNA says,"
13 Ibid.
14 Curran, "Something Alarming about the Scope of Hospital Cuts."

15 Hamilton and Riga, "Planners Say Glut of Hospitals Means Some Must Close." [Author's emphasis]

16 Amdur, "Defending Medicare."

17 Personal interviews with Pat Titterton, John Hughes, and Fred Weigan.

18 Jackson, "At Debt's Door," 1–2.

19 Ibid., 1.

20 Reid, *Shakedown: How the New Economy Is Changing Our Lives*. See also McQuaig, *Shooting the Hippo*. McQuaig's detailed analysis at the time blamed John Crow, director of the Bank of Canada, for choosing to cut social services instead of raising taxes on the rich in order to deal with the national debt. She also blamed his decision to keep interest rates high; however, she did not have the benefit of seeing that year's IMF Report to Canada, which makes it clear that Crow's decisions also must have been influenced by that organization's orders to the Canadian government. In that book, she tellingly quoted Pierre Fortin, president of the Canadian Economics Assiciation, who charged that Canadian policies "should be more concerned with the welfare of Canadians than with the welfare of foreign investors." See also "Notes on *Shooting the Hippo*," from www.basicincome.com/basic_mcquaig.htm, 3, accessed on 5 January 2007.

21 Derfel, Aaron, "Is Our Health System Failing?" B3.

22 Hamilton, "Local Hospital Closings Done Strictly by the Numbers," A4.

23 Chambers, "It's a Mistake to Close Hospitals with Proven Record of Care."

CHAPTER TWO

1 Heaman, *St. Mary's*, 32.

2 Rosenberg, *The Care of Strangers*, 5.

3 Griffith, A.R., "Some Reminiscences."

4 Griffith, H.R., "Highlights in the Life of Harold Randall Griffith."

5 Ibid.

6 Griffith, H.R., *The Evolution of Modern Anaesthesia*, 32.

7 Griffith, A.R., "Some Reminiscences."

8 Ibid., 75–6.

9 Ibid.

10 Conor, "A Trip to Chinatown,"1892.

11 Rosenberg, *The Care of Strangers*, 15.

12 Ibid., 5.

13 Griffith, A. R. "Some Reminiscences."

14 Ibid.

15 Ibid.

16 Rosenberg. *The Care of Strangers*, 26.

17 Ibid.
18 Heaman, *St. Mary's*, 28.
19 Ibid., 31–2.
20 Ibid., 32.
21 All this may seem laughably primitive, but it's instructive to realize that even with modern antibiotics – or rather because of over-reliance on them – our current neglect of basic cleanliness more than a hundred and thirty years later has resulted in the proliferation of many dangerous pathogens in hospitals, including *Clostridium difficile*, a diarrhea that can destroy whole sections of the colon, causing a very painful death; methicillin-resistant *Staph aureus* (MRSA), which causes blood infections; and vancomycin-reistant *Enterococcus* (VRE), which infects the bladder. All are potentially fatal, especially *C. difficile*, which killed more people in Canada in 2004 than the far more publicized SARS epidemic. These and other hospital-specific infections, as well as emerging pathogens like SARS or various forms of hepatitis spread by infected blood supplies, have again threatened the confidence of the public in the safety of surgical and hospital care.
22 Hanaway and Cruess, *McGill Medicine*, 63–4.
23 Heaman, *St. Mary's*, 29.
24 Hanaway and Cruess, *McGill Medicine*, 84.
25 Griffith, A.R. "Some Reminiscences."
26 Ibid.
27 Rosenberg, *The Care of Strangers*, 43–4, notes 59–69.
28 Duffe, *Diary*.
29 Griffith, A.R., "Some Reminiscences."
30 Rosenberg, *The Care of Strangers*, 23.
31 As the miracles of antibiotics fail, we may find ourselves going back to the stepladder of hospital choices that still obtained while A.R. and Mary worked in New York.
32 Rosenberg, *The Care of Strangers*, 23, 26.
33 Griffith, A.R., "Some Reminiscences."
34 Ibid.
35 Griffith, Harold, *Seventy-Five Years of Service: The Story of the Queen Elizabeth Hospital of Montreal*, 149–50.
36 Griffith, A.R., "Some Reminiscences."
37 Ibid.
38 Ibid.
39 Ibid.
40 Ibid.
41 Rosenberg, *The Care of Strangers*.
42 Ibid.

43 Ibid.

44 Ibid., 6–7.

45 Ibid.

46 Back cover of the *Annual Report of the Homoeopathic Hospital of Montreal, 1926.* This was the last year that governors, as well as doctors, had authority over admissions, although the actual practice had diminished yearly since the turn of the century.

47 Griffith, H.R., *Seventy-Five Years of Service: The Story of the Queen Elizabeth Hospital of Montreal,* 7.

48 Ibid.

49 Gagan, *For Patients of Moderate Means,* 27.

50 Ibid., 27.

51 Griffith, A.R., "Some Reminiscences."

52 Rosenberg, *The Care of Strangers,* 8–9.

53 Griffith, A.R., "Some Reminiscences."

54 Rosenberg, *The Care of Strangers,* 5.

55 Ibid.

56 Ibid., 25.

57 Ibid.

58 Ibid.

59 Ibid., 35–6.

60 Ibid.

60 Ibid., 38–9.

61 Ibid., 39.

62 Philadelphia Almshouse Hospital Committee Minutes, 28 January 1846. In Rosenberg, *The Care of Strangers.*

63 Medical Board Minutes, Episcopal Hospital Archives, 21 May 21 1857, as cited in Rosenberg, *The Care of Strangers,* 40, note 53.

64 Minutes, Almshouse Commissioners, SCHS, 11 May 1842. In Rosenberg, *The Care of Strangers,* 40, note 54.

65 Heamon, St. Mary's, 101–2.

66 Rosenberg, *The Care of Strangers,* 41.

67 Ibid.

68 Arnold, *Memoir of Jonathan Mason Warren, M.D.,* 85. In Rosenberg, *The Care of Strangers,* 41, note 56.

69 Heaman, *St. Mary's,* 31.

70 Ibid.

71 Rosenberg, *The Care of Strangers,* 41.

72 Griffith, H.R., *Seventy-Five Years of Service: The Story of the Queen Elizabeth Hospital of Montreal,* 7.

73 Griffith, A.R., *Medical Superintendent's Annual Report, 1900,* 22.

74 Gagan, *For Patients of Moderate Means*, 24.

75 Ibid., 25.

76 Ibid.

77 Ibid., 26.

78 Copp, *The Anatomy of Poverty*, 88–105. In Shortt, *Medicine in Canadian Society: Historical Perspectives*, 395.

79 Ibid., 399–400.

80 Ibid.

81 Annual Report of the Homeopathic Hospital of Montreal, 1924, "Causes of Death," 22. See also Annual Report of the Homeopathic Hospital of Montreal, 1927, 22 and 24–5.

82 Conversation with Beverley Rowat about her sister Barbara Rowett Flam's maternity experience at the Queen E, 19 Nov. 2004.

83 Copp, *The Anatomy of Poverty*, as cited in Shortt, *Medicine in Canadian Society: Historical Perspectives*, 400–3.

84 Gagan, *For Patients of Moderate Means*, 26.

85 Ibid., 27.

86 Griffith, A.R., Annual Report of the Montreal Homeopathic, 1900, 12.

87 Patton, Annual Report of the Montreal Homeopathic, 1906, 7–8.

88 Gagan, *For Patients of Moderate Means*, 29.

89 Griffith, A.R., Annual Report of the Homeopathic Hospital of Montreal, 1900, 22.

90 "Trained Nurses," *Canadian Lancet*, 17 December 1885, 120, as cited in Gagan, *For Patients of Moderate Means*, 29.

91 Gagan, *For Patients of Moderate Means*, 30.

92 Griffith, H.R. *Seventy-five Years of Service: The Story of the Queen Elizabeth Hospital.* 8–9.

93 Provincial Archives of British Columbia, GR785, Province of British Columbia Royal Commissions and Commissions of Inquiry, Commission of Inquiry, Vancouver General Hospital, 1912, Investigative Proceedings, 297; *Vancouver Daily World*, 14 and 25 February 1911; cited in Gagan, *For Patients of Moderate Means*, 30.

94 Gagan, *For Patients of Moderate Means*, 30.

95 Griffith, H.R., *Seventy-Five Years of Service: The Story of the Queen Elizabeth Hospital*, 11.

96 Godfrey, *A Struggle to Serve*, 15–16.

97 Ibid., 16.

98 Ibid., 16–21.

99 *The Moncton Daily Times*, 2 April 1895, as cited in Godfrey, *A Struggle to Serve: A History of the Moncton Hospital, 1895–1953*, 24–5.

100 Godfrey, *A Struggle to Serve: A History of the Moncton Hospital, 1895–1953,* 30.
101 Ibid.
102 Griffith, H.R., "Highlights in the Life of Harold Randall Griffith."
103 Ibid.

CHAPTER THREE

1 Griffith, Harold, "Highlights in the Life of Harold Randall Griffith."
2 Griffith, Harold. Diary entry, 160.
3 Griffith, Harold. "Highlights in the Life of Harold Randall Griffith," 31.
4 This and all subsequent quotes about Vimy are from Harold Griffith's letter to Mary Griffith, 1918, "Letter from Vimy Ridge," copy housed at the Queen Elizabeth Hospital Archives of McGill University.
5 Griffith, Harold. Diary entry, 104–5.
6 Ibid., 167–8.
7 Griffith, Harold. *"Highlights in the Life of Harold Randall Griffith,"* 40.
8 Ibid., 35.
9 Ibid., 41.
10 Ibid.
11 Ibid., 39.
12 Ibid.
13 Griffith, A.R. "Report of the Medical Superintendent," Annual Report of the Montreal Homeopathic Hospital, 1917–18, 11.
14 Griffith, A.R. "Report of the Medical Superintendent," Annual Report of the Montreal Homeopathic Hospital, 1919, 20–21.
15 Ibid., 12.
16 Griffith, A.R. "Report of the Medical Superintendent," Annual Report of the Montreal Homeopathic Hospital, 1906, 14–15.
17 Bodman and Gillies. *Harold Griffith, The Evolution of Modern Anaesthesia,* 35.
18 Griffith, Harold. "Highlights in the Life of Harold Randall Griffith," 47.
19 Quote from Elizabeth Morton at her husband's gravesite, provided on the official website of the Nurse-Anesthetists of America, www.anesthesia-nursing.com/ether2.html, accessed 04 April 2006.
20 Sykes, *Essays on the First Hundred Years of Anaesthesia,* 105.
21 Ibid.
22 As quoted in Atkinson and Boulton. *The History of Anesthesia,* 43, the great anesthetics pioneer John Snow quotes a Roman text as saying, "'a wine is prepared from the bark of [the] root, without boiling and three pounds are put into a cadus (about 18 gallons) of sweet wine, and 3 cyathea are administered to those requiring to be cut or cauterized: when being thrown into a

deep sleep, they do not feel any pain.' A preparation of mandrake was also taken against sleeplessness."

23 Ibid., 43 and 47.

24 Ibid., 49.

25 Ibid., 43.

26 Description of the discovery of ether, presented on the official website of the Nurse-Anesthetists of America, www.anesthesia-nursing.com/ether.html, accessed on 10 February 2006.

27 www.neurosurgery.mgh.harvard.edu/History the website of the Massachusetts General Neurosurgery Department, as accessed on 10 Feb 2006.

28 Description of the history of neurosurgery on Harvard Univerisity's website, www.neurosurgery.mgh.harvard.edu/History, as accessed on 10 Feb 2006.

29 Duncum, Barbara M., "A Quick Look at the First London Etherists," 76–80.

30 Rupreht, J. "The Knowledge Spreads through Europe," 82–6.

31 Official website3 of Nurse-Anesthetists of America, www.anesthetic-nursing. com/ether.html accessed 11 February 2006.

32 Description of Charles Jackson's experiences with ether, as presented on the official website of the Nurse-Anesthetists of America, www.anesthesia-nursing.com/ether.html, accessed on 11 February 2006.

33 Sykes, *Essays on the First Hundred Years of Anaesthesia*, 105.

34 Ibid., 100–1.

35 According to Sykes, *Essays on the First Hundred Years of Anaesthesia*, 101, *The Lancet* during this early period deserves credit for trying to alter the situation with strong articles. It charged that the "responsibilities of the medical profession on this count" were serious. After all, "It...brought in the agent which caused the deaths; on its recommendation the general public accepted the agent, and by and through its voice declared the anaesthetic beneficent."

36 Sykes, *Essays on the First Hundred Years of Anaesthesia*, 102–3.

37 Ibid., 109.

38 Griffith, Harold, "An Anaesthetist's Valediction," 3.

39 Tirer, Samual. "Metaphysical conclusions derived from a proposed mode of anaesthetic action," 56–63.

40 Bodman and Gillies, *Harold Griffith: The Evolution of Modern Anaesthesia*, 40–1.

41 Sykes, *Essays on the First Hundred Years of Anaesthesiology*.

42 Griffith, Harold, "The Boundless Realm of Anaesthesiology," 2.

43 Sykes, *Essays on the First Hundred Years of Anaesthesia*, 104.

44 Bodman and Gilles, *Harold Griffith: The Evolution of Modern Anesthesia*, 55.

45 Ibid., 43

46 Ibid., 44.

47 Griffith, Harold, "The Boundless Realm of Anaesthesiology," 2.

48 As quoted in Bodman and Gilles, *The Evolution of Modern Anaesthesia*, 45. "[Magill] discovered that when he passed a catheter through the nose, it sometimes went of its own accord through the larynx into the trachea, and by stimulating the breathing with a little carbon dioxide, he could achieve a high rate of success." This technique allowed a large enough tube so the patient could breathe ether and air freely without the need for an insufflation pump. This wide bore tube took Magill's name, as the "Magill endotracheal tube."

49 Ibid., 46.

50 Ibid., 43–8.

51 Hoffman, "Medic Proves Poison Not Best Opiate" [author's emphasis].

52 Sturges, "Cabins on Neversink Produce World's Best Anesthetic."

53 Letter from Karl Connell, Connell Apparatus, Big Indian, New York, to Harold Griffith, available in The Queen Elizabeth Archives, McGill University.

54 Griffith, Harold, "The Pattern of Anesthesia," 2.

55 Ibid. See also The *Canadian Medical Association Journal* 31, 157–160.

56 Bodman and Gillies, *Harold Griffith, The Evolution of Modern Anaesthesia*, 48.

57 According to Bodman and Gillies, *Harold Griffith, The Evolution of Modern Anaesthesia*, 50, "He was attracted to this new anesthetic because it is a sweet-smelling, non-irritating gas, unlike ether, and is more potent than nitrous oxide or ethylene. It produces surgical anesthesia in low concentrations of 10 to 15 percent. Therefore, the percentage of oxygen mixed with it can be raised to 85 or even 90 percent, which gives 'a wide margin of safety' to the patient. Nitrous oxide, which was useful for only minor and superficial surgery, was far more dangerous because it could be diluted with only 10 to 15 percent of oxygen – less than in the air we breathe. The oxygen in ethylene could be slightly higher – 20 percent – but was relatively light in effect."

58 Bodman and Gillies, *Harold Griffith, The Evolution of Modern Anaesthesia*, 51–3.

59 Ibid., 54.

60 Review of Philip Smith's book on curare, *Weekend Magazine*, 10 January 1970.

61 Heim, *Alexander von Humboldt, Life and Work*, 216.

62 Sykes, *Essays on the First Hundred Years of Anaesthesia*, 89–91.

63 Ibid,

64 Von Humboldt, "Curare Report," as cited in Heim, *Alexander von Humboldt, Life and Work*, 211–15.

65 Ibid., 212.

66 Ibid.

67 Ibid., 218–19.

68 Bennett, *Anaesthesia and Analgesia*, 487.

69 Ibid.

70 Smith, Philip, *Arrows of Mercy*.

71 Bodman and Gillies. *Harold Griffith, The Evolution of Modern Anaesthesia*, 60–64.

72 Griffith, H.R. *The Evolution of Modern Anaesthesia*.

CHAPTER FOUR

1 Hammond, "Treasurer's Report," Annual Report of the Homeopathic Hospital of Montreal, 1926.

2 Gagan, *For Patients of Moderate Means*, 182–3.

3 Ibid., 183.

4 Ibid., 175.

5 Ibid.

6 Ibid.

7 Ibid., 162.

8 Ibid., 162, 183.

9 Hammond. "Treasurer's Report," Annual Report of the Homeopathic Hospital of Montreal, 1926.

10 Naylor, *Private Practice, Public Payment*, 47.

11 Ibid., 56–7.

12 Terkel, *Hard Times: An Oral History of the Great Depression*, 142–7.

13 Naylor, *Private Practice, Public Payment*, 58–9.

14 Ibid., 59.

15 Ibid.

16 Survey of Public General Hospitals in Ontario, Part 4, 1; as quoted in Gagan, *For Patients of Moderate Means*, 162.

17 Gagan, *For Patients of Moderate Means*, 151.

18 "Report of the Lady Superintendent," Minutes of the Medical Board of the Homeopathic Hospital of Montreal, 1932–36.

19 Annual Report of the Homeopathic Hospital of Montreal, 1936, 20.

20 Gagan, *For Patients of Moderate Means*, 50–2.

21 W.G. Godfrey. *The Struggle to Serve*, 57.

22 Gagan, *For Patients of Moderate Means*.

23 "Graduate Nurses of the Phillips Training School of the Homeoeopathic Hospital of Montreal," Annual Reports of The Homeopathic Hospital of Montreal, 1920–32.

24 "Report of Lady Superintendent," Annual Report of the Homeopathic Hospital of Montreal, 1932, 19.

25 Gagan, *For Patients of Moderate Means,* 152.
26 Annual Report of the Homeopathic Hospital of Montreal, 1924, 27.
27 Gagan, *For Patients of Moderate Means,* 143.
28 Minutes of the Medical Board of the Homeopathic Hospital of Montreal, 1935, 2.
29 "Report of the Lady Superintendent," Annual Report of the Homeopathic Hospital of Montreal, 1936, 20.
30 Ibid., 18.
31 Minutes of the Medical Board of the Homeopathic Hospital of Montreal, 11 Feb. 1958.
32 Gagan, *For Patients of Moderate Means,* 154, note 169.
33 New CMA ethics code, 1937, as quoted in Naylor, *Canadian Health Care and the State,* 91 [author's emphasis].
34 Minutes of the Medical Board of the Homeopathic Hospital of Montreal, 1937, 5.
35 Ibid.
36 Terkel, *Hard Times: An Oral History of the Great Depression,* 145.
37 Naylor, *Private Practice, Public Payment,* 90.
38 Ibid., 95.
39 "Report of the Committee on Ethics and Credentials," CMAJ 37 (Sept.1937): supplement, 9, as quoted in Naylor, *Private Practice, Public Payment,* 91.
40 Naylor, *Private Practice, Public Payment,* 93.
41 Terkel, *Hard Times: An Oral History of the Great Depression,* 146.
42 Gagan, *For Patients of Moderate Means,* 155.
43 Ibid., 156.
44 Annual Report of the Homeopathic Hospital of Montreal, 1936, 12.
45 Griffith, H.R., "Report of the Superintendent," Annual Report of the Homeopathic Hospital of Montreal, 1947, 19.
46 Gagan, *For Patients of Moderate Means,* 160, footnote 9.
47 "Report of the Medical Superintendent," Annual Report of the Homeopathic Hospital of Montreal, 1952, 28–9.
48 "Report of the Medical Superintendent," Annual Report of the Homeopathic Hospital of Montreal, 1947, 21.
49 Annual Report of the Homeopathic Hospital of Montreal, 1947, 19.
50 Minutes of the Medical Board of the Homeopathic Hospital of Montreal, 15 Oct. 1945.
51 Minutes of the Medical Board of the Homeopathic Hospital of Montreal, 24 Sept.1945.
52 Minutes of the Medical Board of the Homeopathic Hospital of Montreal, 22 Sept.1952 and 20 April 1953.

53 Minutes of the Medical Board of the Homeopathic Hospital of Montreal, 2 and 19 Oct. 1953.

54 Minutes of the Medical Board of the Homeopathic Hospital of Montreal, 1952.

55 Minutes of the Medical Board of the Homeopathic Hospital of Montreal, 13 Nov. 1953.

56 Gagan, *For Patients of Moderate Means,* 172.

57 Minutes of the Medical Board of the Homeopathic Hospital of Montreal, 10 Jan 1961.

58 "Report of the Infection Control Committee," Minutes of the Medical Board of the Homeopathic Hospital of Montreal, 20 Nov 1957.

59 Minutes of the Medical Board of the Homeopathic Hospital of Montreal, 13 Oct 1959; see also Minutes of the Medical Board of the Homeopathic Hospital of Montreal, 15 May 1957.

60 Minutes of the Medical Board of the Homeopathic Hospital of Montreal, 6 Mar 1954.

61 Gagan, *For Patients of Moderate Means,*

62 Oppenhiemer, "Childbirth in Ontario," 66–7. See also *Survey of Public General Hospitals in Ontario,* part 5, 22, as cited in Gagan, *For Patients of Moderate Means,* 172.

63 Minutes of the Medical Board of the Homeopathic Hospital of Montreal, 1955–57.

64 Minutes of the Medical Board of the Homeopathic Hospital of Montreal, 20 Feb 1954.

65 Minutes of the Medical Board of the Homeopathic Hospital of Montreal, 14 Apr 1954.

66 Royal Commission on Health Services, 19 June 1964, as cited in Naylor, *Private Practice, Public Payment,* 214. For the complete brief of the Commission, see CMAJ 86, (19 May 1962): 895–926. Also see Gruending, *Emmett Hall: Establishment Radical,* 14, 17, 52–67, 70, 78–83.

67 Naylor, *Private Practice, Public Payment,* 98.

68 Ibid., 99.

69 Ibid., 100.

70 Ibid.

71 Ibid., 151.

72 Ibid., 252.

73 Vayda and Deber, "The Canadian Health-Care System," as cited in Naylor. *Canadian Health Care and the State,* 125–40.

74 Naylor, *Canadian Health Care and the State,* 126.

75 Vayda and Deber. "The Canadian Health-Care System," as cited in Naylor. *Canadian Health Care and the State,* 126–7.

76 Unwin, Annual Report of the Homeopathic Hospital of Montreal, 1952, 14–15.

77 Unwin, Annual Report of the Homeopathic Hospital of Montreal, 1953, 13.

78 Berton, *The Invasion of Canada,* 313–14.

79 Boychuk, *The Making and Meaning of Hospital Policy in the United States and Canada,* vii.

80 Ibid., viii.

81 Ibid., ix, viii.

82 Ibid. [author's emphasis].

83 "Medical Superintendent's Report," Annual Report of the Queen Elizabeth Hospital of Montreal, 1962, 28.

84 Annual Report of the Homeopathic Hospital of Montreal, 1954, 12.

85 Minutes of the Medical Board of the Queen Elizabeth Hospital of Montreal, motion made 10 Jan. and passed 14 Feb. 1961.

86 Minutes of the Medical Board of the Queen Elizabeth Hospital of Montreal, 1963–1967, 8–9.

87 Minutes of the Medical Board of the Queen Elizabeth Hospital of Montreal, 10 Oct. 1961.

88 Minutes of the Medical Board of the Queen Elizabeth Hospital of Montreal, 9 Oct. 1962.

89 Hectman, unpublished study of the Minutes of the Medical Board of the Queen Elizabeth Hospital of Montreal, 1957–67, 6.

90 Minutes of the Medical Board of the Queen Elizabeth Hospital of Montreal, 10 Nov. 1964.

91 Annual Report of the Queen Elizabeth Hospital of Montreal, 1961.

92 Barlow, *Profit Is Not the Cure,* 19.

93 Naylor, C. David, *Canadian Health Care and the State,* 251.

94 Marden, "Report of the President," Annual Report of the Queen Elizabeth Hospital of Montreal, 1970. [author's emphasis].

95 Ibid.

96 Annual Report of the Queen Elizabeth Hospital of Montreal, 1974, 7.

97 Medical Economics and Administrative Boards, Queen Elizabeth Hospital of Montreal, 24 Oct. 1972.

98 Nixon, Minutes of the Medical Board of the Queen Elizabeth Hospital of Montreal, 197.

99 As quoted from Dressel. "Has Canada Got the Cure?", 24.

100 Boychuk, *The Making and Meaning of Hospital Policy in the United States and Canada,* 23.

101 See Elizabeth Warren et al, in *Norton's Bankruptcy Advisor,* May 2000, http://papers.ssrn.com/sol3/ paper.cfm?abstract_id=224581, accessed 27

July 2007, and Araminta Wordsworth, "US Study: Medical Bills Main Culprit in Bankruptcies – Americans are 'One Illness Away from Financial Collapse," *The National Post,* April 27, 2000.

102 Cassel, *Medicare Matters,* 3–9, 120–2, 159.

103 Dunnigan and Pollock, "Downsizing of acute inpatient beds associated with private finance initiative: Scotland's case study." See also Dodd and Leeder, Ringen, Sawyer, Harris, and Boyd, "Public Patients, Private Profit," 1–2, 5–11.

104 ABC News/Washington Post Poll, cited in www.harpers.org/subjects/ HealthCare/SubjectOf/Fact, accessed 27 July, 2007.

105 Reams of articles and reports in the media, from mainstream press to specialized studies, should have made these increased health dangers amply familiar to the reader. Two of the most recent articles would be D'Aliesio and Brooymans, "Alberta Rivers Flood with Pollutants: Report," reporting how "several massive rainstorms in 2005 turned many Alberta rivers into polluted stews of bacteria, metals and pesticides, a newly released government report shows." A similar article by Darier, entitled "Algues blues: Greenpeace accuse l'industrie agricole," concerns the highly toxic blue algae problem in Quebec lakes and rivers caused by industrial farming. Chapin, Rule et.al, "Airborne Multi-drug Resistant Bacteria Isolated from a Contaminated Swine Feeding Operation." And Otte, Roland-Holst et. al, "Industrial Livestock Production and Global Health Risks," about avian flu.

106 Health Science Center, University of Texas, Austin, cited at www.harpers. org/subjects/HealthCare/SubjectsOf/Fact, accessed 27 July 2007.

107 Fraser Institute. "How Private Hospital Competition Can Improve Canadian Health Care," as cited in Taft and Steward, *Clear Answers: The Economics and Politics of For-Profit Medicine.* 27.

108 MacBeth, as quoted in Taft and Steward, *Clear Answers: The Economics and Politics of For-Profit Medicine,* 23–4. This and the following quote are part of a Question Period that took place in the Alberta legislature, 1 Dec. 1999.

109 Klein, as quoted in Taft and Steward, *Clear Answers: the Economics and Politics of For-Profit Medicine,* 27.

110 *Harper's Magazine,* "Harper's Index," Feb., 2006 at www.harper's.org/ archive/2006/02/008090, accessed 20 July 2007 ; see also Prof James Kahn, University of California at San Francisco on the above website.

111 Hewitt Associates LLC (Lincolnshire, ILL), source quoted for "Harper's Index," Harper's Magazine, Feb. 2006 www.harpers.org/subjects/ HealthCare/SubjectOf ; see also ww.cms.hhs.gov/National Health Expend Data/downloads/tables.pdf.

112 Barlow, review of the article in *Profit Is Not the Cure,* 52.

113 Devereaux, "A Systematic Review and Meta-Analysis of Studies Comparing Mortality between Private For-Profit and Private Not-For-Profit Hospitals," 1–5. See also the May 2002 issue of the *Canadian Medical Association Journal.*

114 Ross et al. "Relation between income inequality and mortality in Canada and in the United States: cross sectional assessment using census data and vital statistics," 109–17, 111, 113.

115 Altmayer et.al, "Geographical disparity in premature mortality in Ontario, 1992–1996." See also Jennissen, "Health Issues in Rural Canada."

116 Trovato, "Mortality differentials in Canada, 1951–1971: French, British and Indians," 459–77.

117 These statistics are a conservative compilation from the most accepted sources. See Trovato, above, Chandrakant, below, and CIA World Fact Book, Centers for Disease Control, World Health Organization, http://hdr.undp.org/hdr2006/pdfs/report/HDR06.

118 Chandrakant, *Public Health and Preventative Medicine in Canada,* 139–40.

119 Ibid.,139; Statistics and charts are from Health Field Indicators, Health and Welfare Canada, and Statistics Canada.

120 Ibid., and *National Vital Statistic Reports,* Vol. 53, No. 5, 12 Oct. 2004, www.cdc.gov/nchs/fastats , as accessed 3 July 2007.

121 See www.mchb.hrsa.gov/chusa03 for *Child Health USA 2003, Health Status – Infants;* Health Resources and Services Administration (HRSA), with graphs illustrating "Breastfeeding Rates, by Race/Ethnicity, 2001"; "Very Low Birth Weight among Infants, by Race/Ethnicity 1985–2001," where the line for black babies is in a separate section right off the charts.

122 Jasmer, "Racial Disparity and Socioeconomic Status in Association with Survival in Older Men with Local/Regional Stage Prostate Carcinoma Findings from a Large Community-based Cohort."

123 See www.mchb.hrsa.gov/chusa03 for *Child Health USA 2003, Health Status – Infants;* Health Resources and Services Administration (HRSA), with graphs illustrating "Breastfeeding Rates, by Race/Ethnicity, 2001"; Very Low Birth Weight among Infants, by Race/Ethnicity 1985–2001"

124 Marmot et al., "Disease and Disadvantage in the United States and in England."

125 Barlow, *Profit Is Not the Cure,* 59.

126 www.legermarketing.com/eng/tencom.asp, "Les Quebecois et l'acces aux soins de sante," accessed 27 July, 2007; see also www.cbc.ca/homerun, 9 July 2007.

127 Veda and Deber, "The Canadian Health-Care System," 135–6 [author's emphasis].

128 Garrett, *Betrayal of Trust: The Collapse of Global Public Health*, 572.

CHAPTER FIVE

1 "Report of the President," Annual Report of the Queen Elizabeth Hospital of Montreal, 1973, 7.
2 "Minutes," Medical Board of the Queen Elizabeth Hospital of Montreal, 3 Nov. 1970.
3 Ibid., 2 Nov. 1971.
4 Ibid., 4 June 1974.
5 Ibid., 6 Nov. 1979.
6 Ibid., 20 Sept. 1974. See also, Zacharia, "Tears Flow as Emergency Ward Packs Up."
7 Letter sent to Medical Board and entered in the Minutes, 5 May 1975.
8 "Minutes," Medical Board of the Queen Elizabeth Hospital of Montreal, 4 Mar. 1980.
9 Ibid., 5 Jan. 1982.
10 Ibid., 6 Dec. 1983; see also 3 Jan. 1984.
11 Ibid., 7 June 1988 and letter written 5 Dec. 1988.
12 Ibid., 4 Jan. 1977.
13 Ibid., 5 April 1977.
14 Ibid., 6 Mar. 1979.
15 Mair, "President's Report," 2.
16 "Minutes," Medical Board of the Queen Elizabeth Hospital of Montreal, 6 Dec. 1983.
17 Ibid., 6 July 1982.
18 Ibid., July, 1982.
19 Ibid., 1 Nov. 1988 and letter from ICU Committee Chair, 5 Dec. 1988.
20 Ibid., 2 Nov. 1989.
21 Ibid., 7 Jan. and 1 April 1986.
22 Ibid., 9 May 1989.
23 Ibid., 5 June 1990.
24 Ibid., 4 Sept. 1990.
25 Ibid., 3 Oct. 1989.
26 Findley, *Writing Home*, 67.
27 "Minutes," Medical Board of the Queen Elizabeth Hospital of Montreal, 3 Apr. 1990.
28 Ibid., 8 Jan. and 5 Feb. 1991.
29 Ibid., 4 Jun. and 5 Nov. 1991.
30 Ibid., 3 Dec. 1991, 7 Jan. and 4 Feb. 1992.

31 Ibid., 20 Jan. and letter, 2 Feb. 2, 1993.
32 Ibid., 5 Mar. 1991.
33 Ibid., 2 Apr. 1991.
34 Ibid., 2 Nov. 1992.
35 Ibid., 7 Mar. and 5 May 1992.
36 Ibid., 1 June 1993.
37 Ibid., 7 Mar. 1995; See also Canadian Institute for Health Information stats on hospital stays, www.cihi.ca.
38 Ibid., 12 Apr. and 6 Dec. 1994.
39 Ibid., 7 Feb. 1995.
40 Ibid., 2 May 1995.
41 Ibid., 6 June 1995.
42 Adolph and Sutherland, "Fighting for survival."
43 Robinson, "Planned Hospitals Closing Leave Loyal Volunteers Feeling Betrayed."
44 Curran, "Queen E's Backers Haven't Forgotten That David Beat Goliath."
45 Hamilton and Riga, "Planners Say Glut of Hospitals Means Some Must Close."
46 "Minutes," Medical Board of the Queen Elizabeth Hospital of Montreal, 18 July 1995.
47 Ibid.
48 Cellini and Katz, "Hundreds rally to save hospitals; showdowns, cuts done in a 'savage way,' radiologist."
49 "Minutes," Medical Board of the Queen Elizabeth Hospital of Montreal, 5 Sept. 1995.
50 Katz, "Toronto Firm Recruiting MDS from Doomed Hospitals."
51 "Minutes," Medical Board of the Queen Elizabeth Hospital of Montreal, 5 Sept. 1995.
52 Ibid., 10 Oct. 1995.
53 Ibid., 9 Jan. 1996.
54 Ibid.
55 Ibid., 7 May 1996.
56 Ibid.
57 Levy, Letter to the Editor, *The Monitor.*
58 Abley, Letter to the Editor, *The Montreal Gazette,* 31 May 1995.
59 Taft and Steward, *Clear Answers: The Economics and Politics of For-Profit Medicine,* 44.
60 Ibid., 38–9.
61 Robinson, "Planned Hospitals Closing Leave Loyal Volunteers Feeling Betrayed."

62 Article on the World Socialist website, www.wsws.org, "Tories Oust Liberals in Nova Scotia election," 29 July 1999. Accessed April 2006.

63 Curran, "Queen E's Backers Haven't Forgotten that David Beat Goliath."

64 HEN, "What Are the Lessons Learnt by Countries That Have Had Dramatic Reductions of Their Hospital Bed Capacity?"

65 May and Weinman, "Wrong Medicine; Technocratic Vision, Not Reality, Is Behind Closures."

66 Hamilton, "Many Ask, 'Who'll Take Care of Us?' Health-care Goes under the Knife."

67 Derfel, "The super-hospital ... will it really offer better service?" See also Taft and Steward, *Clear Answers: The Economics and Politics of For-Profit Medicine*, 38.

68 Taft and Steward, *Clear Answers: The Economics and Politics of For-Profit Medicine*, xx.

69 *Hospital Trends in Canada 2005*, from the Canadian Institute for Health Information website, http://secure.cihi.ca/cihiweb/dispPage.jsp?cw_page= PG_374_E&cw_topic=374&cw_rel=AR_1215_E.s emphasis.] Accessed March 2006. [Author's emphasis]

70 Ibid.

71 Ibid., 2 [author's emphasis].

72 See "Trends in Hospital Beds" 1976–2002, Fig 1, 3; "Response Rates," Fig 2, 4; "Admissions," Fig3, 6; "Separations and Admissions," Fig 4, 6; "Hospital Beds Staffed and in Operation," Fig 7, 9 in *Hospital Trends in Canada 2005*, from the Canadian Institute for Health Information website, http://secure.cihi.ca/cihiweb/dispPage.jsp?cw_page=PG_374_E&cw_topic= 374&cw_rel=AR_1215_E, accessed on 14 March 2006.

73 Ibid., 2–3.

74 HEN, "What Are the Lessons Learnt by Countries that Have Had Dramatic Reductions of Their Hospital Bed Capacity?

75 Ibid.

76 Ibid.

77 Ibid.

78 Ibid.

79 Roos and Shapiro, "Using the Information System to Assess Change: The Impact of Downsizing the Acute Sector." 1995, 33, 12: DS109–126, as quoted on the WHO European Regional Office website, www.euro.who.int/HEN/ Syntheses/20030820_1 [author's italics].

80 Bagust, Place, and Posnet, "Dynamics of Bed Use in Accommodating Emergency Admissions: Stochastic Simulation Model" [author's emphasis].

81 Beech and Larkinson, "Estimating the Financial Savings from Maintaining the Level of Acute Services with Fewer Hospital Beds," [author's emphasis].

82 Shepard, "Estimating the Effect of Hospital Closure on Area Wide Inpatient Hospital Costs: A Preliminary Model and application." See also Shanahan, Bownell, and Roos, "The Unintended and Unexpected Impact of Downsizing: Costly Hospitals Become More Costly" and Zwanziger et al. "Comparison of Hospital Cost in California, New York, and Canada."

83 Liu L. et al., "Impact of rural hospital closures in Saskatchewan, Canada." [author's emphasis].

84 Reiff, DesHarnais, and Bernard. "Community Perceptions of the Effects of Rural Hospital Closure on Access to Care." 15:202–209.

85 Ibid.; See also: McKay, and Coventry, "Access Implications of Rural Hospital Closures and Conversions." See also: Hart, Pirani, and Rosenblatt. "Causes and Consequences of Rural Small Hospital Closures from the Perspectives of Mayors."

86 Interview with a public health employee [name withheld by request], 2005.

87 The Canadian Institute for Health Information Report 6, as on their website: www.cihi.ca.

88 Findley. *Writing Home*, 67.

89 Korten, *The Post-Corporate World*, 43, 56–7. See also Karlinger, *The Corporate Planet*, 23, 43, and especially Cavanagh et al., *Alternatives to Economic Globalization*, 37–43.

90 See Mander et al., *The Case Against Globalization*, 82–3, 89, 292–3, 301; and Chossudovsky, *The Globalization of Poverty*, 111–15, 117–20. Suzuki and Dressel, *From Naked Ape to Super-species*, 262–4.

91 Article IV, Statement of the Fund Mission, Ottawa, 7 Dec. 1995. Obtained by the Halifax Initiative under the Access to information Act, 30 Sept. 1999. www.halifaxinitiative.org

92 Ibid.

93 Statement by the Fund Mission to the Minster of Finance, 9 Dec. 1994, 12 [author's emphasis].

94 Ibid., 15.

95 Ibid., 16, 17.

96 Ibid.

97 O'Connor, "*Report of the Walkerton Inquiry, The Events of May 2000 and Related Issues.*" See especially sections 10.4 and 10.5, "The Move to Privatization in 1995–96" and "Concerns About the Lack of Notification Before, During and After Privatization," 374–88.

98 Dinner at the Queen Elizabeth Hotel in Montreal, December 2004, reported by Dr John Hughes.

99 From "The Future of Medicare," one of Douglas' last speeches, as found on www.healthcoaltion.ca/tommy.html, accessed 24 January 2007.

100 Taft and Steward, *Clear Answers: The Economics and Politics of For-Profit Medicine*, 2.

101 Ibid., 3.

102 Gratzer, *Code Blue*, 118, 137.

103 Cassel, *Medicare Matters*, 8.

104 Gratzer, *Code Blue*. 118, 137.

105 Taft and Steward, *Clear Answers: The Economics and Politics of For-Profit Medicine*, 7.

106 Gratzer, *Code Blue*, 171–3.

107 Cassel, *Medicare Matters*, 7.

108 Ibid.

109 Ibid.

110 Taft and Steward, *Clear Answers: The Economics and Politics of For-Profit Medicine*, 8–9.

111 Ibid., 11.

112 Woolhandler and Himmelstein. "Costs of Care and Administration at For-Profit Hospitals in the United States." See also Relman, "What Market Values Are Doing to Medicine," 99–106.

113 Silverman, Skinner, and Fisher, "The Association Between For-Profit Hospital Ownership and Increased Medicare Spending."

114 Consumers' Association of Canada (Alberta Branch) "Patient Charges for 'Enhanced' Cataract Lens," and "Waiting Times for Publicly Insured Cataract Surgery." See also Consumers' Association of Canada, "Provincial Consumer Survey on Access to Cataract Surgery Casts Doubt on Claims by Private Health Interests." See also Taft and Stewart, *Clear Answers: The Economics and Politics of For-Profit Medicine*, 14.

115 Himmelstein et al., "Quality of Care in Investor-Owned vs. Not-for-Profit HMOs," 162–3.

116 William Hsiao, "Medical Savings Accounts."

117 See also Elizabeth Warren et al, in *Norton's Bakruptcy Advisor*, May 2000, http://papers.ssrn.com/sol3/paper.cfm?abstract _id=224581, accessed 27 July 2007. See also Zeldin, "Health Debtor Accounts."

118 Glennester, "Internal Markets: Context and Structure."

119 *The Economist*, "Grappling with Deficits." Also available at www.liberty-page.com/issues/healthcare/ukdeficit.html.

120 Zelder, "Take a Queue from Canada!" 9–10.

121 Shaker, "Public-Private Partnerships Would Open a Trade Treaty Door That Might Prove Impossible to Close."

122 Barlow, "Tipping Point on Public Health? – Creeping Privatization Threatens to Trigger NAFTA Lawsuits," [author's emphasis].

123 Barlow, *Profit Is Not the Cure*, 196.

124 Ibid.

125 "2001 *Annual Report* of the CIHI," as cited in Barlow, *Profit Is Not the Cure,* 198. See also, under year, www.cihi.ca.

126 Gibson "Goodbye, Europe. Hello, USA."

127 Guyatt, "Beware P3 Hospitals: It's a Matter of Accounting."

128 Pollock, "How Private Finance Is Moving Primary Care into Corporate Ownership."

129 Guyatt, "Beware P3 Hospitals: It's a Matter of Accounting," and "For-profit hospitals: A government giveaway."

130 Ibid.

CHAPTER SIX

1 Official Eli Lilly site for the anti-depressant Cymbalta, www.cymbalta.com, accessed 13 July 2007.

2 U.S. government website on Ritalin, www.nida.nih.gov/Infofacts/ Ritalin.html, accessed 13 July 2007.

3 Garrett, *Betrayal of Trust,* 572 [author's emphasis].

4 For ranking of drug companies by income, see: en.wikipedia.org/wiki/ list_of_pharmaceutical_companies [author's emphasis].

5 Hsiao, "Medical Savings Accounts."

6 Washburn, *University, Inc.: The Corporate Corruption of Higher Education,* 122.

7 Ibid., 120.

8 Ibid., 121.

9 Ibid.

10 Ibid., 121–2. See also Relman, "What Market Values Are Doing to Medicine" and Taft and Stewart, *Clear Answers: The Economics and Politics of For-Profit Medicine.* 76–84.

11 Washburn, *University, Inc.: The Corporate Corruption of Higher Education,* 122–3. See also Keung, "MD Settles Lawsuit with U of T over Job," A23, and Healy, "Conflicting Interests in Toronto: Anatomy of a Controversy at the Interface of Academia and Industry."

12 Washburn, *University, Inc.: The Corporate Corruption of Higher Education,* 123. See a full review of this case by Thompson, Baird, et al., *The Oliveri Report: The Complete Text of the Report of the Independent Inquiry Commissioned by the Canadian Association of University Teachers.*

13 Washburn, *University, Inc.: The Corporate Corruption of Higher Education,* 123–4. See also Phillips and Hoey, "Constraints of Interest: Lessons at the Hospital for Sick Children," 955–957 and Shuchman, "Legal Issues Surrounding Privately Funded Research Cause Furore in Toronto."

14 For details of a scandal that rocked the Canadian medical establishment and has largely destroyed the reputation of one of the world's most prestigious

medical journals, see Hooey, "The editorial autonomy of CMAJ," Branswell, "The Lancet Calls CMAJ Firings 'Deeply Troubling,'" 2 March 2006, and for the full chronology, "The CMAJ Firings: Crisis at Canada's Most Influential Medical Journal, www.tribemagazine.com/board/showthread.php?t=113033.

15 Deverell, "U of T Appeals to Ottawa to Help Generic Drug Firms."

16 Washburn, *University, Inc.: The Corporate Corruption of Higher Education*, 123.

17 Ibid., 116–7.

18 Ibid., 112–14.

19 Ibid.

20 Ibid., 134; also Kong and Bass, "Case at Brown Leads to Review; NIMH Studies Tighter Rules on Conflicts."

21 Washburn, *University, Inc.: The Corporate Corruption of Higher Education*, 114–15. See also Keller, ISI author publication A03902003-H at http//:hcr3.isiknowledge.com.

22 Washburn, *University, Inc.: The Corporate Corruption of Higher Education*, 112–13.

23 Eichenwald and Kolata, "A Doctor's Drug Trials Turn into Fraud," A1. See also Larkin, "Clinical Trials: What Price Progress?" 1534.

24 Washburn, *University, Inc.: The Corporate Corruption of Higher Education*, 116, note 50. See also Mundy, *Dispensing with the Truth*, 164.

25 Washburn, *University, Inc.: The Corporate Corruption of Higher Education*, 128, n106. Note that 70 percent of total grant spending in 2002 on clinical trials involving humans in the U.S. was paid for by the biopharmaceutical industry and according to Getz, "Clinical Grants Market Decelerates," "If device manufacturers are included, the total fraction of grant support rises to 80 percent, with the remainder ... supplied primarily by the National Institutes of Health." *Center Watch* 7, 11 (Nov. 2000). See www.centerwatch.com/bookstore/pubs_profs_periodicals.html.

26 CBC, "Heart of the Matter," Part 2, 29.

27 "Drugs for Money," as posted on www.tompaine.com/articles/2006/05/11/drugs_for_money.php; accessed 11 May 2006.

28 See the Canadian Health Coalition website, www.healthcoalition.ca; The Council of Canadians, especially "Putting Our Food at Risk: The Security and Prosperity Partnership Is Lowering Food Standards in Canada." www.canadians.org/integratethis/backgrounder/food, html; Transition= Abdication, A Citizen's Guide to the Health Protection branch Transition Consultations," Sept 1998; www.healthcoaltion.ca/abdication.html#Anchor-Table–59724; and also "Missing Information and Secret Tabling," "Keeping Parliament and Canadians in the Dark," "Quebec Dodges Health Canada," at www.healthcoalition.ca/wheresthemoney.html.

29 Harold Griffith, "Some Reminiscences."

30 Bueckert, "Scientist Gets Congratulatory Letter from Health Canada after Being Fired," as posted on www.healthcoalition.org.

31 Caplan, "Indicting Big Pharma."

32 Ibid.

33 Canadian Health Coalition, "Transition = Abdication – A Citizen's Guide to the Health Protection branch Transition Consultations," Sept 1998. See also "Missing Information and Secret Tabling," "Keeping Parliament and Canadians in the Dark," "Quebec Dodges Health Canada," at www.healthcoalition.ca/wheresthemoney.html; accessed 25 May 2007.

34 Canadian Health Coalition website, www.healthcoalition.ca and the Council of Canadians, especially "Putting Our Food at Risk: The Security and Prosperity Partnership is Lowering Food Standards in Canada. www.canadians. org/integratethis/backgrounder/food. html; accessed 12 June 2007.

35 Common Dreams website, "Stripping Away Big Pharma's Figleaf," posted on June 13, 2002, www.commondreams.org/views/02/0613–07.htm; accessed 7 July, 2007.

36 Angell, "The Truth about the Drug Companies," www.nybooks.com/articles/ 17244; accessed 10 Aug 2005.

37 Angell. *The Truth about the Drug Companies.*

38 Ibid.

39 McKinnell, *"A Call To Action: Taking Back Healthcare for Future Generations,"* 46.

40 See www.pharmopoly.org/blog/2005/07/mea-culpa-by-big-pharma-ceo. html, accessed on 15 Jan 2006.

41 Levine, "Eli Lilly, Zyprexa & the Bush Family."

42 See p. 335 for a list of current attacks on the pharmacology industry by doctors and other medical insiders.

43 Cassel, *Medicare Matters,* 148.

44 Caplan, "Indicting Big Pharma."

45 Ibid.

46 Wazana, "Physicians and the Pharmaceutical Industry: Is a Gift Ever Just a Gift?" [author's emphasis].

47 Caplan, "Indicting Big Pharma."

48 McBane, "Ill-Health Canada," as posted on www.healthcoalition.ca. See also "Smart Regulation Puts Profit before Health," Canadian Health Coalition Media Release, 29 March 2005, as posted on www.medicare.ca and www.healthcoaltion.ca/102.pdf+Ill+Health.

49 CBC, "Heart of the Matter, Part #1."

50 Ibid. See also Ravnskov, "High cholesterol may protect against infections and atherosclerosis," and Jacobs et.al, "Report of the conference on low blood cholesterol: mortality associations."

51 Ibid.

52 Ibid.

53 Ibid.

54 Ibid. See also Mozaffarian, Rimm, and Harrington, "Dietary Fats, Carbo-hydrates, and Progression of Coronary Atherosclosis in Postmenopausal Women."

55 CBC. Ibid., Parts #1 and 2.

56 Ibid., Part 2" [author's emphasis]. See also Abramson, *Overdosed America: The Broken Promise of American Medicine.*

57 CBC, "Heart of the Matter, Part 2."

58 Ibid., [author's emphasis].

59 Ibid.

60 Ibid.

61 "On a per person basis, the U.S. has three times as many ... lithotripsy units (which destroy kindney stones and gallstones) according to the National Center for Policy Analysis: A Leader in Providing Private Alternatives to Government Programs. See also Trautwein, "A Look at Single Payer Systems Around the World," as posted on www.niahu.org/laws/legislative_analysis/single_ payer_systems.pdf .

62 Heptinstall, *Pathology of the Kidney*, 1592. See also *Nephron*, 63, no. 2 (1993): 242–3; *Journal of Endourology*, 8, no. 1 (1994): 15–19; *Journal of Urology*, 150, no. 6 (1993): 1765–7; and McTaggart, *What Doctors Don't Tell You*, 322–5.

63 CBC, "Heart of the Matter, Part 2."

64 Ibid., Part 3."

65 Priest, "A Boy's Plight, A Nation's Problem."

66 Priest, "His Cancer Couldn't Wait, Panel Rules." See also Fekete, "Need Surgery? Here's How Long You'll Wait."

67 Canadian Health Coalition website, "Missing Information and Secret Tabling," "Keeping Parliament and Canadians in the Dark," and "Quebec Dodges Health Canada," as posted on www.healthcoaltion.ca; accessed 15 Sept. 2006.

68 Ibid. [author's emphasis].

69 Chua, "Waiting Lists in Canada." See also Sanmartin et al., "Waiting for Medical Services in Canada." The Canadian debate about access to care, and waiting lists in particular, is characterized by disturbing chasms between widely held views and evidence from research.

70 McDonald et al. "Waiting Lists and Waiting Times for Health Care in Canada: More Management!! More Money?"

71 Ibid.

72 Chua, "Waiting Lists in Canada: Reality or Hype?," 4.

73 Ibid.

74 Blendon et al. "Common Concerns Amid Diverse Systems: Health Care Experiences in Five Countries." 19–31, [author's emphasis].

75 see www.Canadians.org/DI/issues/guide/healthcare.html; accessed 15 June 2006.

76 see www.canadians.org/DI/issues/TILMA/index.html; accessed 15 June 2006.

77 Ibid. [author's emphasis].

78 Ministry of Employment and Solidarity, High Committee on Public Health. *Health in France 2002,* 27.

79 Ibid., 146 and 151 [author's emphasis].

80 Kulik, GRAIN "Fowl play: The poultry industry's central role in the bird flu crisis." See also "Avian influenza goes global, but don't blame the birds," *The Lancet Infectious Diseases,* 6 (2006): 185 and "Where's the Bird Flu Pandemic?" ISIS Press Release 11/05/06; www.i-sis.org.uk; etc.

81 Personal interview, July, 2005 Hopital Publique Bichat, Paris.

CHAPTER SEVEN

1 Griffith, H.R "Medical Superintendent's Report," Annual Report of the Homeopathic Hospital of Montreal, 1955, 21.

2 Griffith, H.R. "Medical Superintendent's Report," Annual Report of the Queen Elizabeth Hospital, 1954, 26–7.

3 HEN, Annex 1, "Defining Primary and Specialist Care," as found in "What Are the Advantages and Disadvantages of Restructuring a Health Care System to Be More Focused on Primary Care Services?" 16–17; see also Orton. "Shared Care."

4 Fyke, *Evaluating Solutions and Building Consensus: A Roundtable of Health Care Reform Commissions,* 2.

5 May and Weinman, "Wrong Medicine; Technocratic Vision, Not Reality, Is Behind Closures."

6 HEN, "What Are the Advantages and Disadvantages of Restructuring a Health Care System to Be More Focused on Primary Care Services?", 1 and 10 [author's emphasis].

7 Nelson, "Bad Practice: How Developing Nations Are Suffering from Canada's Band-Aid Solutions to Our Own Doctor Shortage," 17–19.

8 Shi, "The Relationship between Primary Care and Life Chances"; Shea et al. "Predisposing Factors for Severe, Uncontrolled Hypertension"; Schroeder and Sandy. "Specialty Distribution of US Physicians"; Mark et al. "Medicare costs in urban areas and the supply of primary care physicians"; Moore. "The Case of the Disappearing Generalist"; Franks, Cloancy, and Nutting. "Gate-keeping revisited" [author's emphasis].

9 HEN, "What Are the Advantages and Disadvantages of Restructuring a Health Care System to Be More Focused on Primary Care Services?" 7, 18.

10 Ibid., 9 [author's emphasis]; see also Gervas, Fernadez, and Starfield. "Primary Care, Financing and Gate-keeping in Western Europe"; Delnoji et al. "Does General Practitioner Gate-keeping Curb Health Expenditure?"

11 HEN, Annex 1, "Defining Primary and Specialist Care," as found in ibid., 16–17; see also Orton, "Shared Care"; Hughes and Gordon. *Hospitals and Primary Care*; Avery and Pringle. "Emergency Care in General Practice."

12 Speigel and Yassi, "Lessons from the Margins of Globalization: Appreciating the Cuban Health Paradox"; see also Gallup, consultoria Interdisciplinaria en Desarrollo, "Cubans Show Little Satisfaction with Opportunities and Individual Freedom Rare, Independent Survey Finds Large Majorities Are Still Proud of Island's Health Care and Education."

13 Speigel and Yassi, "Lessons from the Margins of Globalization" [author's emphasis].

14 DePalma. "Sicko, Castro and the '120 Years Club.'"

15 U.S. government, CIA website, cited on: www.cia.gov/cia/publications/factbook/rankorder/209/rank.html, accessed on 14 June 2007.

16 Banks, Marmot, et al., "Disease and Disadvantage in the United States and England"; see Table 1, Prevalence of diabetes among high-income Americans (8.2 per thousand) and low-income Britons (7.3).

17 For this information and much of what follows, unless otherwise indicated, see Dresang, Brebrick, Murry, Shallue, and Sullivan-Vedder "Family Medicine in Cuba: Community-Oriented Primary Care and Complementary and Alternative Medicine," 10.

18 Reed. "Challenges for Cuba's Family Doctor-and-Nurse Program."

19 Ibid.

20 Ibid.

21 Private interviews with public health care employees and researchers; names withheld by request. 2005–06.

22 Chaplowe, "Havana's Popular Gardens: Sustainable Urban Agriculture;" see also www.foodfirst.org/cuba; and www.cityfarmer.org/cuba, accessed on 17 May 2007.

23 Reed. "Challenges for Cuba's Family Doctor-and-Nurse Program."

24 U.S. government National Health Institutes website on CAM; also the Canadian Institute of National and Integrative Medicine website, www.cinim.org.

25 Interview with Adam Gavsie, 25 February 2006.

26 American College of Physicians. "The Impending Collapse of Primary Care Medicine and Its Implications for the State of the Nation's Health Care."

27 Ibid.

28 Ibid.

29 Canadian Institute of Health Information website.

30 American College of Physicians. "The Impending Collapse of Primary Care Medicine and Its Implications for the State of the Nation's Health Care."

31 Ibid. See also the international studies mentioned previously and for the U.S., Nelson, Zubkoff, Manning, Rogers, Kravitzl et al. "Variations in Resource Utilization among Medical Specialties and Systems of Care"; Parchman and Culler. "Primary Care Physicians and Avoidable Hospitalizations."

32 Bindman A.B. et al. "Preventable Hospitalizations and Access to Health Care."

33 American College of Physicians. "The Impending Collapse of Primary Care Medicine and Its Implications for the State of the Nation's Health Care" [author's emphasis].

34 Ibid., 14 [author's emphasis].

35 Green and Nguyen, "Strategies for Cutting Hospital Beds: The Impact on Patient Service," 439.

36 Ibid., 421.

37 Conference Transcripts, "Beyond the Water's Edge: European Comparisons," 1–5. See www.misc-iecm.mcgill.ca/HCC/hlthpub.htm.

38 Figures cited are from OECD, 2005, available at www.nchc.org.

39 HEN, Annex 1, "Defining Primary and Specialist Care," as found in "What Are the Advantages and Disadvantages of Restructuring a Health Care System to Be More Focused on Primary Care Services?" 16–17

40 HEN, Diagnostics and Solutions; Building Consensus for Health care Reform in Canada, 2002/02/14–16, as found in ibid., 1–2, and also at www.misc-iecm.mcgill.ca/HCC/hlthpub.htm.

41 Pollock, "How Private Finance Is Moving Primary Care into Corporate Ownership." See also Guyatt "Beware P3 hospitals: It's a Matter of Accounting," and "For-profit Hospitals a Government Giveaway."

42 The San Diego Union Tribune, "Doctor Lets Patient Die, Is Rewarded with Raise."

43 Peeno, "Managed Care Ethics: The Close View Prepared for U.S. House of Representatives Committee on Commerce, Subcommittee of Health and Environment."

44 See www.uow.edu.au/arts/sts/bmartin/dissent/documents/health/quotes.html

45 Creuss in Evaluating Solutions and Building Consensus: A Roundtable of Health Care Reform Commissions.

46 Ibid., 2.

47 Griffith, Harold. "Medical Superintendent's Report," Annual Report of the Homeopathic Hospital of Montreal,1955, 22.

48 Ibid., 21.

49 *What Doctors Don't Tell You* 13, no. 9 (2003): 7.

50 Griffith, H.R. Lay sermon, private papers, ca. 1960.

51 Many gene therapy subjects have died horribly, and many "once high-flying" gene therapists have found their research severely restricted by the FDA. For an overview of the many issues, see Thompson, "Human Gene Therapy, Harsh Lessons, High Hopes." [author's emphasis].

52 Griffith, H.R., "Retirement Speech, 1964, in private papers [author's emphasis].

53 *Harrisons; Principles of Internal Medicine.*

Bibliography

Abley, Mark. Letter to the Editor. *The Montreal Gazette,* 31 May 1995.

Abramson, John. *Overdosed America: The Broken Promise of American Medicine.* New York: Harper Collins, 2004.

Adolph, Caroline, and Anne Sutherland. "Fighting for Survival." *The Montreal Gazette,* 11 May 1995.

Altmayer, Chris A., et.al. "Geographical Disparity in Premature Mortality in Ontario, 1992–1996." *International Journal of Health Geographics.* Posted on pubmedcentral.nih.gov/articlerender.fcgi?artid=222916.

Amdur, Reuel. "Defending Medicare." *Straight Goods,* 19 April 2006.

American College of Physicians, "The Impending Collapse of Primary Care Medicine and Its Implications for the State of the Nation's Health Care." Posted on http:www.acponline.org/hpp/statehco6_1.pdf. Accessed 14 March 2006.

Angell, Marcia. *The Truth About the Drug Companies.* New York: Random House, 2004.

– "The Truth about the Drug Companies." *The New York Review of Books* 51, no. 12 (15 July 2004).

Atkinson, R.S., and T.B. Boulton, eds. *The History of Anesthesia.* London, New York: Royal Society of Medicine Services and The Parthenon Publishing Group, 1989.

Avery A., and M. Pringle. "Emergency Care in General Practice." *British Medical Journal* 310 (1995): 6.

Bagust A., M. Place, and J.W. Posnet. "Dynamics of Bed Use in Accommodating Emergency Admissions: Stochastic Simulation Model." *British Medical Journal* 319 (1999): 155–8.

Banks, James, Michael Marmot, et al., "Disease and Disadvantage in the United States and England." *Journal of the American Medical Association* 295 (2006): 2037–45.

Barlow, Maude. "Tipping Point on Public Health: Creeping Privatization Threatens to Trigger NAFTA Lawsuits." *Straight Goods*, 4 November 2005. Posted on www/straightgoods/ca/ViewFeature5.cfmposted04Nov.05 or list.web.ca/archives/straight-good_l/2005-November/00302.html.

– *Profit Is Not the Cure* Toronto. McClelland and Stewart, 2002.

Beech, R., and J. Larkinson. "Estimating the Financial Savings from Maintaining the Level of Acute Services with Fewer Hospital Beds." *International Journal of Health Planning and Management* 5 (1990): 89–103.

Bennett, Abram Elting. Letter to Squibb & Sons, as cited in "The History of the Introduction of Curare into Medicine." *Anaesthesia and Analgesia ... Current Researches* 47, no. 5 (Sept-Oct., 1968).

Berton, Pierre. *The Invasion of Canada.* Toronto: McClelland and Stewart, 1980.

Bindman, A.B. et al. "Preventable Hospitalizations and Access to Health Care." *Journal of the American Medical Association* 274 (1995): 305–11.

Blendon, Robert J. et al. "Common Concerns amid Diverse Systems: Health Care Experiences in Five Countries." *Health Affairs* (May/June 2003).

Board of Directors, Homeopathic Hospital of Montreal. "Annual Reports." Available at the Queen Elizabeth Archives, McGill University.

– Homeopathic Hospital of Montreal. "Minutes." Available at the Queen Elizabeth Archives, McGill University.

– Queen Elizabeth Hospital of Montreal. "Annual Reports." Available at the Queen Elizabeth Archives, McGill University.

– Queen Elizabeth Hospital of Montreal. "Minutes." Available at the Queen Elizabeth Archives, McGill University.

Bodman, Richard, and Dierdre Gillies. *Harold Griffith, The Evolution of Modern Anaesthesia.* Toronto: Dundurn Press, 1992.

Boychuk, Terry. *The Making and Meaning of Hospital Policy in the United States and Canada.* Ann Arbor, Michigan: University of Michigan Press, 1999.

Branswell, Helen. "The Lancet Calls CMAJ Firings 'Deeply Troubling.'" 2 March 2006. Posted on cnews.canoe.ca/CNEWS/MediaNews/2006/03/02/pf-1470179.html.

Bueckert, Dennis. "Scientist Gets Congratulatory Letter from Health Canada after Being Fired." 4 August 2004. Posted on www.healthcoalition.org. Accessed 12 June 2007.

Canadian Auto Workers Union. "Campaigns & Issues, Conservative Government Record on Health Care." Posted on www.caw.ca/campaigns&issues/pastcampaigns/elections1999. Accessed 10 June 2006.

CBC. "The Heart of the Matter." Three-hour radio series for the on-going program Ideas, first broadcast 7, 14, and 21 June 2005, produced by Jill Eisen.

Canadian Health Coalition. "Transition = Abdication – A Citizen's Guide to the Health Protection Branch Transition Consultations." Sept 1998. Posted on www.healthcoaltion.ca/abdication.html#Anchor-Table–59724. Accessed 6 May 2007.

– "Missing Information and Secret Tabling." posted on www.healthcoaltion.ca/wheresthemoney.html. Accessed 25 May 2007.

– "Keeping Parliament and Canadians in the Dark." posted on www.healthcoalition.ca/wheresthemone.html. Accessed 25 May 2007.

– "Quebec Dodges Health Canada." posted on www.healthcoalition.ca/wheresthemone.html. Accessed 25 May 2007.

Canadian Institute for Health Information (a division of Statistics Canada). *Hospital Trends in Canada: Results of a Project to Create a Historical Series of Statistical and Financial Data for Canadian Hospitals over Twenty-seven Years.* Accessible at http://secure.cihi.ca/cihiweb/ dispPage.isp.cw.page=media_11jan2006. Accessed 16 April 2007.

Canadian Institute of National and Integrative Medicine. www.cinim.org. Accessed on 17 May 2007.

Caplan, Arthur. "Indicting Big Pharma." American Scientist Online, January-February, 2005. Posted on www.americanscientis.org/template/ BookReviewTypeDetail. Accessed 10 May 2006.

Cassel, Christine. *Medicare Matters: What Geriatric Medicine Can Teach American Health Care.* Berkeley: University of California Press, 2005.

Cavanagh, John, et al. *Alternatives to Globalization.* San Francisco: Berrett-Koehler, 2002.

Cellini, Adelia, and Helena Katz. "Hundreds Rally to Save Hospitals; Showdowns, Cuts Done in a 'Savage Way,' Radiologist." *The Montreal Gazette,* 26 May 1995.

Chambers, Greta. "It's a Mistake to Close Hospitals with Proven Record of Care." Editorial page, *The Montreal Gazette,* 27 May 1995.

Chandrakant P. Shah. *Public Health and Preventative Medicine in Canada.* Toronto: Elesvier Canada, 2003.

Chapin, Amy, Ana Rule, et.al. "Airborne Multi-drug Resistant Bacteria Isolated from a Contaminated Swine Feeding Operation." Johns Hopkins Bloomberg School of Public Health Online, 22 Nov. 2004. Posted on http://dx.doi.org/.

Chaplowe, Scott G. "Havana's Popular Gardens: Sustainable Urban Agriculture." *WSAA Newsletter* 5, no.22 (Fall, 1996).

Chossudovsky, Michel. *The Globalization of Poverty*. Penang: Third World Network, 1997.

Chua, Kao-Ping, "Waiting Lists in Canada: Reality or Hype?" 22 Aug. 2005; available at: http://www.amsa.org/studytours/WaitingTimes_primer.pdf

Conor, Harry. *A Trip to Chinatown*. (A Musical), 1892.

Consumers Association of Canada (Alberta Branch). "Patient Charges for 'Enhanced' Cataract Lens," and "Waiting Times for Publicly Insured Cataract Surgery," *Information Bulletin*. May, 1999.

– "Provincial Consumer Survey on Acces to Cataract Surgery Casts Doubt on Claims by Private Health Interests." Press Release and Backgrounder, March 1999.

Copp, Terry. *The Anatomy of Poverty: The Condition of the Working Class in Montreal, 1897–1929*. Toronto: McClelland and Stewart, 1974.

Cruess, Barbara. "Evaluating Solutions and Building Consensus: A Roundtable of Health Care Reform Commissions." Transcripts of the 7th Annual Conference, available from the McGill Institute for the Study of Canada, www.arts.mcgill.ca/program/misc/ and at www.misc-iecm. mcgill.ca/HCC/hlthpub.htm.

Curran, Peggy. "Don't Tell Mrs. Taylor That Cutbacks Won't Hurt." *The Montreal Gazette*, 9 June 1995.

– "Something Alarming about the Scope of Hospital Cuts." *The Montreal Gazette*, 11 May 1995.

– "Queen E's Backers Haven't Forgotten That David Beat Goliath." *The Montreal Gazette*, 2 Sept. 1995.

D'Aliesio, Renata, and Hanneke Brooymans. "Alberta Rivers Flood with Pollutants: Report." *Calgary Herald* and *The Edmonton Journal*, 19 July 2007.

Darier, Eric. "Algues blues: Greenpeace accuse l'industrie agricole." *Le Devoir*, 25 July 2007.

Delnoji, D., et al. "Does General Practitioner Gate-keeping Curb Health Expenditure? *Journal of Health Services Research and Policy* 5 (2000): 22–6.

DePalma, Anthony. "Sicko, Castro and the '120 Years Club.'" *The New York Times*, 27 May 2007. Posted on www.nytimes.com/2007/05/27.

Derfel, Aaron. "Is Our Health System Failing?" *The Montreal Gazette*, 13 January 2007.

– "The Super-hospital …Will It Really Offer Better Service?" *The Montreal Gazette*, 19 February 2000.

Devereaux, P.J., et al. "A Systematic Review and Meta-Analysis of Studies Comparing Mortality between Private For-Profit and Private Not-For-Profit Hospitals." *Clinical Epidemiology and Biostatistics* (May, 2002).

Deverell, John. "U of T Appeals to Ottawa to Help Generic Drug Firms." *Toronto Star*, 4 September 1999.

Dodd, Leeder, Ringen, Sawyer, Harris, and Boyd. "Public Patients, Private Profit." Posted on www.abc.net.au/rn/talks/bbing/stories/s10626.htm.

Dranove, David. *The Economic Evolution of American Health Care: From Marcus Welby to Managed Care.* Princeton, NJ: Princeton University Press, 2000.

Dresang, Lee T., Laurie Brebrick, Danielle Murray, Ann Shallue, and Lisa Sullivan-Vedder. "Family Medicine in Cuba: Community-Oriented Primary Care and Complementary and Alternative Medicine." *The Journal of the American Board of Family Practice* (2005). Posted on www.fabfm.org/cgi/content/full/a8/4/297.

Dressel, Holly. "Has Canada Got the Cure?" *Yes! Magazine* (Fall 2006): 24–8.

Duffe, John. "Diary." Ms. Div., New York Historical Society, 24 March and 12 June 1844.

Duncan, Barbara M. "A Quick Look at the First London Etherists." In Atkinson and Boulton, *The History of Anesthesia.*

Dunnigan, Matthew G., and Allyson M. Pollock. "Downsizing of Acute Inpatient Beds Associated with Private Finance Initiative: Scotland's Case Study." University College London. Posted on http://bmj.bmjjournals.com/ cgi/content/abridged/326/7395/905,

Economist. "Grappling with Deficits," 11 March 2006.

Eichenwald, Kurt, and Gina Kolata. "A Doctor's Drug Trials Turn into Fraud." *New York Times*, 17 May 1999.

Eisler, Dale. "An Unprecedented Hospital Closing in Calgary." *Maclean's*, 28 April 1997.

Fekete, Jason. "Need Surgery? Here's How Long You'll Wait." *Calgary Harold*, 28 July 2004.

Findley, Timothy, In Constance Rooke, *Writing Home.* Toronto: McClelland and Stewart, 1997.

Franks P, C.M. Cloancy, P.A. Nutting. "Gate-keeping Revisited: Protecting Patients from Over-treatment." *New England Journal of Medicine* 328 (1993): 621–7.

Fyke, Ken. "Evaluating Solutions and Building Consensus: A Roundtable of Health Care Reform Commissions." Transcripts of the 7th Annual Conference, available from the McGill Institute for the Study of Canada, www.arts.mcgill.ca/program/misc/ and at www.misc-iecm.mcgill.ca/HCC/hlthpub.htm.

Gagan, Rosemary, and David Gagan. *For Patients of Moderate Means: A Social History of the Vountary Public General Hospital in Canada, 1890–1950.* Montreal: McGill-Queen's University Press, 2002.

Gallup/consultoria Interdisciplinaria en Desarrollo, "Cubans Show Little
    Satisfaction with Opportunities and Individual Freedom Rare,
    Independent Survey Finds Large Majorities Are Still Proud of Island's
    Health Care and Education," 10 January 2007. Posted on
    www.worldpublicopinion.org/ [pipa/articles/briatinamericara/
    300.php?nid=&id=&pnt=3—$ib-bria. Accessed 5 May 108-/
Garrett, Laurie. *Betrayal of Trust: The Collapse of Global Public Health.* New York:
    Hyperion, 2000.
Gervas, J. Fernadez, B. Perez, B. Starfield. "Primary Care, Financing and
    Gate-keeping in Western Europe." *Family Practice* 11 (1994): 307–17.
Getz, Ken. "Clinical Grants Market Decelerates." *CenterWatch* 10, no. 4
    (2003). Posted on www.center-watch.com/bookstore/ pubs_profs_
    periodical.html.
– "Grant Market to Exceed $4 Billion in 2000." *CenterWatch* 7, no. 11
    (November 2000). Posted on www.center-watch.com/bookstore/
    pubs_profs_periodical.html.
Gibson, Diana. "Goodbye, Europe. Hello, USA." Posted on the website of
    Straight Goods, www.straightgoods.ca. Accessed 6 June 2006.
Glennester, Howard. "Internal Markets: Context and Structure," as cited in
    Jerome-Forget, Monique, Joseph White, and Joshua M. Wiener, eds., *Health
    Care Reform Through Internal Markets*, 17–26. Montreal/Washington:
    The Institute for Research on Public Policy/The Brookings Institution,
    1995.
Godfrey, W.G. *A Struggle to Serve: A History of the Moncton Hospital, 1895–1953.*
    Montreal: McGill-Queen's University Press, 2004.
Green, Linda V., and Vien Nguyen. "Strategies for Cutting Hospital Beds:
    The Impact on Patient Service." Posted on the Health Services Research
    website: www.pubmedcentral.nih.gov/articlerender.fcgi?artid=1089232.
Grieshaber-Otto, Jim, and Scott Sinclair. "*Bad Medicine: Trade Treaties, Priva-
    tization and Health Care Reform in Canada.*" Posted on policyalternatives.ca/
    index.cfm?at=news&call=809&do=article&pA=BB736455.
Griffith, A. R. "Diary." Conserved in the Queen Elizabeth Hospital Archives,
    McGill University.
– "Medical Superintendent's Annual Report," 1900–1936. Available at the
    Queen Elizabeth Hospital Archives, McGill University.
– "Some Reminiscences." Conserved at the Queen Elizabeth Hospital
    Archives, McGill University.
Griffith, Harold R. *1894–1969: Seventy-five Years of Service. The Story of the
    Queen Elizabeth Hospital of Montreal.* Available at the Queen Elizabeth
    Hospital Archives, McGill University.

– "An Anaesthetist's Valediction." Available at the Queen Elizabeth Hospital Archives, McGill University.
– Annual Reports of the Homeopathic Hospital of Montreal, 1936–1974. Available at the Homeopathic Hospital Queen Elizabeth Hospital Archives, McGill University.
– "The Boundless Realm of Anaesthesiology." Available at the Queen Elizabeth Hospital Archives, McGill University.
– *The Evolution of Modern Anaesthesia.* Toronto: Dundurn Press, 1992.
– "Highlights in the Life of Harold Randall Griffith." Available at the Queen Elizabeth Hospital Archives, McGill University.
– "The Pattern of Anesthesia." Available at the Queen Elizabeth Hospital Archives, McGill University.
– Personal diary. Conserved in the Queen Elizabeth Hospital Archives, McGill University.
– "The Story of the Queen Elizabeth Hospital of Montreal." Available at the Queen Elizabeth Hospital Archives, McGill University.
Gruending, Dennis. *Emmett Hall: Establishment Radical.* Toronto: Macmillan, 1985.
Guyatt, Gordon. "Beware P3 Hospitals: It's a Matter of Accounting." *Straight Goods.* Posted on www.straghtgoods.ca. Accessed 5 May 2006.
Guyatt, Gordon. "For-profit Hospitals a Government Giveaway." *Straight Goods.* Posted on www.straghtgoods.ca. Accessed 5 May 2006.
Hamilton, Graeme. "Many Ask, 'Who'll Take Care of Us?' Health-care Goes Under the Knife." *The Montreal Gazette,* 20 May 1995.
– "Reprieve for Hospitals Seems Unlikely." *The Montreal Gazette,* 6 June 1995.
Hamilton, Graeme, and Michelle Lalonde. "Seven Local Hospitals Slated to Close, MNA says." *The Montreal Gazette,* 10 May 1995.
Hamilton, Graeme, and Andy Riga, "Planners Say Glut of Hospitals Means Some Must Close." *The Montreal Gazette,* 11 May 1995.
Hammond, S.B. "Treasurers Report." Annual Report of the Homeopathic Hospital of Montreal, 1926. Available at the Queen Elizabeth Hospital of Montreal Archives, McGill University.
Hanaway, Joseph, and Richard Creuss. *McGill Medicine, Volume I: The First Half Century.* Montreal: McGill-Queen's University Press, 1996.
Harrison's Principles of Internal Medicine. New York: McGraw-Hill, 2005.
Hart, L.G., M.F. Pirani, and R.A. Rosenblatt. "Causes and Consequences of Rural Small Hospital Closures from the Perspectives of Mayors." *Journal of Rural Health* 7 (1991): 22–45.
Healy, David. "Conflicting Interests in Toronto: Anatomy of a Controversy at the Interface of Academia and Industry." *Perspectives in Biology and Medicine* 45, no. 2 (spring 2002): 250–63.

Health Resources and Services Administration (HRSA). *Child Health USA 2003, Health Status – Infants.* Posted on www.mchb.hrsa.gov/chusa03.

Heim, Wolfgang-Hagen, ed. *Alexander von Humboldt, Life and Work.* Ingelheim am Rhein: C.H. Boehringer Sohn, 1987.

HEN (The Health Evidence Network branch of the World Health Organization Regional Office for Europe). "What Are the Lessons Learnt by Countries That Have Had Dramatic Reductions of Their Hospital Bed Capacity?" Hen Report published 29 August 2003. Posted on www.euro.who.int/HEN/Syntheses/20030820_1. Accessed 11 October 2005.

– "What Are the Advantages and Disadvantages of Restructuring a Health Care System to Be More Focused on Primary Care Services?" Posted on www.euro.who.int/HEN/Synthesis/primaryvspecialist/20040115_2. Accessed 8 July 2006.

Henman, E.A. *St. Mary's: The History of a London Teaching Hospital.* Montreal: McGill-Queen's University Press, 2003.

Heptinstall, Robert H. *Pathology of the Kidney.* Boston: Little, Brown and Company, 1992.

Himmelstein, David U., et al. "Quality of Care in Investor-Owned vs. Not-for-Profit HMOs." *Journal of the American Medical Association* 282, no. 2 (14 July 1999).

Hoffman, Fergus. "Medic Proves Poison Not Best Opiate." *The Montreal Star,* 7 October 1956. Available at the Queen Elizabeth Hospital of Montreal archives, McGill University, Harold Griffith papers.

Hooey, John. "The Editorial Autonomy of CMAJ." 21 February 2006. Posted on www.canada.com/components/print.aspx?id=1a628873–8a46–42e0-aa8e-cf12bbob264d.

Hsiao, William. "Medical Savings Accounts." *Health Affairs* 14, no. 2 (Summer 1995): 260–6.

Hughes, J., and P. Gordon. *Hospitals and Primary Care – Breaking the Boundaries.* London: King's Fund Centre, 1993.

Institute of Science in Society. "Where's the Bird Flu Pandemic?" ISIS Press Release, 11 May 2006. Posted on www.i-sis.org.uk.

Jackson, Dale. "At Debt's Door." *Trade by Numbers* 4, no. 6 (July 2007). Posted on http://magazine.globeinvestor.com.

Jacobs, D., et. al., "Report of the Conference on Low Blood Cholesterol: Mortality Associations." *Circulation* 86 (1992): 1046–60.

Jasmer, Robert. "Racial Disparity and Socioeconomic Status in Association with Survival in Older Men with Local/Regional Stage Prostate Carcinoma: Findings from a Large Community-based Cohort." Reviewed on *MedPage*

Today at www.medpagetoday.com/HematologyOncology/ProstateCancer, 13 Feb 2006.

Jennisen, Therese. "Health Issues in Rural Canada." Ottawa: Government of Canada, 1992. Available at Statistics Canada, dsp-psd.pwgsc.gc.ca/Collection-R/LoPBdP/BP/bp325.e.htm.

Karlinger, Joshua. *The Corporate Planet.* San Francisco: Sierra Club Books, 1997.

Kassirer, Jerome. *On the Take: How Medicine's Complicity with Big Business Can Endanger Your Health.* New York: Oxford University Press, 2006.

Katz, Helena. "Toronto Firm Recruiting MDs from Doomed Hospitals." *The Montreal Gazette,* 23 May 1995.

Keller, Martin B. ISI Author Publication A03902003-H, last updated 24 June 2003. Thompson Scientific ISIHighlyCited.com, Philadelphia. Posted on http//:hcr3.isiknowledge.com.

Keung, Nicolas. "MD Settles Lawsuit with U of T over Job." *Toronto Star,* 1 May 2002.

Kong, Dolores, and Alison Bass. "Case at Brown Leads to Review; NIMH Studies Tighter Rules on Conflicts." *Boston Globe,* 8 October 1999.

Korten, David. *The Post-Corporate World.* San Francisco: Bennett-Koehler, 1999.

Kulik, Devlin. "Fowl Play: The Poultry Industry's Central Role in the Bird Flu Crisis." Feb, 2006. Posted on the GRAIN website, www.grain.org.

Lancet. "Avian Influenza Goes Global, but Don't Blame the Birds." *Lancet Infectious Diseases* 6 (2006):185. Posted on http://www.greenpartysask.ca/GPS_Principles_Platform/Backgrounder_Articles/Health/Avian_Flu_Global_Spread_Factors.htm

Larkin Marilynn. "Clinical Trials: What Price Progress?" *The Lancet,* 30 October 1999.

Law, Jackie. *Big Pharma: How Modern Medicine Is Damaging Your Health.* New York: Carroll and Graf, 2006.

Levine, Bruce. "Eli Lilly, Zyprexa and the Bush Family." *Z Magazine* 17, no.5 (May, 2004). Posted on http://zmagsite.zmag.org/May2004/levine0504.html. Accessed 15 June 2004.

Levy, Samuel. Letter to *The Monitor,* 12 July 1995, included in "Clippings on Closure – an incomplete selection and condensation of press clippings relevant to the slated closure of the Queen Elizabeth Hospital." Available in the Queen Elizabeth Archives, McGill University.

Levy, Samuel. Letter to *The Montreal Suburban,* 9 August 1995, included in "Clippings on Closure – an incomplete selection and condensation of press clippings relevant to the slated closure of the Queen Elizabeth Hospital." Available in the Queen Elizabeth Archives, McGill University.

Liu L, et al. "Impact of Rural Hospital Closures in Saskatchewan, Canada."
Social Science and Medicine 52 (2001): 1793–1804.

Mair, Ian D. "President's Report," 94th Annual Meeting of the Queen
Elizabeth Hospital of Montreal, Thursday, 1 June 1989. Available at the
Queen Elizabeth Hospital Archives, McGill University.

Mander, J., et al. *The Case Against Globalization.* San Francisco: Sierra Club
Books, 1996.

Mark, D.H., et al. "Medicare Costs in Urban Areas and the Supply of Primary
Care Physicians." *Journal of Family Practice* 43 (1996): 33–9.

Marmot, et al. "Disease and Disadvantage in the United States and in England."
Journal of the American Medical Association 295 (2006):2037–45. Posted on
www.hdr.undp.org/hdr2006/pdfs/report/ HDR06-complete.pdf.

May, and Weinman. "Wrong Medicine: Technocratic Vision, Not Reality, Is
Behind Closures." *The Montreal Gazette,* 18 May 1995.

McBane, Michael. "Ill-Health Canada." Ottawa: CCPA, 2005. Posted on
www.healthcoalition.ca.

McBane, Michael. "'Smart Regulation' Puts Profit before Health." Canadian
Health Coalition Media Release, 29 March 2005. Posted on
www.medicare.ca and www.healthcoalition.ca/102.pdf+Ill+Health.

McDonald P., et al. "Waiting Lists and Waiting Times for Health Care in
Canada: More Management!! More Money??" *Health Canada,* July 1998.
Posted on www.hc-sc.gc.ca/english/media/releases/waiting_list.html.
Accessed 30 June 2007.

McGuire, Susan. Letter to the *Westmount Examiner,* 27 July 1995.

McKay, N.L., and J.A. Coventry. "Access Implications of Rural Hospital
Closures and Conversions." *Hospital and Health Service Administration* 40
(1995): 227–46.

McKinnell, Hank. *A Call To Action: Taking Back Healthcare for Future
Generations.* New York: McGraw-Hill, 2005.

McTaggart, Lynn. *What Doctors Don't Tell You.* London: HarperCollins, 2005.

McQuaig, Linda. *Shooting the Hippo.* Toronto: Random House, 1995.

Ministry of Employment and Solidarity, High Committee on Public Health.
Health in France 2002. Montrouge, France: Editions John Libbey Eurotext,
2002.

Minutes, Hospital Committee, Board of Guardians, PCA. Entry for 28 January
1846.

Montreal Gazette. "Local Hospital Closings Done Strictly by the Numbers." *The
Montreal Gazette,* 16 May 1995.

Moore, G.T. "The case of the Disappearing Generalist: Does It Need to Be
Solved?" *Milbank Quarterly* 1992.

Mozaffarian, Dariush, Eric Rimm, and David Harrington. "Dietary Fats, Carbohydrates, and Progression of Coronary Atherosclerosis in Postmenopausal Women." *The American Journal of Clinical Nutrition* 80, n. 5 (November, 2004): 1102–84.

Mundy, Alicia. *Dispensing with the Truth*. New York: St Martin's Press, 2001.

National Academy of Enginering and Institute of Medicine. *Building a Better Delivery System: A New Engineering/Healthcare Partnership*. Washington, DC: National Academies Press, 2005.

National Vital Statistic Reports 53, no. 5 (12 Oct. 2004). Posted on www.cdc.gov/nchs/fastats.

Naylor, C. David, ed. *Canadian Health Care and the State*. Montreal: McGill-Queen's University Press, 1992.

– *Private Practice, Public Payment* Montreal: McGill-Queen's University Press, 1986.

Nelson, Greenfield S., M. Zubkoff, W. Manning, W. Rogers, R.I. Kravitz, et al. "Variations in Resource Utilization among Medical Specialties and Systems of Care." *Journal of the American Medical Association* (1992).

Nelson, Kristin. "Bad Practice: How Developing Nations Are Suffering from Canada's Band-aid Solutions to Our Own Doctor Shortage." *This Magazine* 267 (May/June, 2007): 1624–30.

O'Connor, Dennis R. "*Report of the Walkerton Inquiry: The Events of May 2000 and Related Issues*." Ottawa: Ontario Ministry of the Attorney General, Queen's Printer for Ontario, 2002.

Oppenheimer, J. "Childbirth in Ontario: The Transition from Home to Hospital in the Early Twentieth Century." In A. Arnup, A. Levesque, and R. Pierson, eds., *Delivering Motherhood: Maternal Ideologies and Practice in the 19th and 20th Centures*. London: Routledge, 1990.

Orton, P. "Shared Care." *Lancet* 344 (1994): 1413–15.

Otte, J., D. Roland-Holst, et. al. "Industrial Livestock Production and Global Health Risks," June 2007. Posted on "archives" of www.rurale.ca.

Province of British Columbia, Royal Commissions and Commissions of Inquiry, Commission of Inquiry, Vancouver General Hospital, 1912, Investigative Proceedings, PABC, GR785, 297. See also *Vancouver Daily World*, 14 and 25 February 1911.

Parchman, M.L., and S. Culler. "Primary Care Physicians and Avoidable Hospitalizations." *Journal of Family Practice* (1994): 123–8.

Patton, Arthur. Annual Report of the Montreal Homeopathic Hospital, 1906. Available at the Queen Elizabeth Archives, McGill University.

Peeno, Linda. "Managed Care Ethics: The Close View Prepared for U.S. House of Representatives Committee on Commerce, Subcommittee of

Health and Environment." Excerpted in *The National Coalition of Mental Health Professionals and Consumers*, 30 May 1996.

Phillips, Robert A., and John Hoey. "Constraints of Interest: Lessons at the Hospital for Sick Children." Editorial; *Canadian Medical Association Journal* 159, no. 8 (20 October 1998): 983–6.

Pollock, Allyson. "How Private Finance Is Moving Primary Care into Corporate Ownership." *British Medical Journal*, 21 April 2001. Posted on bmj.com/cgi/content/full/322/7292/960. Accessed 15 February 2005.

Priest, Lisa. "A Boy's Plight, a Nation's Problem." *The Globe and Mail*, 13 January 2005.

– "His Cancer Couldn't Wait, Panel Rules." *The Globe and Mail*, 28 January 2006.

Ravnskov, Uffe. "High Cholesterol May Protect against Infections and Atherosclerosis." *Quarterly Journal of Medicine* (2003): 927–34.

Reed, Gail. "Challenges for Cuba's Family Doctor-and-Nurse Program." Posted on www.medicc.org/publications/medicc_review/II/primary/slogody.html. Accessed 10 May 2007.

Reid, Angus. *Shakedown: How the New Economy Is Changing Our Lives*, Toronto: Seal Books, Doubleday Canada, 1997.

Reiff, S.S., S. DesHarnais, and S. Bernard. "Community Perceptions of the Effects of Rural Hospital Closures on Access to Care." *Journal of Rural Health* 15 (1999): 202–9.

Relman, Arnold. "What Market Values Are Doing to Medicine," *Atlantic Monthly*, March 1992, 99–106

Riga. Included in "Clippings on Closure – an incomplete selection and condensation of press clippings relevant to the slated closure of the Queen Elizabeth Hospital." Available in the Queen Elizabeth Archives, McGill University.

Robinson, Jennifer. "Planned Hospitals Closing Leave Loyal Volunteers Feeling Betrayed," *The Montreal Gazette*, 22 June 1995.

Roos, N. P., and E. Shapiro. "Using the Information System to Assess Change: The Impact of Downsizing the Acute Sector." *Medical Care* (1995).

Rosenberg, Charles E. *The Care of Strangers*. New York: Basic Books, 1987.

Ross, Nancy A., et al. "Relation between Income Inequality and Mortality in Canada and in the United States: Cross Sectional Assessment Using Census Data and Vital Statistics." Statistics Canada, originally published in the *British Medical Journal* (2005); reprinted in Nancy Ross, ed., *Health Geography*, GEOG–303, McGill University, 2005.

Ruprecht, J. "The Knowledge Spreads through Europe." In Atkinson and Boulton, ed., *The History of Anesthesia*.

San Diego Union Editorial Staff. "Doctor Lets Patient Die, Is Rewarded with Raise." *The San Diego Union Tribune*, 19 Jan 1997.

Sanmartin, Claudia, et al. "Waiting for Medical Services in Canada: Lots of Heat but Little Light." *Canadian Medical Association Journal* 162 (2000).

Saul, John Ralston. *The Doubter's Companion: A Dictionary of Aggressive Common Sense.* Toronto: Penguin, 1995.

Schroeder, S.A., and Sandy L.G. "Specialty Distribution of US Physicians – the Invisible Driver of Health Care Costs." *New England Journal of Medicine* 328 (1993): 961–3.

Shah, Chandrakant P. *Public Health and Preventative Medicine in Canada.* Toronto: Elesvier Canada, 2003.

Shaker, . "Public-private Partnerships Would Open a Trade Treaty Door That Might Prove Impossible to Close." *Straight Goods*, 27 July 2004. Accessed 28 July 2007.

Shanahan, M., M.D. Bownell, and N.P. Roos. "The Unintended and Unexpected Impact of Downsizing: Costly Hospitals Become More Costly." *Medical Care* 37, no. 6 (1999): 123–34.

Shea, S., et al. "Predisposing Factors for Severe, Uncontrolled Hypertension. *New England Journal of Medicine* 327 (1997): 776–81.

Shepard, D.S. "Estimating the Effect of Hospital Closure on Area-wide Inpatient Hospital Costs: A Preliminary Model and Application." *Health Services Research* 18 (1983): 513–49.

Shi, L. "The Relationship between Primary Care and Life Chances." *Journal of Health Care for the Poor and Underserved* 3 (1992): 321–3.

Shortt, S.E.D., ed. *Medicine in Canadian Society: Historical Perspectives.* Montreal: McGill-Queen's University Press, 1992.

Shuchman, Miriam. "Legal Issues Surrounding Privately Funded Research Cause Furore in Toronto." *Canadian Medical Association Journal* 159, no. 8 (20 Oct. 1998): 983–6.

Silverman, Elaine M., Jonathan Skinner, and Elliot S. Fisher, "The Association between For-Profit Hospital Ownership and Increased Medicare Spending." *New England Journal of Medicine* 341, no. 6 (5 August 1999): 420–6.

Smith, Philip. *Arrows of Mercy.* Toronto: Doubleday Canada, 1969, as excerpted in *Weekend Magazine*, 10 January 1970.

Speigel, J.M., and A.Yassi, "Lessons from the Margins of Globalization: Appreciating the Cuban Health Paradox." *Journal of Public Health Policy* 25, no. 1 (2004): 85–110.

StratCom (Strategic Market Research and Communications). "Health Care in Canada." Posted on www.pagebleu.com/stratcom/level1/care1198.htm.

Sturges, Paul M. "Cabins on Neversink Produce World's Best Anesthetic."
    Ulster County Press, 20 August 1937.

Sutherland, Anne, Kate Stewart, and Philip Authier. "Marchers Decry
    Hospital Closings." *The Montreal Gazette*, 6 June 1995.

Suzuki, David, and Holly Dressel, *From Naked Ape to Super-species*. Toronto:
    Stoddart, 1999.

– *Good News for a Change*. Vancouver, Greystone, 2002.

Sykes, W. Stanley. *Essays on the First Hundred Years of Anaesthesia*. Huntingdon,
    NY: Robert E. Krieger, 1972.

Taft, Kevin, and Gillian Steward. *Clear Answers: The Economics and Politics of
    For-Profit Medicine*. Edmonton: Duval House of Publishing, University of
    Alberta Press and the Parkland Institute, 2000.

Thompson, Jon, and Patricia Baird, et al. *The Oliveri Report: The Complete Text
    of the Report of the Independent Inquiry Commissioned by the Canadian Association
    of University Teachers*. Toronto: James Lorimer, 2001.

Thompson, Larry. "Human Gene Therapy, Harsh Lessons, High Hopes." *FDA
    Consumer Magazine*, Sept-Oct., 2000. Posted on www.fda.gov/fdac/
    features/2000/500_gene.html. Accessed 14 September 2006.

Terkel, Studs. *Hard Times: An Oral History of the Great Depression*. New York:
    Pantheon Books, Random House, 1970.

Tirer, Samual. "Metaphysical Conclusions Derived from a Proposed Mode of
    Anaesthetic Action." In Atkinson and Boulton, *The History of Anesthesia*.

Trautwein, Janet. "A Look at Single Payer Systems Around the World." Posted
    on www.niahu.org/laws/legislative_analysis/ single_payer_systems.pdf.

Trovato, F. "Mortality Differentials in Canada, 1951–1971: French, British
    and Indians." *Culture, Medicine and Psychiatry* 12, no. 4 (Dec 1988).

Unwin, L.B. "Annual Report of the Homeopathic Hospital of Montreal,
    1952." Available in the Queen Elizabeth Hospital Archives, McGill
    University.

– Annual Report of the Homeopathic Hospital of Montreal, 1953." Available
    in the Queen Elizabeth Hospital Archives, McGill University.

US Government National Health Institute website on CAM,
    www.nccam.nih.gov.health.

Vayda, Eugene, and Raisa Deber. "The Canadian Health-Care System." In C.
    David Naylor, ed., *Canadian Health Care and the State*.

Washburn, Jennifer. *University, Inc.: The Corporate Corruption of Higher
    Education*. New York: Basic Books, 2006.

Wazana, Ashley. "Physicians and the Pharmaceutical Industry: Is a Gift Ever
    Just a Gift?" *Journal of the American Medical Association* 283, no.3 (19 Jan
    2000): 769–74.

What Doctors Don't Tell You 13, no. 9 (Dec 2002).

Woolhandler, Steffie, and David U. Himmelstein. "Costs of Care and Administration at For-Profit Hospitals in the United States." *New England Journal of Medicine* 336 (1997): 769–74.

Zacharia, Yvonne. "Tears Flow as Emergency Ward Packs Up." *The Montreal Gazette,* 1 June 1996.

Zelder, Martin. "Take a Queue from Canada!" *Fraser Forum,* Feb. 1999.

Zeldin, Cindy. "Health Debtor Accounts." Posted on www.tompaine.com/articles/20060130/health_debtor_accounts.php, 30 January 2006. Accessed 16 February 2006.

Zwanziger, J., et al. "Comparison of Hospital Cost in California, New York, and Canada." *Health Affairs* 12 (1993): 130–9.

Index

223–5, 227–9, 230, 233–8, 240, 255; controlling costs, 241, 275–6, 310, 312; privatization, 292, 305, 307–9, 355, 360; for profit, 241–2, 297, 302, 303–4. *See also* hospital costs; public/private partnerships
health insurance: doctor-initiated, 210 (*see also* Andreas, Lewis); for profit, 223, 225, 302 (*see also* Blue Cross; employment insurance plans)
Healy, David, 317–18, 321
heart disease, 336, 337, 345–8. *See also* Lown, Bernard
Hechtman, Ken, 248, 254, 266
Heffernan, Tom, 97
HEN (Health Evidence Network), 2004 study, 372–3, 377, 378–9; recommendations, 276–7, 278–9, 280,
HMO (Health Maintenance Organizations): contemporary, 210, 211–12, 216, 223, 228, 301; effects of, 303–4, incursions into Canada, 306
Hoey, John, 319
Holladay, 175
Homeopathic Association, 103
Homeopathic Hospital: culture of, 123; found-

ing of, 103; renaming ceremony, 203
homeopathy: history of, 85–7, 88, 102; Royal Family and, 89
Hôpital Notre-Dame, 191
Hôpital Ste-Justine, 191
hospital closures: Bellechase, 30; in Calgary, 29–30; across Canada, 267–85; Gouin-Rosemont Hospital, 30; Guy Laporte Hospital, 30; in Halifax, 31; Lachine General Hospital, 30; in Montreal, 21, 30; Queen Elizabeth Hospital, 263–6; Reddy Memorial Hospital, 30; Regina Hospital, 31; Riverdale Hospital, 30; Runnymede Hospital, 30; Ste. Jeanne d'Arc Hospital, 30; St. Laurent Hospital, 30; Salvation Army Grace Hospital, 30; in Saskatchewan, 31; in Toronto, 30–1; Villa Medica, 30; Wellesley Hospital, 30, 48
hospital conditions, early history, 92–6, 102–25
hospital costs, 235–7, 255, 273; charitable, 183–4; 217–18; construction, 200; controlling, 241; during depression, 182, 187–8; increasing, 206–7, 209–13, 217,

238, 241–2; technologies, 200
Hospital for Sick Children, 318–19
Hotel Dieu, 102
Houton, J.R., 221
HSAS (Health Savings Accounts). *See* MSAS
Hughes, John: re airway management, 164–5; re closure, 286; re costs, 277–8; re Deidre Gilles, 254–5; re doctor shortages, 246, 259, 373, 374; hospital hierarchy, 18; hospital size, 67; re Larivière, 261; re length of stay, 271; re medical informatics, 405–7; re medical innovations, 67, 256–7; re natural systems, 43–4; patient-centred care, 26, 342; re pharmaceutical companies, 333; selection committee, 35; specialization, 369
Hurley, Michael, 33

IMF (International Monetary Fund), 353; documents, 290–3, 294; community hospital closures, 40, 289; lending practices, 39; *IMF Reports to Canada*, 42, 294, 295–6; origins, 288; recommendations, 293, 294
infant mortality rate: Canadian, 236, 240;